Cancer Cell Signalling

Cancer Cell Signalling

Edited by

Amanda Harvey
Biosciences, Brunel University, London, UK

WILEY Blackwell

Library of Congress Cataloging-in-Publication Data

Cancer cell signalling / edited by Amanda Harvey.

p. ; cm.

Includes bibliographical references and index.

ISBN 978-1-119-96756-9 (cloth) – ISBN 978-1-119-96757-6 (pbk.)

I. Harvey, Amanda, 1970- editor of compilation.

[DNLM: 1. Neoplastic Processes. 2. Signal Transduction. 3. Neoplasms–genetics.

4. Neoplasms–therapy. 5. Protein Kinases–genetics. 6. Receptors, Cell Surface–physiology. QZ 202]

RC268.5

616.99′4–dc23

2013023364

A catalogue record for this book is available from the British Library.

Contents

List of contributors

Andrea R. Daniel

Departments of Medicine (Division of Hematology, Oncology, and Transplantation) and Pharmacology, University of Minnesota, Masonic Cancer Center, 420 Delaware Street, Minneapolis, MN 55455, USA

Christy R. Hagan

Departments of Medicine (Division of Hematology, Oncology, and Transplantation) and Pharmacology, University of Minnesota, Masonic Cancer Center, 420 Delaware Street Minneapolis, MN 55455, USA

Ester M. Hammond

The Cancer Research UK/MRC Gray Institute for Radiation Oncology and Biology, Department of Oncology, The University of Oxford, Oxford, OX3 7DQ, UK

Amanda Harvey

Biosciences, Brunel University, London, Kingston Lane, Uxbridge, UB8 3PH, UK

Christopher Hillyar

The Cancer Research UK/MRC Gray Institute for Radiation Oncology and Biology, Department of Oncology, The University of Oxford, Oxford, OX3 7DQ, UK

Stephen Hiscox

School of Pharmacy and Pharmaceutical Sciences, Cardiff University, CF10 3NB, UK

Emmanouil Karteris

Biosciences, Brunel University, London, Kingston Lane, Uxbridge, UB8 3PH, UK

Todd P. Knutson

Departments of Medicine (Division of Hematology, Oncology, and Transplantation) and Pharmacology, University of Minnesota, Masonic Cancer Center, 420 Delaware Street Minneapolis, MN 55455, USA

Carol A. Lange

Departments of Medicine (Division of Hematology, Oncology, and Transplantation) and Pharmacology, University of Minnesota, Masonic Cancer Center, 420 Delaware Street Minneapolis, MN 55455, USA

Katarzyna Leszczynska

The Cancer Research UK/MRC Gray Institute for Radiation Oncology and Biology, Department of Oncology, The University of Oxford, Oxford, OX3 7DQ, UK

Erald Shehu

Biosciences, Brunel University, London, Kingston Lane, Uxbridge, UB8 3PH, UK

Gudrun Stenbeck

Biosciences, Brunel University, London, Kingston Lane, Uxbridge, UB8 3PH, UK

Maria Thorpe

Biosciences, Brunel University, London, Kingston Lane, Uxbridge, UB8 3PH, UK

David Tree

Biosciences, Brunel University, London, Kingston Lane, Uxbridge, UB8 3PH, UK

Acknowledgements

Having read numerous acknowledgments sections in dissertations and theses over the years, it could be assumed that these should be easy to write. However, this is very clearly not the case!

As can be seen from the numerous chapter contributors, this book has not been a solo effort. A sincere thank you goes to all those who have written the drafts, re-written them and produced figures at the editor's whims. Your perseverance and co-operation has been much appreciated. This has been a team effort; we are, of course, supported by our networks of friends and families and we thank them for their patience.

Personally, as the daughter of a biochemistry technician and a Fellow of the Royal Society of Chemistry, a scientific career was hardly unexpected; however, whether it was 'nature or nurture', or indeed something entirely different, we are all driven and inspired by a diverse range of individuals. Sadly, not all the people who inspire us are still with us and this book is dedicated to them.

Introduction

One of the on-line encyclopaedias that is frequently used by students defines cell signalling as 'part of a complex system of communication that governs basic cellular activities and coordinates cell actions' (Wiki, 2013). As far definitions are concerned, this is a reasonable representation of the role of cell signalling within cells.

Historically, the cell signalling field dates back to the early 1920s when Banting and Best discovered insulin. In the 1950s Italian developmental biologist Rita Levi-Montalcini showed that the chick embryo nervous system was induced to develop by a nerve-growth promoting factor that was released from a transplanted mice tumour. Along with Stanley Cohen the nerve growth promoting factor was subsequently purified, characterised and named nerve growth factor (NGF). Cohen also discovered a second growth factor that promoted opening of the eyelids and tooth eruption. Owing to its action on epithelial cells this factor was termed epidermal growth factor.

This pioneering work paved the way for development of the field we now know as cell signalling, and Stanley Cohen and Rita Levi-Montalcini were jointly awarded Nobel Prizes for their discoveries in 1986 (Nobel Prize Website, 1986). Since then numerous growth factors and their associated receptors have been discovered and their roles in governing the function of normal cells are becoming very well characterised. John Nelson's volume *Structure and Function in Cell Signalling* (Nelson, 2009) provides an excellent foundation for understanding the mechanics of cell signalling. There are some very good definitions and descriptions of the fundamental aspects of ligand–receptor interactions in addition to, in Chapter 6, an introduction to the concept of signalling cross-talk.

As academics and researchers it is easy to place emphasis on our own specific cell-signalling pathway of interest. It is often the centre of our research specialism and, from a teaching viewpoint, focusing on a single pathway keeps information streamlined and simple and, importantly, from the student perspective, easier to understand.

The reality, however, is far from simple. Many signalling pathways share common effector molecules or feed into common signalling foci or hubs. This allows for altered dynamics within a single pathway to have an effect on a separate, alternate, pathway. Such effects underpin the basis of signalling cross-talk. We now know that stimulation of individual pathways has a far more complex biological outcome than first envisaged.

Much of our knowledge relating to signalling cross-talk has come from cancer biology. In order for a cancer cell to survive, and for a tumour to develop, a number of biological processes need to occur. The cells within the tumour display increased proliferative capabilities and replicative immortality, a reduced capacity for cell death and often a decreased reliance on growth factors. There is also an increase in invasion and metastasis as well as the potential for angiogenesis both in the primary and metastatic tumours. These characteristics or 'hallmarks' of cancer cells have been summarised very clearly in Hanahan and Weinberg's reviews of 2000 and 2011 (for those not familiar with cancer biology, these reviews make an excellent starting point for bedtime reading). In both reviews the intracellular circuitry associated with cancer hallmarks has been summarised, although in the decade between the articles the vast increase in knowledge has made it much more difficult to depict the signalling circuits clearly (Hanahan and Weinberg, 2000, 2011).

As our understanding of tumour biology has developed, molecules involved in disrupting normal cell signalling and driving cells towards a more cancerous phenotype have provided the basis for new drug targets, and a number of targeted biological therapies now exist for the treatment of tumours. However, many cancer patients have tumours that are either refractory to treatment or which develop resistance. The amount of research into this area has provided a wealth of information about cross-talk between signalling pathways and compensatory signalling.

This book aims to introduce a number of cell-signalling pathways that are both well characterised and reported to play central roles in the development of a number of different tumour types. Each chapter will focus on an individual pathway, its key components and dysregulation in tumour development. The state of play with respect to current therapies as well as future strategies will also be discussed.

The final chapter of this volume is devoted to signalling cross-talk. Interactions between signalling pathways, compensatory signalling and tumour related issues are discussed with the hope that the reader will not only develop a better appreciation for the role of signalling in disease, but also begin to understand the relevance of cross-talk. The take-home message is intended to be that whilst pathways are important, networks are even more so, especially in the context of cancer development and therapy.

References

Hanahan, D., and Weinberg, R.A. (2000) Hallmarks of cancer. *Cell*, **100** (1), 57–70.

Hanahan, D. and Weinberg, R.A. (2011) Hallmarks of cancer: the next generation. *Cell*, **144** (5), 646–674.

Nelson, J. (2009) *Structure and Function in Cell Signalling*, John Wiley & Sons, Ltd, Chichester.

Nobel Prize Website (1986) http://www.nobelprize.org/nobel_prizes/medicine/laureates/1986/press.html (accessed 10 March 2013).

Wiki (2013) http://en.wikipedia.org/wiki/Cell_signaling (accessed 19 March 2013).

About the companion website

This book is accompanied by a companion website:

www.wiley.com/go/harvey/cancercellsignalling

The website includes:

- Powerpoints of all figures from the book for downloading
- PDFs of tables from the book

1

Epidermal growth factor receptor family

Amanda Harvey

Biosciences, Brunel University, London

ErbB receptor ligands bind to their respective receptors, initiating the formation of homo- or heterodimers. The intracellular kinase domain of one receptor trans-phosphorylates the intracellular tyrosine residues on the opposite receptor thereby activating downstream signalling pathways.

At a cellular level, ErbB receptor ligands control a number of processes, including cell cycle progression, proliferation, cell death, protein synthesis, metabolism and differentiation. Physiologically this results in regulation of wound healing, neonatal growth and development as well as the development of adult tissues. Alterations in ErbB receptor signalling can result in oncogenesis in response to increased proliferation and decreased cell death as well as up-regulation of processes required for cell metastasis, such as adhesion, migration, invasion and neo-angiogenesis.

1.1 ErbB receptors and their structure

The epidermal growth factor receptor (EGFR/HER1) and the other family members (c-ErbB2/HER2/neu, ErbB3/HER3 and ErbB4/HER4) are 160–190 kDa transmembrane (type 1) receptor tyrosine kinases. They each comprise extracellular ligand binding and cysteine-rich domains, a transmembrane region, a kinase domain and an intracellular *C*-terminal tail, which contains the multiple tyrosine phosphorylation sites that are required for regulating receptor activation (reviewed in Ferguson, 2008).

EGFR was the first member of the family to be identified; it is a 170 kDa glycoprotein (Carpenter, 1987). Co-purification of the receptor with its growth factor ligand (epidermal growth factor, EGF) was reported in 1979 (McKanna *et al.*,

1979), which followed the discovery of EGF in 1972 (Savage *et al.*, 1972) and Stanley Cohen's pioneering work showing that EGF bound to the surface of cells (Cohen *et al.*, 1975; Carpenter *et al.*, 1975, 1978). HER2 was characterised in the 1980s as a 185 kDa protein (Schechter *et al.*, 1984) and has been shown to be highly homologous to EGFR (Coussens *et al.*, 1985). There are proto-oncogenic and oncogenic forms of HER2 and these differ in sequence by a single amino acid substitution (Bargmann *et al.*, 1986). HER2 is the preferred dimerisation partner of the other three family members and it is always available for dimerisation, as it largely exists in normal cells in a monomeric state (Weiner *et al.*, 1989a).

ErbB3 and ErbB4 were identified as the third and fourth members of the EGFR/ErbB family in the late 1980s based on their sequence homology with EGFR (Plowman *et al.*, 1990, 1993; Kraus *et al.*, 1989). Much of the sequence is conserved between the family members, with the highest degree of homology between each receptor and EGFR being in the kinase domain.

Of the family, EGFR and ErbB4 are the only fully functional members. ErbB3 has minimal kinase activity so the formation of ErbB3 homodimers does not result in active signalling and, as yet, there has been no ligand identified for HER2.

1.2 ErbB ligands

The monomeric growth factor ligands in this peptide family are 45–60 amino acids and they contain six conserved cysteine residues, which are linked by three disulphide bonds. EGF was the first factor to be characterised over 40 years ago (Savage *et al.*, 1972), followed eight years later by transforming growth factor-α (TGFα) (Roberts *et al.*, 1980; Torado *et al.*, 1980). Shortly following its initial discovery, EGF was shown to stimulate DNA synthesis and cell proliferation (Carpenter and Cohen, 1976).

In the 30 years since the discovery of TGFα, the family has grown to over 12 ligands that have different receptor binding preferences and therefore have the ability to regulate different cellular events (Figure 1.1).

EGF, TGFα, epigen and amphiregulin bind to EGFR; epiregulin and heparin binding EGF-like growth factor (HB-EGF) bind to EGFR and HER4; the neuregulins (1–6) have binding preferences for both HER3 and HER4, and betacellulin (BTC) binds to HER2, HER3 and HER4 (reviewed in Eccles, 2011). What is perhaps most striking is that despite appearing to have a functional ligand-binding domain, no ligand has yet been identified that binds HER2 with high affinity, although HER2 will bind with low affinity to the EGF family of ligands.

1.2.1 Ligand production

EGF family ligands are secreted but often require cleavage, unlike ligands for other receptor tyrosine kinases. The ligands are found tethered to the external

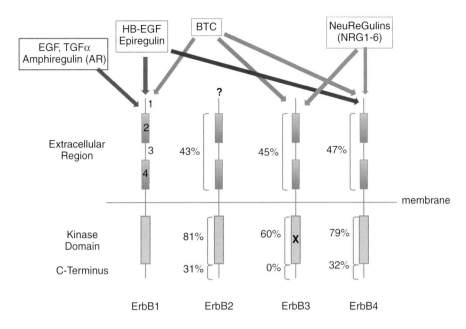

Figure 1.1 **Schematic representation of the ErbB receptors.** All four receptors are depicted and the percentage sequence homology in each domain with the EGFR is indicated. The extracellular region of the receptor has four subdomains, two of which (1 and 3) are involved in ligand binding and two (2 and 4) are cysteine rich and are involved in mediating dimerization. Individual ligands have different binding affinities for specific receptors; note that ErbB2/HER2 does not have a ligand (indicated by ?) and that ErbB3 does not have an active kinase domain (indicated by X), possibly as a result of its reduced homology with EGFR.

surface of the cell membrane in pro-forms and require proteolytic cleavage in order to be released. For many ErbB ligands this is carried out by the disintegrin and metalloproteinase, ADAM17 (Hinkle *et al.*, 2004; Sahin *et al.*, 2004 reviewed in Booth and Smith, 2007) via a process that is known as ectodomain shedding. *In vivo* evidence that ADAM17 acts upstream of EGFR also comes from knockout mice. Both $ADAM17^{-/-}$ and $EGFR^{-/-}$ mice display aberrant developmental phenotypes (Wiesen *et al.*, 1999; Jackson *et al.*, 2003; Yamazaki *et al.*, 2003) and EGFR activation only occurred when ADAM17 and amphiregulin were expressed (Sternlicht *et al.*, 2005).

Once soluble, ligands can activate the receptors in paracrine, autocrine or endocrine fashions. This mechanism forms the basis of some types of signalling cross-talk (Chapter 9).

1.2.2   Effects of ligand binding to receptors

The extracellular domains of the receptors are responsible for ligand binding and facilitate most of the dimerisation events. Many of our insights into the

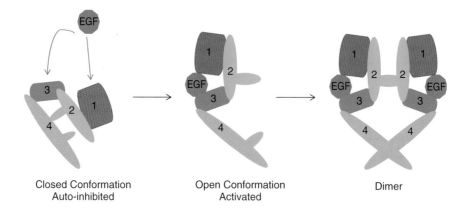

Closed Conformation   Open Conformation   Dimer
Auto-inhibited   Activated

Figure 1.2 **Schematic representation of the extracellular domain rearrangement leading to receptor dimerization.** In a closed confirmation the receptor is inactive. Ligand (EGF) can bind weakly to subdomain 1, which is not enough to induce receptor activation. However on binding to subdomain 3, the receptor confirmation opens up into an extended confirmation allowing ligand binding to both domains 1 and 3 and exposing the dimerization arm. The extended receptor then dimerizes through interactions that are mediated predominantly through subdomain 2 and, to a lesser extent, subdomain 4 (based on Ferguson *et al.*, 2003).

mechanisms of ligand binding and the events involved in receptor dimerisation have come from experimental mutations of the receptors (reviewed in Brennan *et al.*, 2000; Ferguson, 2008). Once the ligand has bound to the receptor, an event that occurs with a 1:1 stoichiometry, a change occurs in the conformation of the receptor that facilitates downstream phosphorylation events and signalling transduction.

A number of groups have presented models for investigating ligand–receptor interactions. When the ligand binds to its receptor, a large domain rearrangement occurs that ultimately results in receptor dimerisation. Dimerisation itself is mediated in part, but not solely, by a dimerisation arm or loop that protrudes from the receptor due to the structural rearrangement that takes place upon ligand binding removing the arm from its intra-molecular tether (Garrett *et al.*, 2002; Ogiso *et al.*, 2002; Ferguson *et al.*, 2003; Greenfield *et al.*, 1989). Exposure of the dimerisation arm initiates the subsequent dimerisation of the receptors with an asymmetric interaction between the intracellular domains (Figure 1.2). In contrast with other signalling pathways (such as IGF, see Chapter 2) ErbB dimerisation involves direct interaction between the receptors, rather than via an association mediated through a divalent ligand that acts as a molecular 'bridge' (reviewed in Ferguson, 2008).

In addition, ligand binding also brings about additional conformational changes that are required for dimerisation including rotation of part of the receptor (Ogiso *et al.*, 2002 and Ferguson *et al.*, 2003). It is clear that the spatial arrangement of the receptors is important in order that additional contact points can be made at the extracellular interface between the two receptors undergoing dimerisation

Table 1.1   Reported ErbB homo- and hetero-dimers.

	ErbB1	ErbB2	ErbB3	ErbB4
ErbB1	1–1	**1–2**	1–3	
ErbB2		$2-2^a$		
ErbB3	3–1	**3–2**	$3-3^b$	3–4
ErbB4		**4–2**		4–4

^{a}With no known ligand ErbB2 homodimerization only contributes to signalling when ErbB2 is over expressed.
^{b}As ErbB3 is kinase inactive, ErbB3 homodimers are not functionally active.

(Ferguson *et al.*, 2003). The arrangement of these contact points could be central in determining the extent of receptor hetero- or homo-dimerisation.

In 2009 Wilson and colleagues hypothesised that different ErbB ligands would stabilise the extracellular regions of the receptors in slightly different conformations (Wilson *et al.*, 2009). This would affect the spatial arrangement of the contact points at the dimer interface, as well as the position of the dimerisation arm. In addition to influencing the 'choice' of dimerisation partner, subtle changes in spatial stabilisation of the extracellular regions of the receptors could also result in altered interactions between the intracellular domains of the two receptors in the dimer.

Unlike other (non-ErbB-related) receptor tyrosine kinases, the EGFR tyrosine kinase domain does not require activation loop trans-autophosphorylation to promote kinase activation (Gotoh *et al.*, 1992). Instead formation of the asymmetric dimer allosterically activates the dimeric kinase domain (Zhang *et al.*, 2006).

Given this asymmetric event, the accessibility of the cytoplasmic tyrosine residues for trans-phosphorylation by the kinase domain of the opposing dimerisation partner will vary depending on the nature of the interaction and the spatial arrangement of the two intracellular domains. Specificity of tyrosine phosphorylation will determine which downstream intracellular effector/adaptor proteins can bind to the activated receptor, resulting in the activation of different downstream pathways.

There are a total of ten possible receptor combinations resulting in dimer formation, although not all result in active signalling complexes (Table 1.1). ErbB3 homodimers have minimal kinase activity, although each monomer highly augments signalling when in a heterodimer with other members of the family.

1.3   Downstream signalling molecules and events

Wilson's hypothesis is supported by our biological knowledge. It has been evident for some time that the different receptors are capable of activating different downstream signalling cascades. When ErbB2/ErbB3 heterodimers form, the cytoplasmic tail of ErbB2 activates the Erk-MAPK pathway and ErbB3 activates PI3K-Akt (phosphatidylinositol 3-kinase, PI3K) signalling pathway (Alimandi *et al.*, 1995). These differences come about, in part, by the specificities of each of the tyrosine phosphorylation events on the *C*-terminal tail of the receptor. The variety of adapter molecules that can then potentially bind to, or dock with, each receptor is summarised in Table 1.2. It can be seen from the table that some signalling effector molecules can dock on all four receptors, potentially at multiple sites, whereas others only have specificity for one receptor or a single site on a limited number of receptors.

Once adapter molecules have bound to the activated receptors, a number of downstream signalling cascades can be induced (Figure 1.3). EGFR activation by EGF, TGFα, amphiregulin, heregulin and HB-EGF, and ErbB3 activation

Table 1.2   Potential docking sites for signaling effectors.

Receptor	Signaling effector	Adaptor docking site[a]
EGFR	Shc	Y703 Y974 Y1086 Y1148 Y1173
	STAT5	Y954 Y974
	Crk	Y954 Y974
	PTP-2c	Y974 Y992
	Src	Y974
	PLC gamma	Y992 Y1173
	Cbl	Y1045
	Grb2	Y1068 Y1086 Y1101 Y1148 Y1173
	SHP1	Y1173
HER2	Shc	Y735 Y1005 Y1196 YY1222 Y1248
	SH3BGRL	Y923 Y1196
	PTP-2c	Y1023
	Grb2	Y1139
HER3	p85 PI3-K	Y1054 Y1197 Y1222 Y1276 Y1289
	Grb2	Y1199 Y1262
	Shc	Y1328
HER4	Shc	Y733 Y1188 Y1258 Y1284
	PLC gamma	Y875
	STAT5	Y984
	PTP-2c	Y984
	Crk	Y1022 Y1150
	STAT1	Y1035
	p85 PI3-K	Y1056
	Abl	Y1056 Y1081 Y1150 Y1162 Y1188 Y1242
	Grb2	Y1162 Y1188 Y1202 Y1208 Y1221 Y1242 Y1268
	Cbl	Y1056
	Src	Y1128
	Syk	Y1150 Y1202
	Ras A1	Y1150
	Vav2	Y1162
	Nck	Y1268

[a]There are numerous potential phosphor-tyrosine (Y) docking sites for signalling effectors (adapted from Wilson *et al.*, 2009). Note the number of putative Grb2 docking sites on both EGFR and HER4, and Shc sites on EGFR, HER2 and HER4, although Grb and Shc potentially dock on four receptors. This contrasts with Abl, which docks exclusively on HER4 and p85 PI3-K that is almost exclusive to HER3.

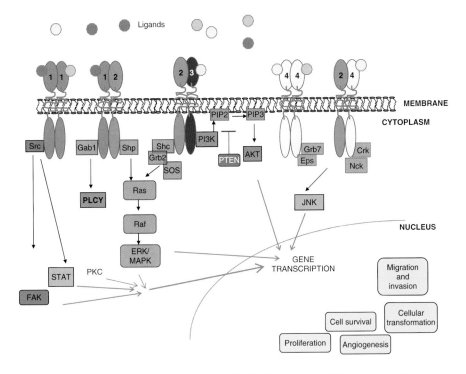

Figure 1.3   Key intracellular binding partners for ErbB receptors. This is a simplistic summary of the key signaling pathways that are initiated on ligand binding and dimerization of ErbB family members. As with subsequent chapters, colour has been used to highlight individual pathways, although it must be noted that many of the adaptor proteins/kinases indicated are frequently shared between different pathways (see Chapters 2, 5, 6, 7 and 9).

via neuregulins leads to the activation of phosphatidylinositol 3-kinases (PI3K), resulting in phosphorylation of phosphotatidylinositol 4,5-bisphosphate (PIP_2) to produce phosphatidylinositol 3,4,5-triphosphate (PIP_3). Akt then translocates to the membrane, and the conformational change that is produced when this happens allows Akt to be activated through phosphorylation of its active sites (threonine 308 and serine 473) by phosphoinositide-dependent protein kinase 1 (PDK1) and the mTOR complex 2 (mTORC2) (Sarbassov *et al.*, 2005). Akt activation results in phosphorylation of key downstream targets such as NF-kB, FOXO family members and mTOR complex 1 (mTORC1 – Chapter 5) (reviewed in Vivanco and Sawyers, 2002). At a cellular level, apoptosis is inhibited and cell proliferation and growth are induced in response to Akt activation (reviewed in Freudlsperger *et al.*, 2011).

Regulation of Akt activation occurs thorough the actions of PTEN (phosphate and tensin homolog deleted on chromosome 10) which antagonises PI3K activity by de-phosphorylating PIP_3 (reviewed in Cully *et al.*, 2006; Carnero *et al.*, 2008).

Docking proteins such as Grb2 and Shc are also capable of binding to phosphorylated residues on the cytoplasmic tail of the receptor (Schulze *et al.*, 2005). This ultimately results in formation of a Grb2/SOS complex initiating removal of GDP from a Ras family member, and activation by substitution with GTP. Ras then activates Raf, which subsequently activates the mitogen-activated-protein-kinase (MAPK) cascade. The outcome of MAPK cascade signaling is increased transcription, as a result of transcriptional activator activation (e.g. myc) (Chuang and Ng, 1994) and increased translation due to phosphorylation of the 40S ribosomal protein S6 kinase (Shahbazian *et al.*, 2006). Interestingly S6 kinase isoforms are also targets of mTOR activation (Chapter 5).

The Janus kinase (JAK)/signal transducers and activators of transcription (STAT) cascade also regulate cell survival. Members of the JAK/STAT pathway also interact with activated receptors to initiate signalling. As their name suggests, the outcome of signalling results in an increase in transcription, especially of target genes whose protein products are involved in increased proliferation and decreased cell death responses.

1.4   Signalling regulation

1.4.1   Regulation of phosphorylation events

Receptor conformation

In normal cells, the activation of signalling cascades is tightly regulated. The relative levels, as well as the combinations of receptors and growth factors that are available will govern specificity of signalling. The result will be that certain pathways will be activated to a higher or lesser extent than the alternatives based on the nature of receptor dimerisations that occur, and by the conformational changes that result from ligand binding, only allowing specific adaptor proteins to have accessibility to the cytoplasmic tail of the activated receptors (see Section 1.2.2).

Action of phosphatases

Control of signalling, where receptors and/or growth factor levels are not limiting, can also occur within the cell by families of lipid phosphatases or serine/threonine phosphoprotein phosphatases. PTEN is a well reviewed example and inhibits PI3-K/Akt signalling by de-phosphorylating PIP_2 and PIP_3 (reviewed in Zhang and Claret, 2012). Given that amongst its many roles PI3K activation results in increased proliferation, cell survival and motility, it is not surprising that PTEN functions as a tumour suppressor protein, inhibiting these actions. It is even less surprising then that PTEN is commonly lost in many tumour types (reviewed in Sansal and Sellers 2004), and individuals with syndromes involving germline mutations in PTEN (e.g. Cowden's Syndrome) are at increased risk of breast tumour development (Liaw *et al.*, 1997).

The 145 kDa protein, SHIP, specifically hydrolyses PIP_3 and is ubiquitously expressed in differentiated cells (reviewed in Zhang and Claret, 2012). As an antagonist of haematopoietic cell proliferation, SHIP is also classed as a tumour suppressor and deletion, especially in conjunction with PTEN, results in the formation of highly aggressive lymphomas (Helgason *et al.*, 1998; Miletic *et al.*, 2010).

Two members of the serine/threonine protein phosphatase family, PP1 and PP2, account for the vast majority of cellular phosphatase activity, despite being present in the cell in low amounts (Lin *et al.*, 1998). This family of proteins exist as heterotrimeric holoenzymes and the range of regulatory subunits that are available increase both the number of phosphoproteins that exist and allow for specificity of the de-phosphorylation reaction (reviewed in Zhang and Claret, 2012). The biological outcome of such specific phosphatases is that distinct pathways such as MAPK cascade, Wnt signalling and PI3K activity can be regulated (reviewed in Mumby, 2007).

1.4.2   Internalisation of receptors

It has been known for over three decades that receptors internalise and our knowledge of EGFR internalisation stems from early work by Stanley Cohen (Carpenter and Cohen, 1976). After internalisation the EGF/EGFR complex is degraded. In normal cells without over-expression of EGFR, this process takes a few hours, however when the receptor is over-expressed the half-life of internalisation increases (reviewed in Sorkin and Goh, 2008). Under normal physiological conditions, the majority of ErbB receptors are in the cell membrane and are internalised into endosomes at a constant rate as the membrane recycles. Inactive receptors are then recycled back to the cell membrane (Wiley, 2003). The constitutive rate of recycling is higher than internalisation, meaning that receptors will mainly be localised at the cell membrane, and this is enhanced by over-expression of receptors as both internalisation and degradation are saturable processes (reviewed in Sorkin and Goh, 2008).

Binding of a ligand to a receptor increases the rate of receptor internalisation via clathrin-coated pits. Here, the receptors are 'pinched' off the cell membrane and internalised into endosomes (reviewed in Sorkin, 2004). Once internalised, receptors are carried in budding vesicles, sorted and then trafficked to alternate cellular localisations including the Golgi, ER and nucleus as well as the mitochondria (reviewed in Wang and Huang, 2012). A number of groups have reported localisation of ErbBs in the nucleus (reviewed in Wang *et al.*, 2010a). Regulation of trafficking is carried out by Rab GTPases, and different Rab proteins are required for specific trafficking 'routes' (Maxfield and McGraw 2004; Grant and Donaldson, 2009; Rink *et al.*, 2005; Ceresa and Bahr, 2006).

PI3K activation has been linked to microtubule-associated vesicle trafficking affecting both receptor turn-over and transport to alternative cellular localisations. The p85 domain has a wide range of binding partners that play central roles in receptor internalisation and vesicle formation (reviewed Mellor *et al.*, 2012).

The evolutionary conserved family of snx-BAR proteins induce deformation of the cell membrane resulting in tubule formation and ultimately endosome production. They regulate sorting in the maturing endosome, where receptors are either degraded or recycled back to the cell membrane (reviewed in van Weering *et al.*, 2010).

Whilst it was initially assumed that receptor internalisation served to terminate signalling, more recent data suggest, at least for EGFR, that endocytosis can be a requirement for full activation of signalling. In some cellular circumstances increased internalisation of EGFR/HER2 complexes was associated with increased proliferation and cell invasion (Gao *et al.*, 2012). It is also becoming clear that the requirements for endocytosis of receptors may differ depending on the stimuli (Grandal *et al.*, 2012).

1.5   Dysregulation of signalling in cancer

Dysregulation of ErbB receptor expression and signalling and has been identified in a number of different cancer types, including tumours from breast, ovary, brain, prostate, GI tract, lung and head and neck (reviewed in Burden and Yarden, 1997; Hynes and Stern, 1994). There are a number of mechanisms through which increased signalling would occur such as mutations, increased receptor, ligand and adaptor protein expression, as well as altered cellular localisation of signalling components.

1.5.1   Receptor over-expression

One of the most well described gene amplifications is that of *ErbB2*, which was first reported in the mid-1980s (Ullrich *et al.*, 1984; King *et al.*, 1985). In high-grade ductal and inflammatory breast cancer the *ErbB2* gene is amplified and over-expressed which contrasts with benign lesions where *ErbB2* is expressed at low levels (Allred, 1992; Gusterson, 1998, reviewed in Freudenberg, *et al.*, 2009).

Overall the *ErbB2* gene is amplified in 25–30% of breast cancers (Slamon *et al.*, 1989), as well as some ovarian, stomach and aggressive uterine tumours, and the elevated HER2 protein that is produced as a result is crucial to driving tumour cell proliferation and migration. The differences in expression levels between benign lesions and higher-grade tumours, along with our knowledge of the cellular events that are regulated by HER2, suggest that HER2 over-expression occurs during disease development. There is also evidence that HER2 increases the metastatic potential of cells that have not been fully transformed, indicating that *ErbB2* amplification and over-expression is a driving force in breast cancer progression (reviewed in Freudenberg *et al.*, 2009).

Increased levels of HER2 will mean that, as the preferred heterodimerisation partner for all the receptors, there will possibly be an increase in heterodimerisation rather than homodimerisation, resulting in increased levels of signalling without the need for elevated ligand levels. Given that the dimerisation arm is constitutively exposed in HER2, high levels of HER2 protein could also result in increased formation of HER2:HER2 homodimers that are constitutively active, even in the absence of ligand. HER2/ErbB2 expression on its own is not sufficient to cause cellular transformation of normal cells and co-expression with ErbB3 is required for pre-neoplastic transformation (Vaught *et al.*, 2012). However in an already partially transformed cell, increased HER2 homodimers could certainly promote proliferation and evasion of apoptosis (reviewed in Freudenberg *et al.*, 2009).

EGFR is over-expressed, with or without gene amplification, in a wide variety of epithelial tumours (reviewed in Arteaga, 2002). In ovarian cancer, at least 70% of tumours are reported to over-express *EGFR* (Kohler *et al.*, 1989), and there is a relationship between *EGFR* expression and decreased survival in both ovarian and cervical cancers (Psyrri *et al.*, 2005a; Perez-Regadera *et al.*, 2011).

However not all ErbB receptors, when elevated, are linked to increased tumour formation. There are reports that in breast cancers ErbB4 over-expression is linked to improved prognosis and increased tumour suppression, as well as a correlation with the positive prognostic indicator, the oestrogen receptor (Fujiwara *et al.*, 2012; reviewed Wang *et al.*, 2010a). However, ErbB4 has also been shown to be oncogenic (reviewed in Burgess, 2008). The relative levels of other family members are likely to be important in governing both ErbB3 and ErbB4 function, as ErbB1 or HER2 are required for ErbB3 and ErbB4 mediated transformation and oncogenesis (Mill *et al.*, 2011; Gilbertson *et al.*, 1998; Zhang *et al.*, 1996). Histopathological analysis of all ErbBs may therefore be required, especially for heterogeneous epithelial tumours.

1.5.2 Activating mutations

Oncogenic HER2 is largely found homodimerised rather than in the 'normal' monomeric state (Weiner *et al.*, 1989b) suggesting that spontaneous ligand-independent dimerisation is occurring in tumours when HER2 is over-expressed (reviewed in Brennan *et al.*, 2000). The amino acid substitution whereby glutamic acid is substituted with valine means that a negative charge on the transmembrane region of the receptor is introduced (Bargmann *et al.*, 1986). Changing the charge on the receptor presumably impacts on the receptor conformation, thereby promoting the formation of homodimers, which is required for the tyrosine kinase activity of the receptor (Weiner and coworkers, 1989a and b).

A subset of extracellular EGFR mutations in glioblastomas enhance receptor activation by destabilising the inactive conformation of the receptor (Ferguson, 2008). In non-small cell lung carcinomas (NSCLC) mutations in components of the EGFR pathway are largely mutually exclusive. That is, in the vast majority of cell lines studied, only one member of the pathway harboured a mutation (Gandhi *et al.*, 2009). These studies in cultured cell lines are also supported by observations from clinical surgical samples (Shigamtsu *et al.*, 2005), suggesting that multiple EGFR pathway mutations are not required to promote tumourigenesis but that single mutations may be sufficient. Interestingly, but not surprisingly in the light of Iressa failure (reviewed in Blagosklonny and Darzynkiewicz, 2003), the component of the pathway that was mutated had a bearing on whether the cells responded to anti-EGFR therapy or were intrinsically resistant to EGFR inhibition (Gandhi *et al.*, 2009).

A number of mutations in the intracellular domains of EGFR, such as in-frame deletions in the catalytic pocket and the L834R missense mutation, result in both increased kinase activity and coupling to Akt and STAT5 phosphorylation (Zhang *et al.*, 2006; Sordella *et al.*, 2004).

1.5.3   Altered cellular localisation

EGFR has been identified in the nucleus of a number of different tumour cells, including breast cancer, ovarian cancer, and oropharyngeal and esophageal squamous cell carcinomas. Localisation to the nucleus appears to be correlated with poorer patient outcomes (Psyrri *et al.*, 2005b; Lo *et al.*, 2005b; Hoshino *et al.*, 2007; Xia *et al.*, 2009), and this is possibly due to its association with STAT3 in the nucleus where it can lead to transcriptional up-regulation of inducible nitric oxide synthase (iNOS) and cyclo-oxygenase-2 (COX-2) (Lo *et al.*, 2005a; Lo *et al.*, 2010). Elevated expression of *iNOS* and subsequent increase in nitric oxide (NO) is common in many tumours (Cianchi *et al.*, 2003; Vakkala *et al.*, 2000). Increased *COX-2* expression is associated with inflammation in a number of tumour types, including breast cancer where it is associated with poorer patient outcomes (Subbaramaiah *et al.*, 2012; Karray-Chouayek *et al.*, 2011). The fact that HER2 can also activate *COX-2* gene expression (Wang *et al.*, 2010b) presumably contributes to the poor prognosis that has previously been associated with HER2 positive breast cancers.

Following internalisation and sorting, EGFR can localise to the mitochondria where it may modulate the function of cytochrome c oxidase subunit II and mito-chondrial functions that are dependent on this enzyme, including regulation of apoptosis (reviewed in Wang and Huang, 2012).

One of the truncated variants of HER2 (p95HER2) can be found in the nucleus and the combination of expression and nuclear localisation is associated with local metastasis and decreased prognosis for breast cancer patients (reviewed in Arribas, 2011).

In contrast nuclear ErbB4 is associated with improved patient outcomes, especially for those treated with tamoxifen.

1.5.4   Changes in ligand levels

One of the simplest ways from a biological perspective for signalling to increase is via increased expression of the relevant ligands. As long as the ligand-binding sites on the receptors are not saturated an increase in ligand concentration is likely to result in increased receptor occupancy and a subsequent increase in activation.

A number of ErbB ligands, especially those that bind to EGFR, are associated with tumour development and progression. TGFα, amphiregulin and HB-EGF are all associated with poorer patient prognosis or resistance to chemotherapeutic agents. In breast cancers, TGFα and EGFR expression are associated with a clinically aggressive tumour subset and EGF expression is linked to poor prognosis (Castellani *et al.*, 1994; Mizukami *et al.*, 1991); in NSCLC serum levels of TGFα and amphiregulin correlate with aggressiveness and poor responses to therapy (Ishikawa *et al.*, 2005). In EGFR positive lung adenocarcinomas, patients with high EGF and TGFα levels had shorter survival times than those with no EGF or TGFα (Tateishi *et al.*, 1990).

1.5.5   Changes in adaptor protein levels

Over-expression or re-localisation of novel adapter proteins can enhance ErbB signalling. For example, Brk/PTK6 is physiologically expressed in a limited number of normal epithelial tissues where it plays a role in regulating differentiation and appears to have a more nuclear localisation. However, during carcinogenesis Brk is found to be cytoplasmic and associated with ErbB receptors where its role is believed to be oncogenic (Aubele *et al.*, 2010; Derry *et al.*, 2003; Petro *et al.*, 2004; reviewed in Harvey and Burmi, 2011).

The effects are more striking in the breast, as Brk is not found in normal mammary tissue (Barker *et al.*, 1997; Llor *et al.*, 1999) but is over-expressed in breast carcinomas with higher mRNA and protein levels correlating with increased tumour grade (Ostrander *et al.*, 2007; Chakraborty *et al.*, 2008; Harvey *et al.*, 2009). Brk augments the mitogenic effects of EGF (Kamalati *et al.*, 1996) and this may well be a result of increasing recruitment of p85 PI3K to ErbB3 (Kamalati *et al.*, 2000).

Brk and other ErbB signalling effector proteins are also implicated in other signalling pathways such as IGF (Irie *et al.*, 2010) (see Chapter 2), suggesting that cross-talk plays a crucial role in signalling regulation (see Chapter 9).

1.6   Therapeutic opportunities

Some breast cancers can express up to 50 copies of the *ErbB2* gene (reviewed in Sørlie, 2004) making HER2 an attractive tumour target, especially given the low expression of HER2 in most adult tissues.

The Greene laboratory were the first to show that targeting a protein involved in the cellular transformation process for degradation could reduce the malignant phenotype of the cells by blocking downstream signalling. Strikingly, this effect was observed both *in vivo*, as well as in *in vitro* studies (Drebin *et al.*, 1985, 1986).

Patients with HER2 positive early stage breast cancer or hyperplasia that has yet to become disseminated or fully transformed should benefit most from HER2 targeted therapies, as the additional changes required for full transformation that are mediated by HER2 have yet to occur and will therefore be prevented. Comparison of clinical trial data from patients with HER2 positive breast cancer that had been surgically removed showed that HER2-targeting improved patient outcomes (Romond *et al.*, 2005). Patients with late stage breast cancer also benefit from HER2 targeted therapy and the guidelines for the HER2 screening of breast cancer patients were updated by the American Society for Clinical Oncology (ASCO) in 1998 and further optimised in 2007 (ASCO, 1998, 2007).

1.6.1   Current strategies

There are a number of therapeutic strategies that can be considered for suppressing ErbB signalling. In addition to blocking receptor function through the use of monoclonal antibodies, or kinase activity with small molecule inhibitors, inhibiting the function of downstream signalling components and molecules involved in stabilising receptor conformation could also be considered.

Monoclonal antibodies

Trastazumab (Herceptin) and Pertuzamab (Perjeta) are the most commonly used monoclonal antibodies directed against HER2 in the clinic. They both prevent HER2 dimerisation but, as they are targeted towards different extra cellular domains of HER2, the nature of the dimer affected by each antibody is different. Trastazumab prevents HER2 homodimerisation, whereas Pertuzamab is more effective against HER2 heterodimerisation with HER3 or EGFR (reviewed in Eccles, 2011). Patients with advanced metastatic breast cancer that had acquired resistance to Herceptin responded to a combination of Herceptin and Pertuzamab (Gelmon *et al.*, 2008). As well as providing benefit to patients by overcoming the adaptive features of Herceptin resistance, these data provide an insight into the mechanisms of acquired resistance and the contribution of signalling cross-talk to therapeutic responses.

Given that only a subset of HER2 positive breast cancer patients reportedly responded to Trastazumab (Nahta *et al.*, 2006), data from the Arteaga laboratory suggest measuring the levels of HER2 homo- and hetero-dimers may be important in stratifying HER2 positive patients for antibody therapy (Ghosh *et al.*, 2011).

Kinase inhibitors

A number of different kinase inhibitors have been developed. Some, such as erlotinib and gefitinib, inhibit EGFR (Zhang *et al.*, 2007) whilst others, such as lapatinib, target both EGFR and HER2 (Rusnak *et al.*, 2001). In breast and in head and neck tumour cells, both MAPK and AKT pathways are inhibited in response to lapatinib treatment resulting in cell death (Xia *et al.*, 2002).

Lapatinib has good clinical efficacy in HER2 positive cancers that have become refractory to treatment with other targeted antibody based agents such as Trastazumab (Olson *et al.*, 2012; Hirano *et al.*, 2012), or in combination with trastazumab to achieve complete HER2 blockade (Wang *et al.*, 2011).

Although early pre-clinical studies with gefitinib were promising, Iressa™ became the first drug to be withdrawn following accelerated approval by the American FDA due to its lack of clinical efficacy (FDA, 2004; Frantz, 2005). This highlights the issues faced with kinase inhibition and the importance of relevant pre-clinical studies.

Destabilising receptor conformations

Many cellular proteins are highly dependent on chaperone proteins for correct folding and cellular localisation. Inhibition of chaperone function would destabilise the conformation of the client protein and target it for proteosomal degradation. HER2 is no exception; it is highly dependent on the chaperone function of Hsp90 for correct folding (Xu *et al.*, 2001 reviewed Buchner, 1999). Inhibition of Hsp90 results in degradation of HER2 both *in vitro* and *in vivo* and convincing antitumour effects have been observed in HER-positive mouse xenograft models (Eccles *et al.*, 2008).

Targeting Hsp90 in HER2 over-expressing tumours could prove to be extremely effective as a number of downstream signalling effectors such as PDK1 and Brk/PTK6 are also reported to be Hsp90 client proteins (Fujita *et al.*, 2002; Kang *et al.*, 2012). In addition, as EGFR is also stabilised by Hsp90 (Ahsan 2012), inhibiting Hsp90 could antagonise EGFR, which would limit the 'options' for compensatory signalling via other members of the ErbB family in HER2/EGFR positive tumours.

Downstream signalling effectors

Downstream of Akt is mTOR. Blocking mTOR signalling is therapeutically very attractive as a number of pathways merge at this signalling 'hub' (Chapters 5 and 9). mTOR inhibitors show antitumour activity in a wide range of different tumour models and some of these are discussed in Chapter 5.

Therapeutic resistance

Signalling cross-talk plays a major role in the development of resistance to targeted anticancer therapies (see Chapter 9).

However, altered cellular localisation of receptors has been gaining more attention in recent years. EGFR has been shown to translocate to the mitochondria following tyrosine kinase inhibition, suggesting that mitochondrial localisation of receptors may play a role in therapeutic responses and resistance (Cao *et al.*, 2011).

Nuclear EGFR has been reported as applying a role in acquired resistance to the anti-EGFR antibody, cetuximab (Li *et al.*, 2009). Both cetuximab and gefitinib inhibit radiation-induced EGFR nuclear transport and sensitises cells to the effects of radiation, suggesting that EGFR may contribute to radio resistance (Dittmann *et al.*, 2005; Bailey *et al.*, 2007). Lapatinib also inhibits the nuclear translocation of EGFR and HER2 sensitising cancer cells to 5-fluorouracil (Kim *et al.*, 2009). These studies are part of a growing body of evidence suggesting that nuclear EGFR may be associated with therapeutic resistance to conventional therapies, and the development of kinase inhibitors and monoclonal antibodies are providing the tools to investigate this further.

1.6.2   Future strategies

Therapeutic combinations and alternative treatments

Using combinations of ErbB targeted therapies with the more conventional anti-cancer drugs is not straightforward.

HER2 positive cancers can be more resistant to some but not all chemotherapy agents (reviewed in Eccles, 2011). Conversely, topoisomerase 2 is co-amplified with the *ErbB2* gene making HER2 positive cancers more sensitive to the topoisomerase inhibitor doxorubicin (reviewed in Bonnefoi, 2011). An obvious combination for treatment would therefore be an HER2-targeted therapy alongside doxorubicin; however, as both approaches result in cardiomyopathies, this strategy is no longer advisable (Procter *et al.*, 2010).

As the scientific knowledge of signalling cross-talk improves alongside greater understanding of the cellular mechanisms that contribute to therapeutic resistance to EGFR- or HER2-targeted therapies, combinatorial approaches to signalling inhibition will no doubt predominate in clinical practice (Chapter 9).

As biochemical technology moves forward it is possible that, in the future, disrupting protein–protein interactions could offer therapeutic benefit by targeting very specific aspects of signalling.

Disease prevention

The Greene laboratory showed that anti-HER2 antibodies can prevent tumours from forming in transgenic mice models. Transgenic mice that over-expressed the activated *neu* oncogene (rat oncogenic HER2) were treated with HER-targeted antibodies at 20 weeks of age, which was before tumours had formed. The study showed that there was a decrease in tumour incidence that was dose-dependent, and mice that remained tumour free appeared to remain protected against tumour development for life (Katsumata *et al.*, 1995). These data suggest that HER2 antibodies could be used to vaccinate against the formation of HER positive tumours.

Other pre-clinical studies are also suggesting that DNA-based vaccines may have benefit in treating HER positive cancers (Whittington *et al.*, 2008). More recent Phase I/II clinical trials have shown efficacy of peptide-based HER2 vaccines in the treatment of cancer with only limited toxicity (reviewed in Baxevanis *et al.*, 2012).

References

Aubele, M., Spears, M., Ludyga, N. *et al.* (2010) In situ quantification of HER2–protein tyrosine kinase 6 (PTK6) protein–protein complexes in paraffin sections from breast cancer tissues. *British Journal of Cancer*, **103** (5), 663–337.

Ahsan, A., Ramanand, S.G., Whitehead, C., *et al.* (2012) Wild-type EGFR is stabilized by direct interaction with HSP90 in cancer cells and tumors. *Neoplasia*, **14** (8), 670–677.

Alimandi, M., Romano, A., Curia, M.C. *et al.* (1995) Cooperative signaling of ErbB3 and ErbB2 in neoplastic transformation and human mammary carcinomas. *Oncogene*, **10**, 1813–1821.

Arribas, J., Baselga, J., Pedersen, K., and Parra-Palau, J.L. (2011) p95HER2 and breast cancer. *Cancer Research*, **71** (5) 1515–1519.

Arteaga, C.L. (2002) Epidermal growth factor receptor dependence in human tumors: more than just expression? *The Oncologist*, **7** (suppl 4), 31–39.

ASCO (1999) American Society of Clinical Oncology 1998 update of recommended breast cancer surveillance guidelines. *Journal of Clinical Oncology*, **17** (3) 1080–1082.

ASCO (2007) Guideline summary: American Society of Clinical Oncology/College of American Pathologists Guideline recommendations for human epidermal growth factor receptor HER2 testing in breast cancer. *Journal of Oncology Practice*, **3** (1) 48–50.

Bailey, K.E., Costantini, D.L., Cai, Z. *et al.* (2007) Epidermal growth factor receptor inhibition modulates the nuclear localization and cytotoxicity of the Auger electron emitting radiopharmaceutical 111In-DTPA human epidermal growth factor. *Journal of Nuclear Medicine*, **48**, 1562–1570.

Bargmann, C.I., Hung, M.C., Weinberg, R.A. *et al.* (1986) The neu oncogene encodes an epidermal growth factor receptor-related protein. *Nature*, **319**, 226–230.

Barker, K.T., Jackson, L.E. and Crompton, M.R. (1997) BRK tyrosine kinase expression in a high proportion of human breast carcinomas. *Oncogene*, **15** (7), 799–805.

Baxevanis, C.N., Papamichail, M., and Perez, S.A. (2012) Toxicity profiles of HER2/neu peptide anticancer vaccines: the picture from Phase/I and II clinical trials. *Expert Review of Vaccines*, **11** (6), 637–640.

Blagosklonny, M.V. and Darzynkiewicz, Z. (2003) Why Iressa failed: toward novel use of kinase inhibitors (outlook). *Cancer Biology and Therapy*, **2** (2) 137–140.

Bonnefoi, H.R. (2011) Anthracyclines, HER2, and TOP2A: the verdict. *Lancet Oncology*, **12** (12), 1084–1085.

Booth, B.W. and Smith, G.H. (2007) Roles of transforming growth factor-alpha in mammary development and disease. *Growth Factors*, **25**, 227–235.

Brennan, P.J., Kumogai, T., Berezov, A. *et al.* (2000) HER2/Neu: mechanisms of dimerization/oligomerization. *Oncogene*, **19** (53), 6093–6101.

Buchner, J. (1999) Hsp90 & Co. – a holding for folding. *Trends in Biochemical Sciences*, **24**, 136–141.

Burden, S. and Yarden, Y. (1997) Neuregulins and their receptors: a versatile signaling module in organogenesis and oncogenesis. *Neuron*, **18** (6), 847–855.

Burgess, A.W. (2008) EGFR family: structure physiology signalling and therapeutic targets. *Growth Factors*, **26**, 263–274.

Cao, X., Zhu, H., Ali-Osman, F. and Lo, H.W. (2011) EGFR and EGFRvIII undergo stress- and EGFR kinase inhibitor-induced mitochondrial translocalization: a potential mechanism of EGFR-driven antagonism of apoptosis. *Molecular Cancer*, **10**, 26.

Carnero, A., Blanco-Aparicio, C., Renner, O. *et al.* (2008) The PTEN/PI3K/AKT signalling pathway in cancer, therapeutic implications. *Current Cancer Drug Targets*, **8** (3), 187–198.

Carpenter, G. (1987) Receptors for epidermal growth factor and other polypeptide mitogens. *Annual Review of Biochemistry*, **56**, 881–914.

Carpenter, G., Lembach, K.J., Morrison, M.M. and Cohen, S. (1975) Characterization of the binding of 125-I-labeled epidermal growth factor to human fibroblasts. *Journal of Biological Chemistry*, **250** (11), 4297–304.

Carpenter, G. and Cohen, S. (1976) Human epidermal growth factor and the proliferation of human fibroblasts. *Journal of Cell Physiology*, **88** (2), 227–237.

Carpenter, G., King, L., Jr, and Cohen, S. (1978) Epidermal growth factor stimulates phosphorylation in membrane preparations in vitro. *Nature*, **276**, 409–410.

Castellani, R., Visscher, D.W., Wykes, S. *et al.* (1994) Interaction of transforming growth factor-alpha and epidermal growth factor receptor in breast carcinoma. An immunohistologic study. *Cancer*, **73** (2), 344–349.

Ceresa, B.P. and Bahr, S.J. (2006) Rab7 activity affects epidermal growth factor:epidermal growth factor receptor degradation by regulating endocytic trafficking from the late endosome. *Journal of Biological Chemistry*, **281**, 1099–1106.

Chakraborty, G., Jain, S. and Kundu, G.C. (2008) Osteopontin promotes vascular endothelial growth factor-dependent breast tumor growth and angiogenesis via autocrine and paracrine mechanisms. *Cancer Research*, **68** (1), 152–161.

Chuang, C.F. and Ng, S.Y. (1994) Functional divergence of the MAP kinase pathway. ERK1 and ERK2 activate specific transcription factors. *FEBS Letters*, **346** (2-3), 229–234.

Cianchi, F., Cortesini, C., Fantappie, O. *et al.* (2003) Inducible nitric oxide synthase expression in human colorectal cancer: correlation with tumor angiogenesis. *American Journal of Pathology*, **162**, 793–801.

Cohen, S., Carpenter, G. and Lembach, K.J. (1975) Interaction of epidermal growth factor (EGF) with cultured fibroblasts. *Advances in Metabolic Disorders*, **8**, 265–284.

Coussens, L., Yang-Feng, T.L., Liao, Y.C. *et al.* (1985) Tyrosine kinase receptor with extensive homology to EGF receptor shares chromosomal location with neu oncogene. *Science*, **230**, 1132–1139.

Cully, M., You, H., Levine, A. and Mak, T. (2006) Beyond PTEN mutations: the PI3K pathway as an integrator of multiple inputs during tumorigenesis. *Nature Reviews Cancer*, **6** (3), 184–192.

Derry, J.J., Prins, G.S., Ray, V. and Tyner, A.L. (2003) Altered localization and activity of the intracellular tyrosine kinase BRK/Sik in prostate tumor cells. *Oncogene.* **22** (27), 4212–4220.

Dittmann, K., Mayer, C. and Rodemann, H.P. (2005) Inhibition of radiation-induced EGFR nuclear import by C225 (Cetuximab) suppresses DNA-PK activity. *Radiotherapy and Oncology*, **76**, 157–161.

Drebin, J.A., Link, V.C., Stern, D.F. *et al.* (1985) Down-modulation of an oncogene protein product and reversion of the transformed phenotype by monoclonal antibodies. *Cell*, **41**, 697–706.

Drebin, J.A., Link, V.C., Weinberg, R.A. and Greene, M.I. (1986) Inhibition of tumor growth by a monoclonal antibody reactive with an oncogene-encoded tumor antigen. *Proceedings of the National Academy of Sciences, USA*, **83**, 9129–9133.

Eccles, S.A. (2011) The epidermal growth factor receptor/Erb-B/HER family in normal and malignant breast biology. *International Journal of Developmental Biology*, **55** (7-9), 685–96.

Eccles, S.A., Massey, A., Raynaud, F.I. *et al.* (2008) NVP-AUY922: a novel heat shock protein 90 inhibitor active against xenograft tumor growth, angiogenesis, and metastasis. *Cancer Research*, **68**, 2850–2860.

Ferguson, K.M., Mitchell, B., Berger, M.B *et al.* (2003) EGF activates its receptor by removing interactions that autoinhibit ectodomain dimerization. *Molecular Cell*, **11**, 507–517.

FDA Website (2004) http://www.fda.gov/newsevents/newsroom/pressannouncements/2004/ucm108383.htm (accessed 8 May 2013).

Ferguson, K.M. (2008) A structure-based view of epidermal growth factor receptor regulation. *Annual Review of Biophysics*, **37**, 353–373.

Frantz, S. (2005) Iressa failure raises fears about accelerated approvals. *Nature, Reviews Drug Discovery*, **4** (94) (News and Analysis).

Freudenberg, J.A., Wang, Q., Katsumata, M. *et al.* (2009) The role of HER2 in early breast cancer metastasis and the origins of resistance to HER2-targeted therapies. *Experimental and Molecular Pathology*, **87** (1), 1–11.

Freudlsperger, C., Burnett, J.R., Friedman, J.A. *et al.* (2011) EGFR-PI3K-AKT-mTOR signaling in head and neck squamous cell carcinomas – attractive targets for molecular-oriented therapy. *Expert Opinion on Therapeutic Targets*, **15** (1), 63–74.

Fujita, N., Sato, S., Ishida, A. and Tsuruo T. (2002) Involvement of Hsp90 in signaling and stability of 3-phosphoinositide-dependent kinase-1. *Journal of Biological Chemistry*, **277** (12), 10346–10353.

Fujiwara, S., Ibusuki, M., Yamamoto, S. *et al.* (2012) Association of ErbB1-4 expression in invasive breast cancer with clinicopathological characteristics and prognosis. *Breast Cancer*, 2012 Epub (PMID: 23100016).

Gandhi, J., Zhang, J., Xie, Y. *et al.* (2009) Alterations in genes of the EGFR signaling pathway and their relationship to EGFR tyrosine kinase inhibitor sensitivity in lung cancer cell Lines. *PLoS ONE*, **4** (2), e4576. doi: 10.1371/journal.pone.0004576.

Gao, M., Patel, R., Ahmad, I. *et al.* (2012) SPRY2 loss enhances ErbB trafficking and PI3K/AKT signalling to drive human and mouse prostate carcinogenesis. *EMBO Molecular Medicine*, **4** (8), 776–790.

Garrett, T., McKern, N., Lou, M. *et al.* (2002) Crystal structure of a truncated epidermal growth factor receptor extracellular domain bound to transforming growth factor-α. *Cell*, **110**, 763–773.

Gelmon, K.A., Fumoleau, P., Verma, S. *et al.* (2008) Results of a phase II trial of trastuzumab (H) and pertuzumab (P) in patients (pts) with HER2-positive metastatic breast cancer (MBC) who had progressed during trastuzumab therapy. *Journal of Clinical Oncology*, *(Meeting Abstracts)*, **26** (15S), 1206.

Ghosh, R., Narasanna, A., Wang, S.E. *et al.* (2011) Trastuzumab has preferential activity against breast cancers driven by HER2 homodimers. *Cancer Research*, **71** (5), 1871–1882.

Gilbertson, R.J., Clifford, S.C., MacMeekin, W. *et al.* (1998) Expression of the ErbB-neuregulin signaling network during human cerebellar development: implications for the biology of medulloblastoma. *Cancer Research*, **58**, 3932–3941.

Gotoh, N., Tojo, A., Hino, M. *et al.* (1992) A highly conserved tyrosine residue at codon 845 within the kinase domain is not required for the transforming activity of human epidermal growth factor receptor. *Biochemical and Biophysical Research Communications*, **186**, 768–774.

Grandal, M.V., Grøvdal L.M., Henriksen, L. *et al.* (2012) Differential roles of Grb2 and AP-2 in p38 MAPK and EGFR induced receptor internalization. *Traffic*, **13** (4), 576–85.

Grant, B.D. and Donaldson, J.G. (2009) Pathways and mechanisms of endocytic recycling. *Nature Reviews Molecular Cell Biology*, **10**, 597–608.

Greenfield, C., Hiles, I., Waterfield, M.D. *et al.* (1989) Epidermal growth factor binding induces a conformational change in the external domain of its receptor. *EMBO Journal*, **8**, 4115–4123.

Harvey, A. and Burmi, R.S. (2011) Future therapeutic strategies: Implications for Brk targeting, in *Breast Cancer - Current and Alternative Therapeutic Modalities* (eds E. Gunduz and M. Gundez), InTech.

Helgason, C.D., Damen, J.E., Rosten, P. *et al.* (1998) Targeted disruption of SHIP leads to hemopoietic perturbations, lung pathology, and a shortened life span. *Genes and Development*, **12** (11), 1610–1620.

Hinkle, C.L., Sunnarborg, S.W., Loiselle, D. *et al.* (2004) Selective roles for tumor necrosis factor alpha-converting enzyme/ADAM17 in the shedding of the epidermal growth factor receptor ligand family: the juxtamembrane stalk determines cleavage efficiency. *Journal of Biological Chemistry*, **279**, 24179–24188.

Hirano, T., Sakurai, K., Fujisaki, S. *et al.* (2012) Lapatinib is useful for metastatic breast cancer patients who cannot be treated with trastuzumab-report of a case. *Gan To Kagaku Ryoho*, **39** (12), 2045–2047.

Hoshino, M., Fukui, H., Ono, Y. *et al.* (2007) Nuclear expression of phosphorylated EGFR is associated with poor prognosis of patients with esophageal squamous cell carcinoma. *Pathobiology*, **74**, 15–21.

Hynes, N.E. and Stern, D.F. (1994) The biology of erbB-2/neu/HER-2 and its role in cancer. *Biochimica et Biophysica Acta*, **1198** (2-3), 165–168.

Irie, H.Y., Shrestha, Y., Selfors, L.M. *et al.* (2010) PTK6 regulates IGF-1-induced anchorage-independent survival. *PLoS ONE*, **5** (7), e11729.

Ishikawa, N., Daigo, Y., Takano, A. *et al.* (2005) Increases of amphiregulin and transforming growth factor-alpha in serum as predictors of poor response to gefitinib among patients with advanced non-small cell lung cancers. *Cancer Research*, **65** (20), 9176–9184.

Jackson, L.F., Qiu, T.H., Sunnarborg, S.W. *et al.* (2003) Defective valvulogenesis in HB-EGF and TACE-null mice is associated with aberrant BMP signaling. *EMBO Journal*, **22**, 2704–2716.

Kamalati T, Jolin, H.E., Mitchell, P.J. *et al.* (1996) Brk, a breast tumor-derived non-receptor protein-tyrosine kinase, sensitizes mammary epithelial cells to epidermal growth factor. *Journal of Biological Chemistry*, **271** (48), 30956–30963.

Kang, S.A., Cho, H.S., Yoon, J.B. *et al.* (2012) Hsp90 rescues PTK6 from proteasomal degradation in breast cancer cells. *Biochemical Journal*, **447** (2), 313–320.

Karray-Chouayekh, S., Trifa, F., Khabir, A. *et al.* (2011) Methylation status and over-expression of COX-2 in Tunisian patients with ductal invasive breast carcinoma. *Tumour Biology*, **32** (3), 461–468.

Katsumata, M., Okudaira, T., Samanta, A. *et al.* (1995) Prevention of breast tumour development in vivo by downregulation of the p185neu receptor. *Nature Medicine*, **1**, 644–648.

Kim, H.P., Yoon, Y.K., Kim, J.W. *et al.* (2009) Lapatinib, a dual EGFR and HER2 tyrosine kinase inhibitor, downregulates thymidylate synthase by inhibiting the nuclear translocation of EGFR and HER2. *PLoS ONE*, **4**, e5933.

King, C.R., Kraus, M.H. and Aaronson, S.A. (1985) Amplification of a novel v-erbB-related gene in a human mammary carcinoma. *Science*, **229**, 974–976.

Kohler, M., Janz, I., Wintzer, H.O. *et al.* (1989) The expression of EGF receptors, EGF-like factors and c-myc in ovarian and cervical carcinomas and their potential clinical significance. *Anticancer Research*, **9**, 1537–1547.

Kraus, M.H., Issing, W., Miki, T. *et al.* (1989) Isolation and characterization of ERBB3, a third member of the ERBB/epidermal growth factor receptor family: evidence for overexpression in a subset of human mammary tumors. *Proceedings of the National Academy of Sciences, USA*, **86**, 9193–9197.

Li, C., Lida, M., Dunn, E.F. *et al.* (2009) Nuclear EGFR contributes to acquired resistance to cetuximab. *Oncogene*, **28** (43), 3801–3813.

Liaw, D., Marsh, D.J., Li, J. *et al.* (1997) Germline mutations of the PTEN gene in Cowden disease, an inherited breast and thyroid cancer syndrome. *Nature Genetics*, **16** (1), 64–67.

Lin, X.H., Walter, J., Scheidtmann, K. *et al.* (1998) Protein phosphatase 2A is required for the initiation of chromosomal DNA replication. *Proceedings of the National Academy of Sciences, USA*, **95** (25), 14693–14698.

Llor, X., Serfas, M.S., Bie, W. *et al.* (1999) BRK/Sik expression in the gastrointestinal tract and in colon tumors. *Clinical Cancer Research*, **5** (7), 1767–1777.

Lo, H.W., Hsu, S.C., Ali-Seyed, M. *et al.* (2005a) Nuclear interaction of EGFR and STAT3 in the activation of the iNOS/NO pathway. *Cancer Cell*, **7**, 575–589.

Lo, H.W., Xia, W., Wei, Y. *et al.* (2005b) Novel prognostic value of nuclear epidermal growth factor receptor in breast cancer. *Cancer Research*, **65**, 338–348.

Lo, H.W., Cao, X., Zhu, H. and Ali-Osman, F. (2010) Cyclooxygenase-2 is a novel transcriptional target of the nuclear EGFR-STAT3 and EGFRvIII-STAT3 signaling axes. *Molecular Cancer Research*, **8** (2), 232–243.

Maxfield, F.R. and McGraw, T.E. (2004) Endocytic recycling. *Nature Reviews Molecular Cell Biology*, **5**, 121–132.

McKanna, J.A., Haigler, H.T. and Cohen, S. (1979) Hormone receptor topology and dynamics: morphological analysis using ferritin-labeled epidermal growth factor. *Proceedings of the National Academy of Sciences, USA*, **76** (11), 5689–5693.

Mellor, P., Furber, L.A., Nyarko, J.N. and Anderson, D.H. (2012) Multiple roles for the p85α isoform in the regulation and function of PI3K signalling and receptor trafficking. *Biochemical Journal*, **441** (1), 23–37.

Miletic, A.V., Anzelon-Mills, A.N., Mills, D.M. *et al.* (2010) Coordinate suppression of B cell lymphoma by PTEN and SHIP phosphatases. *Journal of Experimental Medicine*, **207** (11), 2407–2420.

Mill, C.P., Zordan, M.D., Rothenberg, S.M. *et al.* (2011) ErbB2 is necessary for ErbB4 ligands to stimulate oncogenic activities in models of human breast cancer. *Genes and Cancer*, **2** (8), 792–804.

Mizukami, Y., Nonomura, A., Noguchi, M. *et al.* (1991) Immunohistochemical study of oncogene product ras p21, c-myc and growth factor EGF in breast carcinomas. *Anticancer Research*, **11**, 1485–1494.

Mumby, M. (2007) PP2A: unveiling a reluctant tumor suppressor. *Cell*, **130** (1), 21–24.

Nahta, R., Yu, D., Huang, M.-C. *et al.* (2006) Mechanisms of disease: understanding resistance to HER2-targeted therapy in human breast cancer. *Nature Clinical Practice Oncology*, **3**, 269–280.

Ogiso, H., Ishitani, R., Nureki, O. *et al.* (2002) Crystal structure of the complex of human epidermal growth factor and receptor extracellular domains. *Cell*, **110**, 775–787.

Olson, E.M., Lin, N.U., DiPiro, P.J. *et al.* (2012) Responses to subsequent anti-HER2 therapy after treatment with trastuzumab-DM1 in women with HER2-positive metastatic breast cancer. *Annals of Oncology*, **23** (1), 93–97.

Ostrander, J.H., Daniel, A.R., Lofgren, K. *et al.* (2007) Breast tumor kinase (protein tyrosine kinase 6) regulates heregulin-induced activation of ERK5 and p38 MAP kinases in breast cancer cells. *Cancer Research*, **67** 9, 4199–4209.

Pérez-Regadera, J., Sánchez-Muñoz, A., De-la-Cruz, J. *et al.* (2011) Impact of epidermal growth factor receptor expression on disease-free survival and rate of pelvic relapse in patients with advanced cancer of the cervix treated with chemoradiotherapy. *American Journal of Clinical Oncology*, **34** (4), 395–400.

Petro, B.J., Tan, R.C., Tyner, A.L. *et al.* (2004) Differential expression of the non-receptor tyrosine kinase BRK in oral squamous cell carcinoma and normal oral epithelium. *Oral Oncology*, **40** (10), 1040–1047.

Plowman, G.D., Culouscou, J.M., Whitney, G.S. *et al.* (1993) Ligand-specific activation of HER4/p180erbB4, a fourth member of the epidermal growth factor receptor family. *Proceedings of the National Academy of Sciences, USA*, **90**, 1746–1750.

Plowman, G.D., Whitney, G.S., Neubauer, M.G. *et al.* (1990) Molecular cloning and expression of an additional epidermal growth factor receptor-related gene. *Proceedings of the National Academy of Sciences, USA*, **87**, 4905–4909.

Procter, M., Suter, T.M., De Azambuja, E. *et al.* (2010) Longer-term assessment of trastuzumab-related cardiac adverse events in the Herceptin Adjuvant (HERA) trial. *Journal of Clinical Oncology*, **28**, 3422–3428.

Psyrri, A., Kassar, M., Yu, Z. *et al.* (2005a) Effect of epidermal growth factor receptor expression level on survival in patients with epithelial ovarian cancer. *Clinical Cancer Research*, **11** (24), 8637–8643.

Psyrri, A., Yu, Z., Weinberger, P.M. *et al.* (2005b) Quantitative determination of nuclear and cytoplasmic epidermal growth factor receptor expression in oropharyngeal squamous cell cancer by using automated quantitative analysis. *Clinical Cancer Research*, **11**, 5856–5862.

Rink, J., Ghigo, E., Kalaidzidis, Y. and Zerial M. (2005) Rab conversion as a mechanism of progression from early to late endosomes. *Cell*, **122**, 735–749.

Roberts, A.B., Lamb, L.C., Newton, D.L. *et al.* (1980) Transforming growth factors: isolation of polypeptides from virally and chemically transformed cells by acid/ethanol extraction. *Proceedings of the National Academy of Sciences, USA*, **77**, 3494–3498.

Romond, E.H., Perez, E.A., Bryant, J. *et al.* (2005) Trastuzumab plus adjuvant chemotherapy for operable HER2-positive breast cancer. *New England Journal of Medicine*, **353**, 1673–1684.

Rusnak, D.W., Affleck, K., Cockerill, S.G. *et al.* (2001) The characterization of novel, dual ErbB-2/EGFR, tyrosine kinase inhibitors: potential therapy for cancer. *Cancer Research*, **61**, 7196–7203.

Sahin, U., Weskamp, G., Kelly, K. *et al.* (2004) Distinct roles for ADAM10 and ADAM17 in ectodomain shedding of six EGFR ligands. *Journal of Cell Biology*, **164** (5), 769–779.

Sansal, I. and Sellers, W.R. (2004) The biology and clinical relevance of the PTEN tumor suppressor pathway. *Journal of Clinical Oncology*, **22** (14), 2954–2963.

Sarbassov, D., Guertin, D., Ali, S. and Sabatini, D. (2005) Phosphorylation and regulation of Akt/PKB by the rictor-mTOR complex. *Science*, **307** (5712), 1098–1101.

Savage, C.R. Jr, Inagami, T. and Cohen, S. (1972) The primary structure of epidermal growth factor. *Journal of Biological Chemistry*, **247**, 7612–7621.

Schechter, A.L., Stern, D.F., Vaidyanathan, L. *et al.* (1984) The neu oncogene: an erb-B-related gene encoding a 185,000-Mr tumour antigen. *Nature*, **312**, 513–516.

Schulze, W.X., Deng, L. and Mann, M. (2005) Phosphotyrosine interactome of the ErbB-receptor kinase family. *Molecular Systems Biology*, **1**, 2005.0008.

Shahbazian, D., Roux, P.P., Mieulet, V. *et al.* (2006) The mTOR/PI3K and MAPK pathways converge on eIF4B to control its phosphorylation and activity. *EMBO Journal*, **25** (12), 2781–2791.

Shigematsu, H., Takahashi, T., Nomura, M. *et al.* (2005) Somatic mutations of the HER2 kinase domain in lung adenocarcinomas. *Cancer Research*, **65**, 1642–1646.

Slamon, D.J., Godolphin, W., Jones, L.A. *et al.* (1989) Studies of the *HER-2/neu* proto-oncogene in human breast and ovarian cancer. *Science*, **244**, 707–712.

Sordella, R., Bell, D.W., Haber, D.A. and Settleman, J. (2004) Gefitinib-sensitizing EGFR mutations in lung cancer activate anti-apoptotic pathways. *Science*, **305**, 1163–1167.

Sorkin, A. (2004) Cargo recognition during clathrin-mediated endocytosis: a team effort. *Current Opinion in Cell Biology*, **16** (4), 392–399.

Sorkin, A and Goh, L.K. (2008) Endocytosis and intracellular trafficking of ErbBs. *Experimental Cell Research*, **314** (17), 3093–3106.

Sørlie, T. (2004) Molecular portraits of breast cancer: tumour subtypes as distinct disease entities. *European Journal of Cancer*, **40** (18), 2667–2675.

Sternlicht, M.D., Sunnarborg, S.W., Kouros-Mehr, H. *et al.* (2005) Mammary ductal morphogenesis requires paracrine activation of stromal EGFR via ADAM17-dependent shedding of epithelial amphiregulin. *Development*, **132**, 3923–3933.

Subbaramaiah, K., Morris, P.G., Zhou, X.K. *et al.* (2012) Increased levels of COX-2 and prostaglandin E2 contribute to elevated aromatase expression in inflamed breast tissue of obese women. *Cancer Discovery*, **2** (4), 356–365.

Tateishi, M., Ishida, T., Mitsudomi, T. Kaneko, S. and Sugimahi, K. (1990) Immuno-histochemical evidence of autocrine growth factors in adenocarcinoma of the human lung. *Cancer Research*, **50**, 7077–7080.

Todaro, G.J., Fryling, C. and De Larco, J. E. (1980) Transforming growth factors produced by certain human tumor cells: polypeptides that interact with epidermal growth factor receptors. *Proceedings of the National Academy of Sciences, USA*, **77**, 5258–5262.

Ullrich, A., Coussens, L., Hayflick, J.S. *et al.* (1984) Human epidermal growth factor receptor cDNA sequence and aberrant expression of the amplified gene in A431 epidermoid carcinoma cell. *Nature*, **309**, 418–425.

Vakkala, M., Kahlos, K., Lakari, E. *et al.* (2000) Inducible nitric oxide synthase expression, apoptosis, and angio- genesis in in situ and invasive breast carcinomas. *Clinical Cancer Research*, **6**, 2408–2416.

Van Weering, J.R., Verkade, P. and Cullen, P.J. (2010) SNX-BAR proteins in phosphoinositide-mediated, tubular-based endosomal sorting. *Seminars in Cell and Developmental Biology*, **21** (4), 371–380.

Vaught, D.B., Stanford, J.C., Young, C. *et al.* (2012) HER3 is required for HER2-induced preneoplastic changes to the breast epithelium and tumor formation. *Cancer Research*, **72** (10), 2672–2682.

Vivanco, I. and Sawyers C. (2002) The phosphatidylinositol 3-kinase AKT pathway in human cancer. *Nature Reviews Cancer*, **2** (7, July), 489–501.

Wang, Y.-N., Yamaguchi, H., Hsu, J.-M. and Hung, M.-C. (2010a) Nuclear trafficking of the epidermal growth factor receptor family membrane proteins. *Oncogene*, **29** (28), 3997–4006.

Wang, K.H., Kao, A.P., Chang, C.C., *et al.* (2010b) Increasing CD44+/CD24(−) tumor stem cells, and upregulation of COX-2 and HDAC6, as major functions of HER2 in breast tumorigenesis. Molecular Cancer, doi: 10.1186/1476-4598-9-288.

Wang, Y.C., Morrison, G., Gillihan R. *et al.* (2011) Different mechanisms for resistance to trastuzumab versus lapatinib in HER2-positive breast cancers–role of estrogen receptor and HER2 reactivation. *Breast Cancer Research*, **13** (6), R121.

Wang, Y.-N. and Hung, M.-C. (2012) Nuclear function and subcellular trafficking mechanisms of the epidermal growth factor receptor family. *Cell and Bioscience*, **2**, 13.

Weiner, D.B., Liu, J., Cohen, J.A. *et al.* (1989a) A point mutation in the neu oncogene mimics ligand induction of receptor aggregation. *Nature*, **339**, 230–231.

Weiner, D.B., Kokai, Y., Wada, T. *et al.* (1989b) Linkage of tyrosine kinase activity with transforming ability of the p185neu oncoprotein. *Oncogene*, **4**, 1175–1183.

Whittington, P.J., Piechocki, M.P., Heng, H.H. *et al.* (2008) DNA vaccination controls Her-2+ tumors that are refractory to targeted therapies. *Cancer Research*, **68** (18), 7502–7511.

Wiesen, J.F., Young, P., Werb, Z. and Cunha, G.R. (1999) Signaling through the stromal epidermal growth factor receptor is necessary for mammary ductal development. *Development*, **126**, 335–344.

Wiley, H.S. (2003) Trafficking of the ErbB receptors and its influence on signaling. *Experimental Cell Research*, **284** (1), 78–88.

Wilson, K.J., Gilmore, J.L. Foley, J. *et al.* (2009) Functional selectivity of EGF family peptide growth factors: implications for cancer. *Pharmacology and Therapeutics*, **122** (1), 1–8.

Xia, W., Mullin, R.J., Keith, B.R. *et al.* (2002) Anti-tumor activity of GW572016: a dual tyrosine kinase inhibitor blocks EGF activation of EGFR/erbB2 and downstream Erk1/2 and AKT pathways. *Oncogene*, **21**, 6255–6263.

Xia, W., Wei, Y., Du, Y. *et al.* (2009) Nuclear expression of epidermal growth factor receptor is a novel prognostic value in patients with ovarian cancer. *Molecular Carcinogenesis*, **48** (7), 610–617.

Xu, W., Mimnaugh, E., Rosser, M.F. *et al.* (2001) Sensitivity of mature ErbB2 to geldanamycin is conferred by its kinase domain and is mediated by chaperone protein Hsp90. *Journal of Biological Chemistry*, **276**, 3702–3708.

Yamazaki, S., Iwamoto, R., Saeki, K. *et al.* (2003) Mice with defects in HB-EGF ectodomain shedding show severe developmental abnormalities. *Journal of Cell Biology*, **163**, 469–447.

Zhang, H., Berezov, A., Wang, Q. *et al.* (2007) ErbB receptors: from oncogenes to targeted cancer therapies. *Journal of Clinical Investigation*, **117**, 2051– 2058.

Zhang, Q. and Claret, F.X. (2012) Phosphatases: the new brakes for cancer development? *Enzyme Research*, doi:10.1155/2012/659649.

Zhang, K., Sun, J., Liu, N. *et al.* (1996) Transformation of NIH 3T3 cells by HER3 or HER4 receptors requires the presence of HER1 or HER2. *Journal of Biological Chemistry*, **271** (7), 3884–3890.

Zhang, X., Gureasko, J., Shen, K. *et al.* (2006) An allosteric mechanism for activation of the kinase domain of epidermal growth factor receptor. *Cell*, **125**, 1137–49.

2

Insulin and the insulin-like growth factor (IGF) family

Maria Thorpe, Erald Shehu and Amanda Harvey
Biosciences, Brunel University, London

Understanding the complex signalling generated from the binding of insulin (IGF) and the two known insulin-like growth factors (IGF1 and IGF2) to their respective ligands has been the subject of extensive research over many years due to their recognised involvement in many fundamental physiological as well as pathological processes. These hormones are critical for many functions such as cell growth, development and DNA synthesis and are ubiquitously expressed across all cell and tissue types.

2.1 Receptors

Insulin, IGF1 and IGF2 signal across the cell membrane via the insulin-like growth factor 1 receptor (IGF1R) and the insulin receptor (IR), which are members of the tyrosine kinase type II class of membrane receptor family (RTK), consisting of an extracellular ligand binding domain, a transmembrane domain, and intracellular tyrosine kinase domain. Uniquely to this class of receptor, unlike other receptors that are present as monomers and dimerise following ligand binding, IFG1R and IR are presented on the membrane as complete dimeric units termed hemireceptors. IR and IGF1R exist as heterotetrameric complexes comprising two α-subunits and two β-subunits covalently linked by disulphide bonds. The α-subunits are the ligand binding domains that are extracellular and the β-subunits span the membrane and contain the tyrosine kinase domain (Figure 2.1) (Belfiore *et al.*, 2009; Ward and Lawrence 2011). The third receptor in the pathway is the insulin-like growth factor receptor 2 (IGF2R) (also known as the mannose-6-phosphate receptor), which is structurally and functionally distinct from the first two because it lacks kinase activity and has not been shown to positively participate in signal

Cancer Cell Signalling, First Edition. Edited by Amanda Harvey.
© 2013 John Wiley & Sons, Ltd. Published 2013 by John Wiley & Sons, Ltd.

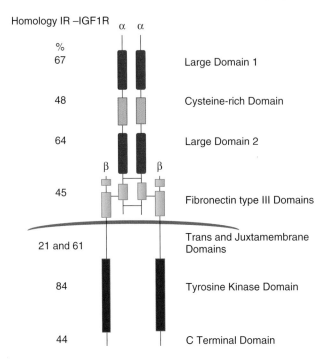

Figure 2.1 **Schematic representation of the IGF receptor (IGFR).** Receptors have extracellular ligand binding domains, trans and juxtamembrane domains as well as a tyrosine kinase domain and a C-terminus for substrate binding. The percentage homology between IGF1R and the insulin receptor (IR) is indicated.

transduction (Martin-Kleiner and Troselj, 2010). The human gene for *IGF2R* is located on chromosome 6q26 and it encodes a glycoprotein of 2491 amino acids, which has a large extracellular domain (2264 amino acids in size) comprising 15 homologous structural repeats. IGF2R sequesters its ligand, IGF2, from the extracellular milieu with high affinity, preventing it binding to either IR or IGF1R, and therefore is considered to act with tumour suppressor activity (De Souza *et al.*, 1995; reviewed in Pollak 2008).

The *IR* and *IGF1R* genes are conserved, and are thought to have originated from the same ancestral gene due to extensive sequence homology in the ligand binding and tyrosine kinase domains (Brogiolo *et al.*, 2001; Hernandez-Sanchez *et al.*, 2008; reviewed in Pollak 2012a). The human gene for *IR* is located on chromosome 19p13.3 and encodes a 1382 amino acid protein; the gene for *IGF1R* is on chromosome 15q26.3, encoding a protein of 1367 amino acids. The ligand-binding domain of IR protein is up to 64% similar to that of IGF1R (Figure 2.1), whilst their kinase and substrate domains can be up to 84% homologous (Mynarcik *et al.*, 1997; Ullrich *et al.*, 1986).

IR and IGF1R have different but complimentary tissue expression. IGF1R expression is found in many tissues, except for adipose and liver where IR is commonly found. Binding of a ligand to the receptor leads to autophosphorylation and the initiation of kinase activity. The regions phosphorylated on these receptors are the juxtamembrane domain, the catalytic domain, and the carboxyterminal regions. Kinase activity correlates with phosphorylation of tyrosine residues in the catalytic domain region. In the IR this is on amino acids 1146, 1151 and 1152 (reviewed in Belfiore *et al.*, 2009); and on IGF1R this is on amino acids 1250, 1251 and 1316 (Blakesley *et al.*, 1996). The three phosphorylated clusters act as docking sites for Src homology 2 (SH2) containing substrates such as the four insulin receptor substrates (IRS1-4) (White, 1998).

There are two functionally and structurally different isoforms of IR: IRA and IRB. *IRA* lacks exon 11 (36 nucleotides), which translates to 12 amino acid residues found on the carboxy-terminus of the receptor's extracellular α-subunit (Seino *et al.*, 1989; Hubbard, 2013). *IRB* expression differs from that of IRA, which is found mainly in the spleen, brain and lymphocytes (Mosthaf *et al.*, 1990). *IRA* expression in foetal tissues was discovered indirectly from a study on IGF signalling during mouse foetal development. Mice lacking *IGF1R* and *IGF2* displayed a developmental retardation phenotype indistinguishable from those lacking *IR* and *IGF1R*, which was in turn more severe than those lacking just *IGF1R* (Louvi *et al.*, 1997). The study concluded that IR mediates, at least in part, IGF2 signalling during foetal development. However, only IRA binds tightly to IGF2, suggesting high IRA expression is required during foetal development. IRA ligand binding kinetics, recycling time and kinase activity may also be different from those of IRB. Contentiously, Mosthaf and colleagues reported that IRA binds insulin faster, but for a shorter time than IRB; Belfiore and colleagues (2009) suggest that when making this observation that a higher rate of internalisation/recycling of IRA was not taken into account and may have contributed to the original findings. IRB displays increased kinase activity and has an additional phospho-peptide region believed to provide other autophosphorylation or binding sites (Yamaguchi *et al.*, 1993; Kosaki *et al.*, 1995).

Studies have revealed that downstream signalling of IRA and IRB are different and are also dependent on which ligand binds to each receptor. IRA activates the PI3K (phosphatidylinositol 3-kinase) class Ia/Akt pathway and preferentially stimulates anti-apoptotic and mitogenic responses. Additionally, IRA also initiates the transcription of the insulin gene forming an autocrine positive-feedback loop. IRB activates the PI3K class II/Akt pathway, leading generally to cellular differentiation, but more specifically to the transcription of the enzyme glucokinase in pancreatic β-cells (Leibiger *et al.*, 2001). The balance between IRA and IRB expression on the cell membrane is essential for normal functioning and an abnormally high expression has been implicated with diseases as diverse as myotonic dystrophy to cancer (Belfiore *et al.*, 2009). Imbalances in receptor levels are also likely to be critical in disease development. IRA is the dominant isoform of IR in breast cancer (Sciacca *et al.*, 1999; Yang and Yee, 2012; Hermani *et al.*, 2013), and it is likely to mediate many oncogenic effects via its association with the PI3K/Akt pathway. At the cellular level, IRA stimulates growth in response to

IGF2, while IRB induces mainly metabolic and differentiation effects (Sciacca *et al.*, 2003; Belfiore *et al.*, 2009).

The extensive homology between the IGF1R and IR hemireceptors permits the formation of IR/IGF1R hybrid receptors. Three hybrid receptors are possible depending on which two hemireceptors dimerise. These are IRA/IGF1R, IRB/IGF1R and IRA/IRB, each with properties relating to its hemireceptor content. IRA/IRB studies indicate that the formation of hybrid receptors is randomly dependent on hemireceptor availability, and that affinity of IRA/IRB for IGF2 is similar to that of IRA homodimers (Blanquart *et al.*, 2008).

The expression pattern and ligand specificity of IRA/IGF1R and IRB/IGF1R were assessed in different tissues by bioluminescence resonance energy transfer, utilising yellow fluorescent proteins, as well as immunoblotting with both anti-IR and anti-IGF1R antibodies, and subsequently estimating their co-localisation or co-expression in a number of different types of cancer cell (Blanquart *et al.*, 2008). Significant fractions of IR and IGF1R were found as hybrid receptors in all tissues studied, including tissues targeted by insulin and IGF ligands. Atypical IR and IGF1R receptors are thought to exist as a result of post-translational modifications, and their expression is likely to be pertinent to the biology of cancer development (Brierley *et al.*, 2010).

There is also much debate about a nuclear role for both IR and IGF1R suggesting that both receptors can translocate to the nucleus and act as transcription factors (Sarfstein and Werner, 2013). This is a new paradigm in signal transduction and would add an additional stratum into what is already considered a highly complicated pathway.

2.2   Ligands

2.2.1   Types of ligands

Insulin

Insulin is produced by the pancreatic cells known as islets of Langerhans, which are also responsible for the production of another hormone, glucagon. Insulin production is well characterised and starts with the synthesis of a single polypeptide chain called preproinsulin. The *N*-terminal end contains a hydrophobic 19 amino acid signal sequence, which is essential for the polypeptide to be delivered to the endoplasmic recticulum. Proteolytic cleavage removes the 19 amino acid sequence in the lumen of the endoplasmic recticulum to produce proinsulin. Proinsulin is then passed to the Golgi apparatus of the cell and enters into secretory granules. This is where a 33 amino acid section of the polypeptide is cleaved by proteolysis leaving, an α-chain of 21 amino acids and a β-chain of 30 amino acids. These two subunits are then reconnected by two disulphide bridges, with a third bridge spanning across the α-chain (Sanger and Thompson, 1953; Adams *et al.*, 1969; reviewed in Ward and Lawrence, 2011).

Insulin-like growth factors (IGFs)

Insulin-like growth factors are also single-chain polypeptides with a high structural homology to proinsulin. Unlike insulin, IGF1 and IGF2 are produced at varying levels by multiple tissue types and are abundant in the blood circulation (Cohick and Clemmons, 1993). Originally named sulphation factors, because the molecules were initially identified as being responsible for the transfer of sulphate into cartilage (Salmon and Daughaday, 1957), they were eventually called IGF once their similarity to insulin became apparent (Rinderknecht and Humbel, 1978). IGF1 is a 70 amino acid polypeptide and IGF2 contains 67 amino acids. Unlike proinsulin where a mid-section of the polypeptide is totally removed, this section becomes an active third subunit for both IGF1 and IGF2, together with an additional fourth carboxyterminal domain (Bonefeld and Moller, 2011). Elevated levels of IGF have been implicated with the development of different types of cancer such as breast (Lann and LeRoith, 2008), prostate (Roddam *et al.*, 2008) and colon cancer (Jenkins *et al.*, 2000; Brierley *et al.*, 2010).

2.2.2   Ligand binding affinities

Ligand binding affinity is different for IR and IGF1R. The IGF1R receptor binds insulin with 100-fold lower affinity than either IGF1 or IGF2, while IR binds tightly to insulin, but has 100-fold lower affinity for IGF1. This structural difference between the two IR isoforms (IRA and IRB) results in crucial functional divergence in their binding interaction with IGF2 ligands. IRB has very low affinity for IGF2, while IRA exhibits IGF2 affinity similar to IGF1R (Frasca *et al.*, 1999). Additionally, IRA affinity for insulin is approximately 1.7-fold higher than that of IRB (Mosthaf *et al.*, 1990). Peculiarities were found with the binding dynamics of insulin and IGF1 to hybrid receptors. Autophosphorylation in response to IGF or insulin binding is similar in both IRA/IGF1R and IRB/IGF1R but their affinity for these ligands differs (Soos *et al.*, 1993a). The association of labelled IGF1 ligand (used as a tracer) with receptors was easily disrupted by low concentrations of unlabelled IGF1, but required high concentrations of insulin to achieve the same effect. In contrast, removal of labelled insulin required low amounts of either unlabelled insulin or IGF1, suggesting that the binding affinity IGF is greater than that of insulin to hemireceptors. From a structural viewpoint, it is believed that IGF1 binding to the α-subunit of the IGF1R hemireceptor inhibits insulin association with the IR counterpart. These results indicate an overall preference of hybrid receptors for IGF1 instead of insulin, and indicate that IRA/IGF1R and IRB/IGF1R behave similar to IGF1R and not IR (Langlois *et al.*, 1995; Brierley *et al.*, 2010).

   Other studies suggest the existence of IR and IGF1R receptors with abnormal binding affinity for IGF1 and IGF2. Transfection of Chinese hamster ovary cells with an IRB cDNA-expressing plasmid resulted in the expression of IRB with weak affinity for both IGF1 and IGF2 (Jonas *et al.*, 1990). Atypical IGF1R with preferential binding to IGF2 was found in mouse myoblasts and human breast cancer cells (Milazzo *et al.*, 1992; Alexandrides and Smith, 1989).

2.2.3   Insulin growth factor binding proteins (IGFBPs)

Insulin growth factor binding proteins (IGFBP) are important in controlling the activity of IGF and bind with high affinity to both IGF1 and IGF2. There are seven human homologues of IGFBP: IGFBP1–6 physically sequester IGF1 and IGF2 and this results in the growth factors becoming inactivated, which also prolongs the half-life of IGF (Pollak, 2012b). IGFBP7 acts in a different manner. It has been shown that this protein antagonises the action of IGF by binding directly to IGF1R (Evdokimova *et al.*, 2012). The complete story surrounding IGFBP has yet to be fully elucidated, however, it is known that proteins such as p53 and TGFβ can increase secretion of IGFBP into the extracellular space.

2.3   Downstream signalling molecules and events

Insulin receptor substrate (IRS) molecules are docking proteins that carry out signal transduction from the IGF system of receptors to downstream intracellular signalling pathways. The IRS family consists of six members (IRS1–6). IRS1 and IRS2 are expressed in many human tissues, including mammary gland, ovary, adipocyte, heart and muscle (Harbeck *et al.*, 1996; Hadsell *et al.*, 2001; Sun *et al.*, 1992); and IRS4 expression, in normal tissue, is limited to the thymus and the brain (Chan and Lee, 2008). IRS3 does not yet have a human homologue but is expressed in rodents, while IRS5 and IRS6 are considered distant relatives as they display little homology with the earlier discovered IRS proteins (Cai *et al.*, 2003; Chan and Lee, 2008). These molecules do not have kinase activity, but act instead as scaffolding proteins for complexes that connect IGF1R and IR signalling to intracellular signalling pathways. IRS proteins recognise the Asn-Pro-Glu-Tyr motif found in the juxtamembrane domain of either IR or IGF1R. The catalytic domain carries out phosphorylation of the IRS on tyrosine residues when docking proteins are bound to one of these regions (Copps and White, 2012). Phosphorylated IRS forms complexes with additional adaptor molecules, such as phosphatidylinositol 3-kinase (PI3K) and growth factor receptor-bound protein 2 (Grb2), mediating further signalling towards the Akt and Ras pathways (Hanke and Mann, 2009) (Figure 2.2).

IRS and Shc proteins can form competing receptor/IRS/Grb2 and receptor/Shc/Grb2 complexes, that are able to bind Son of Sevenless (Sos) and activate the Ras pathway. Ras signalling releases extracellular signal-regulated

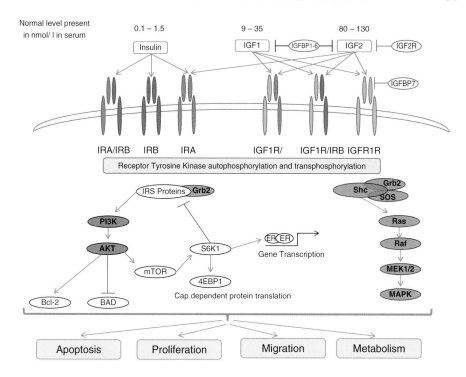

Figure 2.2 **Key signalling pathways downstream of IR and IGFR.** This is a simplistic summary of the key signaling pathways that are initiated on ligand binding to IGFR family members and the cellular outcomes.

kinases 1/2 (ERK1/2), which mediate a variety of cell processes and are implicated in breast cancer (Gee *et al.*, 2001). PI3K converts phosphatidylinositol 4,5-bisphosphate (PIP$_2$) into phosphatidylinositol 3,4,5- triphosphate (PIP$_3$), which is bound by proteins containing a pleckstrin homology (PH) domain. Activation of Akt begins with the recruitment of both phosphoinositide-dependent kinase-1 (PDK1) and Akt at the cell membrane via their PH domains (Stephens *et al.*, 1998; Alessi *et al.*, 1997). PDK1 phosphorylates Akt on threonine 308, while both protein kinase-C (PKC) and the Rictor/mammalian target of rapamycin complex 2 (mTORC2) (Chapter 5) can perform a necessary second phosphorylation of Akt on serine 473, which results in complete activation (Kawakami *et al.*, 2004; Sarbassov *et al.*, 2005). IGF and insulin signalling is therefore closely connected to Akt activity, which in turn mediates a large number of important cellular processes, including protein synthesis via the mTOR pathway (Markman *et al.*, 2010), survival by inhibiting Bcl-2 antagonist of cell death (BAD) (Datta *et al.*, 1997) and the Forkhead transcription factor proteins (Brunet *et al.*, 1999), and glucose metabolism by inhibiting glycogen-synthase-kinase 3 (GSK3) (Cross *et al.*, 1995).

2.4   Dysregulation of signalling in cancer

2.4.1   Over-expression and activation of receptors

Insulin receptor

Initial studies of IR in breast cancer found that the receptor was, on average, up to sevenfold more abundant than in healthy mammary tissue. In addition, IR was primarily localised in neoplastic epithelial tissue (Papa *et al.*, 1990). Subsequent studies established IRA as the predominant isoform of IR in malignant tissues, and attributed its oncogenic activity to its ability to bind IGF2 (Frasca *et al.*, 1999; Sciacca *et al.*, 1999). The high expression of IRA in some breast cancers highlights the importance of the IRA–IGF2 interaction in initiating and sustaining tumour formation. The IRA/IGF1R ratio is also important because IRA–IGF2 may constitute the major pathway for IGF2 dependent proliferation instead of IGF1R–IGF2. IR and IGF1R have similar expression in around half of breast cancer samples studied, but up to 40% of the cases exhibited high and 15% exhibited low IR/IGF1R ratios (Papa *et al.*, 1993). IRA over-expression may result from increased gene copies, the expression of different oncogenes, or over-expression of a high mobility group of proteins characterised by an AT-hook (HMGA), which are a specialised group of proteins responsible for chromosome condensation during cell cycle progression as well as gene transcription, recombination and maintaining the chromatin structure (De Martino *et al.*, 2009). Multiple copies of the IR gene are present in up to only 8% of breast cancer cases and are therefore not likely to be the major cause of IRA over-expression (Papa *et al.*, 1997). IR is found over-expressed in breast cancers initiated by oncogenes such as *Wnt-1*, *HER2* and *Ret* (rearranged during transfection) (Frittitta *et al.*, 1997). Although a causal link between oncogene initiated malignancies and IR over-expression was not shown, IR is likely to enhance growth of these tumours. HMGA proteins act through various transcription factors to activate IR gene expression, which can lead to IRA over-expression in breast cancer (Paonessa *et al.*, 2006). High IGF1R and IR expression in breast cancers allows for the formation of a large number of HRA receptors. In one study, the hybrid receptor content was shown to surpass that of IGF1R in 75% of breast cancer specimens (Pandini *et al.*, 1999), and its autophosphorylation surpassed that of IGF1R when cells were stimulated with IGF1. Insulin binding to IRA/IGF1R could result in phosphorylation of the β-subunit on the IGF1R moiety thus initiating IGF1R downstream events (Pandini *et al.*, 1999).

IGF1R

IGF1R was over-expressed up to 10-fold higher in a study of 449 breast cancer specimens than normal tissues (Papa *et al.*, 1993). The kinase activity of IGF1R was found increased up to fourfold in other studies, additionally enhancing the growth stimulating effect of over-expressed IGF1R (Resnik *et al.*, 1998).

Transgenic mice over-expressing *IGF1R* experience enhanced mammary tumour formation indicating a role for IGF1R in tumour initiation, while IGF1R expressing nodal metastasis suggests a role for IGF1R in tumour migration (Koda *et al.*, 2003; Jones *et al.*, 2007). IGF1 signalling through the IGF1R receptor and IRS2 substrate aids migration by coordinating Rho and integrin signalling (Zhang *et al.*, 2005). Specifically, IGF1R is involved in cell migration by modulating α5β1 in a PI3K dependent manner, and the formation of a complex with CXCR4 and G-protein α- and β-subunits (Lynch *et al.*, 2005; Akekawatchai *et al.*, 2005). Breast cancer growth in response to the insulin ligand can also be attributed to atypical IGF1R that displays a higher affinity for insulin. Atypical IGF1R expression has been found in several breast cancer samples (Soos *et al.*, 1993b; Peyrat *et al.*, 1988). This finding provides an alternative explanation for the sensitisation of breast malignancies to insulin. In addition, IGF1R boosts malignant cell proliferation and survival by activating the PI3K/mTOR and ERK1/2 pathways in order to counteract endoplasmic reticulum induced apoptosis (Novosyadlyy *et al.*, 2008). Gene over-expression and anti-oncogene deactivation, rather than gene amplification, are believed to be the events leading to IGF1R oncogenesis. The *IGF1R* gene itself has only been found to be amplified in just 2% of 975 breast cancer samples studied (Berns *et al.*, 1992). BRCA1 reduces the amount of IGF1R by interacting with the Sp1 transcription factor, which activates the *IGF1R* promoter (Maor *et al.*, 2007). Loss of BRCA1 can therefore result in IGF1R over-expression in the absence of gene amplification. Studies show that both IGF1 and IGF1R are up-regulated in cancers with mutated BRCA1, highlighting the importance of the IGF1–IGF1R interaction in some breast cancers (Hudelist *et al.*, 2007), as well as the central role that BRCA plays as tumour suppressor through down-regulating IGF1R expression. P53 is another tumour suppressor protein that is thought to down-regulate *IGF1R* transcription by interacting with the Sp1 transcription factor, preventing binding to gene promoters (Ohlsson *et al.*, 1998). Overall, both IR and IGF1R play a crucial role in the initiation and progression of breast malignancies.

IGF2R

As alluded to earlier in this chapter, several lines of evidence implicate *IGF2R* in tumour suppression. Breast, ovarian and lung cancer cases were found to contain mutations in at least one copy of the gene (Yamada *et al.*, 1997). Reduction in protein levels or loss of *IGF2R* results in increasingly available IGF2 in cells, and a reduction in the active form of TGF-β, which can induce cell cycle arrest (Oates *et al.*, 1998). Loss of *IGF2R* is believed to result in a pro-invasive cellular phenotype. Reduction in IGF2R correlates with the release of lysosomal proteases such as the aspartyl protease, cathepsin D, into the extracellular space, which in turn can promote tumour invasion via basement membrane degradation (Mathieu *et al.*, 1991; Seino *et al.*, 1989). IGF2R has been shown to act as a tumour suppressor in breast cancer. In one study, transgenic mice constitutively expressing IGF2R were crossed with mice prone to mammary tumour formation due to IGF2 over-expression. The result was slower onset, and reduction in the number of tumours, highlighting the importance of IGF2 recycling by IGF2R in delaying breast cancer initiation and confirming its role as a tumour suppressor gene (Wise and Pravtcheva, 2006).

2.5   Therapeutic opportunities

2.5.1   Targeting receptors

Targeting IGF1R

Targeting IGF1R activity through the use of monoclonal antibodies, tyrosine kinase inhibitors and anti-ligand antibodies has provided promise but, in many cases the compounds have been disappointing in large scale clinical trials (Gombos *et al.*, 2012). There was much enthusiasm when the first Phase I trial for a human monoclonal antibody, Ganitumab/AMG479, led to complete remission for Ewing sarcoma patients and *in vivo*, Ganitumab efficacy was enhanced significantly when used in combination with rapamycin (Beltran *et al.*, 2011). Figitumumab (CP751,871), a monoclonal antibody from Pfizer, entered Phase II trials in metastatic non-small cell lung cancer patients. The data, originally published in 2009, were retracted in 2012 (Karp *et al.*, 2009; Karp *et al.*, 2012). The fundamental reason for the retraction was due to miscalculations suggesting a significant increase in progression-free survival compared with controls, as well as other operational anomalies and serious adverse events (e.g. death) during the trial.

The major patient-focussed issues surrounding the drugs targeting IGF1R to date include severe hyperglycaemia, fatigue and nausea. At a cellular level, when trialled in multiple types of combination therapy, one of the greatest pitfalls has been failure of cell cycle specific chemotherapy to work effectively alongside IGFR inhibition because the IGF1R monoclonal antibody disrupted cell cycle progression, thereby preventing the chemotherapeutic drugs from working in their specific phase. Additionally, IGF1R blockades can result in an increase in insulin production, causing hyperinsulinaemia, which in turn enhances the proliferative rate of IR over-expressing tumour cells (Lee and Yee, 2011).

There are a number of potential therapeutic drugs that are currently in clinical trial involving either monoclonal antibodies or tyrosine kinase inhibitors, most of which are currently being investigated as combination therapies with other, more conventional chemotherapeutic drugs (Table 2.1). Given the difficulty in generating therapeutic success with IGF1R inhibition the results of these trials are awaited with interest.

Targeting other receptors

Aside from IGF1R, other members of the IGF family have been implicated in the development and progression of many cancers. These include IR, IR-A and IGF2

Table 2.1 Summary of on-going and recruiting clinical trials.

Cancer/novel drug	Disease stage	Treatments	Phase
Cixutumumab (C)			
Monoclonal antibody IGF1R			
Adrenocortical carcinoma	Recurrent and stage III/IV	C + mitotane instead of mitotane alone	II/active
Liver	Advanced	C + sorafenib tosylate	I/active
Endocrine	Recurrent and metastatic disease	C + octreotide acetate + everolimus	I/active
Solid tumours	Relapsed or refractory solid tumours in children	C alone	II/active
Solid tumours	Advanced/Adult	C + selumetinib	I/recruiting
Thymoma and thymic carcinoma	Where disease has progressed despite intervention	C alone	II/recruiting
Dalotuzumab (D)			
Monoclonal antibody IGF1R (MK-0646)			
Pancreatic	Advanced	D plus gemcitabine +/− erlotinib	II/active
Non-squamous lung	Stage IIIb/IV metastatic	Pemetrexed/cisplatin +/− D	II/active
Linsitnib (L)			
Dual kinase inhibitor IGF1R and IR (OSI-906)			
Colorectal	Advanced	L +/− irinotecan	I/recruiting
Ovarian	Recurrent	L +/− paclitaxel	I-II/recruiting
Prostate	Recurrent/IV	L alone	II/active
Breast	Metastatic	L +/− erlotinib in combination with letrozole or goserelin	II/withdrawn

Source: Clinical Trials (2013).

and the IGFBP. Therapies directed towards these proteins are currently being investigated and there are several drugs that are undergoing development, which include anti-sense oligonucleotides (Section 2.5.3) and peptides, but these are still at the pre-clinical stage (King and Wong, 2012).

2.5.2 Targeting ligands

It has been proposed that IGF1R monoclonal antibody therapies are insufficient in isolation to inhibit the growth of many cancers. This is in part caused by cross-talk between signalling pathways as well aberrant levels of IGF1 and IGF2 in some patients, especially in the young (Feng and Dimitrov, 2012; King and Wong, 2012).

Additionally, it has been reported that the use of an IGF1R monoclonal antibody (SCH717454) in human umbilical vein endothelial cell cultures and transgenic mice models resulted in the inhibition of angiogenesis. However, when IGF2 was present in the microenvironment, the anti-angiogenic properties of SCH717454 were reversed and this is thought to be mediated by the effects of IGF2 binding to IR (Bid *et al*., 2012). Using MCF-7 breast cancer cells, Dimitrov and his team have proposed that a novel engineered anti-IGF2 antibody, m660, is capable of binding with high affinity to IGF2, ameliorating its effects. When m660 is bound to IGF2 it is thought that large complexes are formed that are eventually phagocytosed by macrophages (Chen *et al*., 2012). Combination of m660 with compounds such as SCH717454 could be very powerful anti-IGF signalling therapies in the future.

2.5.3 Anti-sense oligonucleotides as therapeutics

Second generation anti-sense oligonucleotides to target IGF1R are currently in development. They are short single-stranded DNA or RNA molecules that are designed to be complementary to a target RNA (for example IGFR or IR). On delivery into the cell they bind to the target sequence, signalling its degradation. Both *in vivo* and *in vitro* ATL1101 (an anti-sense oligonuecleotide that targets IGF1R) induced growth inhibition in both prostate cancer models as well as a paclitaxel resistant prostate cancer model (Heidegger *et al*., 2012; King and Wong 2012).

Both anti-sense oligonucleotides and short interfering RNA sequences have potential benefit to cancer patients, and have shown promise in *in vivo* and *in vitro* experiments, but one of the main challenges, that have yet to be consistently overcome, is the delivery of such agents to solid tumours in patients.

2.5.4 Plant compounds as therapeutic alternatives

Ovarian and colon cancer cell lines treated with a phytoalexin (resveratrol), a compound originally extracted from the skin of red grapes, is currently under investigation and showing potential anticancer action. Resveratrol suppresses proliferation of ovarian and colon cancer cell lines by targeting IGF1R and up-regulating p53 (Vanamala *et al*., 2010; Aires *et al*., 2013; Stakleff *et al*., 2012), again highlighting the balance between IGF1R and tumour suppressor gene expression. Recently, this substance was used in a Phase I/II trial in multiple myeloma patients in combination with another multiple myeloma treatment, bortezomib, which is a proteasomal inhibitor (Kapoor *et al*., 2012). Unfortunately, many of the patients developed kidney failure and the trial was halted, however, the reasons/mechanisms underlying the kidney failure are still not fully understood (Popat *et al*., 2012).

2.5.5 Treatment limitations

The biggest barrier to successful clinical outcomes relates to the lack of appropriate biomarkers or access to a reliable diagnostic tool for the IGF signalling family members (Gombos *et al.*, 2012; King and Wong 2012; Pollak, 2012a, 2012b). It is argued that using an 'unselected population' to test the efficacy of any drug means that it is entirely possible to gain a disappointing set of results and overlook a potentially beneficial therapy that could be administered to just a sub-group of the same population. Breast cancer therapies are a prime example, as biomarkers are available for both the oestrogen receptor (ER) and human epidermal growth factor receptor 2 (HER2). If an unselected population was to be included in a trial testing the efficacy of trastuzumab (Herceptin), then the response rate would only be about 7%, as approximately 20% of breast cancer patients are HER2+ve, of which only 30% respond to trastuzumab as a single therapy. Therefore, this demonstrates why it is critical to develop appropriate biomarkers with much urgency (Lee and Yee, 2011; Golan and Javie; 2011).

References

Adams, M.J., Blundell, T.L., Dodson, E.J. *et al.* (1969). Structure of rhombohedral 2-zinc insulin crystals. *Nature*, **224**, 491–495; as cited in Ward and Lawrence, 2011.

Aires, V., Limagne, E., Cotte, A.K. *et al.* (2013) Resveratrol metabolites inhibit human metastatic colon cancer cells progression and synergize with chemotherapeutic drugs to induce cell death. *Molecular Nutrition and Food Research*, **March**, Epub, in press.

Akekawatchai, C., Holland, J.D., Kochetkova, M. *et al.* (2005) Transactivation of CXCR4 by the insulin-like growth factor-1 receptor (IGF-1R) in human MDA-MB-231 breast cancer epithelial cells. *The Journal of Biological Chemistry*, **280** (48), 39701–39708.

Alessi, D.R., Deak, M., Casamayor, A. *et al.* (1997) 3-Phosphoinositide-dependent protein kinase-1 (PDK1): structural and functional homology with the Drosophila DSTPK61 kinase. *Current Biology*, **7** (10), 776–789.

Alexandrides, T.K. and Smith, R.J. (1989) A novel fetal insulin-like growth factor (IGF) I receptor. Mechanism for increased IGF I- and insulin-stimulated tyrosine kinase activity in fetal muscle. *Journal of Biological Chemistry*, **264** (22), 12922–12930.

Belfiore, A., Frasca, F., Pandini, G. *et al.* (2009) Insulin receptor isoforms and insulin receptor/insulin-like growth factor receptor hybrids in physiology and disease. *Endocrine Reviews*, **30** (6), 586–623.

Beltran, P.J., Chung, Y.A., Moody, G. *et al.* (2011) Efficacy of ganitumab (AMG 479), alone and in combination with rapamycin, in Ewing's and osteogenic sarcoma models. *Journal of Pharmacology and Experimental Therapeutics*, **337** (3), 644–654.

Berns, E.M., Klijn, J.G., van Staveren, I.L. *et al.* (1992) Sporadic amplification of the insulin-like growth factor 1 receptor gene in human breast tumors. *Cancer Research*, **52** (4), 1036–1039.

Bid, H.K., Zhan, J., Phelps, D.A. *et al.* (2012) Potent inhibition of angiogenesis by the IGF-1 receptor targeting antibody SCH717454 is reversed by IGF-2. *Molecular Cancer Therapeutics*, **11** (3), 649–659.

Blanquart, C., Achi, J. and Issad, T. (2008) Characterization of IRA/IRB hybrid insulin receptors using bioluminescence resonance energy transfer. *Biochemical Pharmacology*, **76** (7), 873–883.

Bonefeld, K. and Moller, S. (2011) Insulin like growth factor 1 and the liver. *Liver International*, **31** (7), 911–919.

Brierley, G.V., Macaulay, S.L., Forbes, B.E. *et al.* (2010) Silencing of the insulin receptor isoform A favors formation of type 1 insulin like growth factor receptor (IGF-IR) homodimers and enhances ligand-induced IGF-IR activation and viability of human colon carcinoma cells. *Endocrinology*, **151** (4), 1418–1427.

Brogiolo, W., Stocker, H., Ikeya, T. *et al.* (2001) An evolutionarily conserved function of the Drosophila insulin receptor and insulin-like peptides in growth control. *Current Biology*, **11** (4), 213–221.

Brunet, A., Bonni, A., Zigmond, M.J. *et al.* (1999) Akt promotes cell survival by phosphorylating and inhibiting a Forkhead transcription factor. *Cell*, **96** (6), 857–868.

Cai, D., Dhe-Paganon, S., Melendez, P.A. *et al.* (2003) Two new substrates in insulin signaling, IRS5/DOK4 and IRS6/DOK5. *Journal of Biological Chemistry*, **278** (28), 25323–253230.

Chan, B.T.Y. and Lee, A.V. (2008) Insulin receptor substrates (IRSs) and breast tumorigenesis. *Journal of Mammary Gland Biology and Neoplasia*, **13** (4), 415–422.

Chen, W., Feng, Y., Zhao, Q. *et al.* (2012) Human monoclonal antibodies targeting nonoverlapping epitopes on insulin-like growth factor II as a novel type of candidate cancer therapeutics. *Molecular Cancer Therapy*, **11** (7), 1400–1410.

Clinical Trials (2013) Bethesda (MD): National Library of Medicine (US), www.clinicaltrials.gov (accessed 21 March 2013).

Cohick, W.S. and Clemmons, D.R. (1993) The insulin-like growth factors. *Annual Review of Physiology*, **55**, 131–153.

Copps, K.D. and White, M.F. (2012) Regulation of insulin sensitivity by serine/threonine phosphorylation of insulin receptor substrate proteins IRS1 and IRS2. *Diabetologia*, **55** (10), 2565–2582.

Cross, D.A., Alessi, D.R., Cohen, P. *et al.* (1995) Inhibition of glycogen synthase kinase-3 by insulin mediated by protein kinase B. *Nature*, **378** (6559), 785–789.

Datta, S.R., Dudek, H., Tao, X. *et al.* (1997) Akt phosphorylation of BAD couples survival signals to the cell-intrinsic death machinery. *Cell*, **91** (2), 231–241.

De Martino, I., Visone, R., Wierinckx, A. *et al.* (2009) HMGA proteins up-regulate CCNB2 gene in mouse and human pituitary adenomas. *Cancer Research*, **69** (5), 1844–1850.

De Souza, A.T., Hankins, G.R., Washington, M.K. *et al.* (1995) M6P/IGF2R gene is mutated in human hepatocellular carcinomas with loss of heterozygosity. *Nature Genetics*, **11** (4), 447–449.

Evdokimova, V., Tognon, C.E., Benatar, T. *et al.* (2012) IGFBP7 binds to the IGF-1 receptor and blocks its activation by insulin-like growth factors. *Science Signalling*, **5** (255), ra92.

Feng, Y. and Dimitrov, D.S. (2012) Antibody-based therapeutics against components of the IGF system. *OncoImmunology*, **1** (8), 1390–1391.

Frasca, F., Pandini, G., Scalia, P. *et al.* (1999) Insulin receptor isoform A, a newly recognized, high-affinity insulin-like growth factor II receptor in fetal and cancer cells. *Molecular and Cellular Biology*, **19** (5), 3278–3288.

Frittitta, L., Cerrato, A., Sacco, M.G. *et al.* (1997) The insulin receptor content is increased in breast cancers initiated by three different oncogenes in transgenic mice. *Breast Cancer Research and Treatment*, **45**, 141–147.

Gee, J.M., Robertson, J.F., Ellis, I O. and Nicholson, R. I. (2001) Phosphorylation of ERK1/2 mitogen-activated protein kinase is associated with poor response to anti-hormonal therapy and decreased patient survival in clinical breast cancer. *International Journal of Cancer*, **95** (4), 247–254.

Golan, T. and Javie, M. (2011) Targetting the insulin growth factor pathway in gastrointestinal cancers. *Oncology*, **25** (6), 518–526.

Gombos, A., Metzger-Filho, O., Dal lago, L. and Awada-Hussein, A. (2012) Clinical development of insulin-like growth factor receptor-1 (IGF-1R) inhibitors: At the crossroads? *Investigational New Drugs*, **30** (6), 2433–2442.

Hadsell, D.L., Alexeenko, T., Klimentidis, Y. *et al.* (2001) Inability of overexpressed des(1-3) human insulin-like growth factor I (IGF-I) to inhibit forced mammary gland involution is associated with decreased expression of IGF signaling molecules 1. *Endocrinology*, **142** (4), 1479–1488.

Hanke, S. and Mann, M. (2009) The phosphotyrosine interactome of the insulin receptor family and its substrates IRS-1 and IRS-2. *Molecular and Cellular Proteomics*, **8** (3), 519–534.

Harbeck, M.C., Louie, D.C., Howland, J. *et al.* (1996) Expression of insulin receptor mRNA and insulin receptor substrate 1 in pancreatic islet beta-cells. *Diabetes*, **45** (6), 711–717.

Heidegger, I., Ofer, P., Doppler, W. *et al.* (2012) Diverse functions of the IGF/insulin signalling in malignant and noncancerous prostate cells: proliferation in cancer cells and differentiation in noncancerous cells. *Endocrinology*, **153** (10), 4633–4643.

Hermani, A., Shukla, A., Medunjanin, S. *et al.* (2013) Insulin-like growth factor binding protein-4 and -5 modulate ligand-independent estrogen receptor α activation in breast cancer cells in an IGF-independent manner. *Cellular Signalling*, **25** (6), 1395–1402.

Hernandez-Sanchez, C., Mansilla, A., de Pablo, F. and Zardoya, R. (2008) Evolution of the Insulin receptor family and receptor isoform expression in vertebrates. *Molecular Biology and Evolution*, **25** (6), 1043–1053.

Hubbard, S.R. (2013) The insulin receptor: both a prototypical and atypical receptor tyrosine kinase. *Cold Spring Harbor Perspectives in Biology*, **5** (3), a008946.

Hudelist, G., Wagner, T., Rosner, M. *et al.* (2007) Intratumoral IGF-I protein expression is selectively upregulated in breast cancer patients with BRCA1/2 mutations. *Endocrine-Rrelated Cancer*, **14** (4), 1053–1062.

Jenkins, P.J., Frajese, V., Jones, A.M., *et al.* (2000) Insulin-like growth factor I and the development of colorectal neoplasia. *Journal of Clinical Endocrinology and Metabolism*, **85** (9), 3218–3121.

Jonas, H.A., Eckardt, G.S. and Clark, S. (1990) Expression of atypical and classical insulin receptors in Chinese hamster ovary cells transfected with cloned cDNA for the human insulin receptor. *Endocrinology*, **127** (3), 1301–1309.

Jones, R.A., Campbell, C.I., Gunther, E.J. *et al.* (2007) Transgenic overexpression of IGF-IR disrupts mammary ductal morphogenesis and induces tumor formation. *Oncogene*, **26** (11), 1636–1644.

Kapoor, P., Ramakrishnan, V. and Rajkumar, S.V. (2012) Bortezomib combination therapy in multiple myeloma. *Seminars in Hematology*, **49** (3), 228–242.

Karp, D.D., Pollak, M.N., Cohen, R.B. *et al.* (2009) Phase II Study of the anti-insulin-like growth factor type 1 receptor antibody CP – 751,871 in combination with paclitaxel and carboplatin in previously untreated, locally advanced, or metastatic non-small-cell lung cancer. *Journal of Clinical Oncology*, **27** (15), 2516–2522.

Karp, D.D., Pollak, M.N., Cohen, R.B. *et al.* (2012) Retraction - Phase II Study of the anti-insulin-like growth factor type 1 receptor antibody CP – 751,871 in combination with paclitaxel and carboplatin in previously untreated, locally advanced, or metastatic non-small-cell lung cancer. *Journal of Clinical Oncology*, **30** (33), 4179.

Kawakami, Y., Nishimoto, H., Kitaura, J. *et al.* (2004) Protein kinase C betaII regulates Akt phosphorylation on Ser-473 in a cell type- and stimulus-specific fashion. *Journal of Biological Chemistry*, **279** (46), 47720–47725.

King, E.R. and Wong, K.K. (2012) Insulin like growth factor: current concepts and new developments in cancer therapy. *Recent Patents on Anti-Cancer Drug Discovery*, **7** (1), 14–30.

Koda, M., Sulkowski, S., Garofalo, C. *et al.* (2003) Expression of the insulin-like growth factor-I receptor in primary breast cancer and lymph node metastases: correlations with estrogen receptors alpha and beta. *Hormone and Metabolic Research*, **35** (11-12), 794–801.

Kosaki, A., Pillay, T.S., Xu, L. and Webster, N.J. (1995) The B isoform of the insulin receptor signals more efficiently than the A isoform in HepG2 cells. *Journal of Biological Chemistry*, **270** (35), 20816–20823.

Langlois, W.J., Sasaoka, T., Yip, C.C. and Olefsky, J.M. (1995) Functional characterization of hybrid receptors composed of a truncated insulin receptor and wild type insulin-like growth factor 1 or insulin receptors. *Endocrinology*, **136** (5), 1978–1986.

Lann, D. and LeRoith, D. (2008) The role of endocrine insulin-like growth factor-1 and insulin in breast cancer. *Journal of Mammary Gland Biology and Neoplasia*, **13** (4), 371–379.

Lee, A.V. and Yee, D. (2011) Targeting IGF-1R: at a crossroad - commentary. *Oncology*, **25** (6), 535–536.

Leibiger, B., Leibiger, I.B., Moede, T. *et al.* (2001) Selective insulin signaling through A and B insulin receptors regulates transcription of insulin and glucokinase genes in pancreatic beta cells. *Molecular Cell*, **7** (3), 559–570.

Louvi, A., Accili, D. and Efstratiadis, A. (1997) Growth-promoting interaction of IGF-II with the insulin receptor during mouse embryonic development. *Developmental Biology*, **189** (1), 33–48.

Lynch, L., Vodyanik, P.I., Boettiger, D. and Guvakova, M. A. (2005) Insulin-like growth factor I controls adhesion strength mediated by alpha5beta1 integrins in motile carcinoma cells. *Molecular Biology of the Cell*, **16** (1), 51–63.

Maor, S., Yosepovich, A., Papa, M.Z. *et al.* (2007) Elevated insulin-like growth factor-I receptor (IGF-IR) levels in primary breast tumors associated with BRCA1 mutations. *Cancer Letters*, **257** (2), 236–243.

Markman, B., Dienstmann, R. and Tabernero, J. (2010) Targeting the PI3K/Akt/mTOR Pathway – beyond rapalogs. *Oncotarget*, **1** (7), 530–543.

Martin-Kleiner, I. and Troselj, K. G. (2010) Mannose-6-phosphate/insulin-like growth factor 2 receptor (M6P/IGF2R) in carcinogenesis. *Cancer Letters*, **289** (1), 11–22.

Mathieu, M., Vignon, F., Capony, F. and Rochefort, H. (1991) Estradiol down-regulates the mannose-6-phosphate/insulin-like growth factor-II receptor gene and induces cathepsin-D in breast cancer cells: a receptor saturation mechanism to increase the secretion of lysosomal proenzymes. *Molecular Endocrinology*, **5** (6), 815–822.

Milazzo, G., Yip, C.C., Maddux, B. A. *et al.* (1992) High-affinity insulin binding to an atypical insulin-like growth factor-I receptor in human breast cancer cells. *Journal of Clinical Investigation*, **89** (3), 899–908.

Mosthaf, L., Grako, K., Dull, T.J. *et al.* (1990) Functionally distinct insulin receptors generated by tissue-specific alternative splicing. *EMBO Journal*, **9** (8), 2409–2413.

Mynarcik, D.C., Williams, P.F., Schaffer, L. *et al.* (1997) Identification of common ligand binding determinants of the insulin and insulin-like growth factor 1 receptors. Insights into mechanisms of ligand binding. *Journal of Biological Chemistry*, **272** (30), 18650–18655.

Novosyadlyy, R., Kurshan, N., Lann, D. *et al.* (2008) Insulin-like growth factor-I protects cells from ER stress-induced apoptosis via enhancement of the adaptive capacity of endoplasmic reticulum. *Cell Death and Differentiation*, **15** (8), 1304–1317.

Oates, A.J., Schumaker, L.M., Jenkins, S.B. *et al.* (1998) The mannose 6-phosphate/insulin-like growth factor 2 receptor (M6P/IGF2R), a putative breast tumor suppressor gene. *Breast Cancer Research and Treatment*, **47** (7), 269–281.

Ohlsson, C., Kley, N., Werner, H. and LeRoith, D. (1998) p53 regulates insulin-like growth factor-I (IGF-I) receptor expression and IGF-I-induced tyrosine phosphorylation in an osteosarcoma cell line: interaction between p53 and Sp1. *Endocrinology*, **139** (3), 1101–1107.

Pandini, G., Vigneri, R., Costantino, A. *et al.* (1999) Insulin and insulin-like growth factor-I (IGF-I) receptor overexpression in breast cancers leads to insulin/IGF-I hybrid receptor overexpression: evidence for a second mechanism of IGF-I signaling. *Clinical Cancer Research*, **5** (7), 1935–1944.

Paonessa, F., Foti, D., Costa, V. *et al.* (2006) Activator protein-2 overexpression accounts for increased insulin receptor expression in human breast cancer. *Cancer Research*, **66** (10), 5085–5093.

Papa, V., Gliozzo, B., Clark, G. M. *et al.* (1993) Insulin-like growth factor-I receptors are overexpressed and predict a low risk in human breast cancer. *Cancer Research*, **53**, 3736–3740.

Papa, V., Pezzino, V., Costantino, A. *et al.* (1990) Elevated insulin receptor content in human breast cancer. *Journal of Clinical Investigation*, **86** (5), 1503–1510.

Papa, V., Milazzo, G., Goldfine, I.D. *et al.* (1997) Sporadic amplification of the insulin receptor gene in human breast cancer. *Journal of Endocrinology Investigation*, **20**, 531–536.

Peyrat, J.P., Bonneterre, J., Beuscart, R. *et al.* (1988) Insulin-like growth factor 1 receptors in human breast cancer and their relation to estradiol and progesterone receptors. *Cancer Research*, **48**, 6429–6433.

Pollak, M. (2008) Insulin and insulin-like growth factor signalling in neoplasia. *Nature Reviews –Cancer*, **8**, 915–928.

Pollak, M. (2012a) Insulin and insulin-like growth factor signalling in neoplasia: an update. *Nature Reviews – Cancer*, **12** (3), 159–169.

Pollak, M. (2012b) The insulin receptor/insulin-like growth factor receptor family as a therapeutic target in oncology. *Clinical Cancer Research*, **18** (1), 40–50.

Popat, R., Plesner, T., Davies, F. *et al.* (2012) A phase 2 study of SRT501 (resveratrol) with bortezomib for patients with relapsed and or refractory multiple myeloma. *British Journal of Haematology*, **160** (5), 714–717.

Resnik, J.L., Reichart, D.B., Huey, K. *et al.* (1998) Elevated insulin-like growth factor I receptor autophosphorylation and kinase activity in human breast cancer. *Cancer Research*, **58**, 1159–1164.

Rinderknecht, E. and Humbel, R.E. (1978) The amino acid sequence of human insulin-like growth factor 1 and its structural homology with proinsulin. *Journal of Biological Chemistry*, **253**, 2769–2776.

Roddam, A. W., Allen, N. E., Appy, P. *et al.* (2008) Insulin-like growth factors, their binding proteins, and prostate cancer risk: analysis of individual patient data from 12 prospective studies. *Annals of Internal Medicine*, **149** (7), 461–471.

Salmon, W.D., Jr, and Daughaday, W.H. (1957) A hormonally controlled serum factor which stimulates sulphate incorporation by cartilage in vitro. *Journal of Laboratory and Clinical Medicine*, **49** (6), 825–836.

Sanger, F. and Thompson, E.O. (1953) The amino acid sequence in the glycyl chain of insulin. I The identification flower peptides from partial hydrolysates. *Biochemical Journal*, **53** (3), 353–366.

Sarbassov, D.D., Guertin, D.A., Ali, S.M. and Sabatini, D.M. (2005) Phosphorylation and regulation of Akt/PKB by the rictor-mTOR complex. *Science*, **307**, 1098–10101.

Sarfstein, R. and Werner, H. (2013) Minireview: Nuclear insulin and insulin like growth factor 1 receptors: A novel paradigm in signal transduction. *Endocrinology*, **154** (5), 672–1679.

Sciacca, L., Costantino, A., Pandini, G. *et al.* (1999) Insulin receptor activation by IGF-II in breast cancers: evidence for a new autocrine/paracrine mechanism. *Oncogene*, **18**, 2471–2479.

Sciacca, L., Prisco, M., Wu, A. *et al.* (2003) Signaling differences from the A and B isoforms of the insulin receptor (IR) in 32D cells in the presence or absence of IR substrate-1. *Endocrinology*, **144**, 2650–2658.

Seino, S., Seino, M., Nishi, S. and Bell, G. I. (1989) Structure of the human insulin receptor gene and characterization of its promoter. *Proceedings of the National Academy of Sciences, USA*, **86**, 114–118.

Soos, M.A., Field, C.E. and Siddle, K. (1993a) Purified hybrid insulin/insulin-like growth factor-I receptors bind insulin-like growth factor-I, but not insulin, with high affinity. *Biochemical Journal*, **290** (Pt 2), 419–426.

Soos, M.A., Nave, B.T. and Siddle, K. (1993b) Immunological studies of type I IGF receptors and insulin receptors: characterisation of hybrid and atypical receptor subtypes. *Advances in Experimental Medicine and Biology*, **343**, 145–157.

Stakleff, K.S., Sloan, T., Blanco, D. *et al.* (2012) Resveratrol exerts differential effects in vitro and in vivo against ovarian cancer cells. *Asian Pacific Journal of Cancer Prevention*, **13** (4), 1333–1340.

Stephens, L., Anderson, K., Stokoe, D. *et al.* (1998) Protein kinase B kinases that mediate phosphatidylinositol 3,4,5-trisphosphate-dependent activation of protein kinase B. *Science*, **279**, 710–714.

Sun, X.J., Miralpeix, M., Myers, M.G., Jr, *et al.* (1992) Expression and function of IRS-1 in insulin signal transmission. *Journal of Biological Chemistry*, **267**, 22662–22672.

Ullrich, A., Gray, A., Tam, A.W. *et al.* (1986) Insulin-like growth factor I receptor primary structure: comparison with insulin receptor suggests structural determinants that define functional specificity. *EMBO Journal*, **5**, 2503–2512.

Vanamala, J., Reddivari, L., Radhakrishnan, S. and Tarver, C. (2010) Resveratrol suppresses IGF-1 induced human colon cell proliferation and elevates apoptosis via suppression of IGF-1R/Wnt and activation of p53 signaling pathways. *BMC Cancer*, **10**, 238.

Ward, C.W. and Lawrence, M.C. (2011) Landmarks in insulin research. *Frontiers in Endocrinology*, **2**, 76.

White, M.F. (1998) The IRS-signalling system: a network of docking proteins that mediate insulin action. *Molecular and Cellular Biochemistry*, **182**, 3–11.

Wise, T.L. and Pravtcheva, D.D. (2006) Delayed onset of Igf2-induced mammary tumors in Igf2r transgenic mice. *Cancer Research*, **66**, 1327.

Yamada, T., DeSouza, A.T., Finkelstein, S. and Jirtle, R.L. (1997) Loss of the gene encoding mannose 6-phosphate/insulin-like growth factor II receptor is an early event in liver carcinogenesis. *Proceedings of the National Academy of Sciences, USA*, **94** (19), 10351–10355.

Yamaguchi, Y., Flier, J.S., Benecke, H. *et al.* (1993) Ligand-binding properties of the two isoforms of the human insulin receptor. *Endocrinology*, **132**, 1132–1138.

Yang, Y. and Yee, D. (2012) Targeting insulin and insulin-like growth factor signalling in breast cancer. *Journal of Mammary Gland Biology and Neoplasia*, **17**, 251–261.

Zhang, X., Lin, M., van Golen, K.L. *et al.* (2005) Multiple signaling pathways are activated during insulin-like growth factor-I (IGF-I) stimulated breast cancer cell migration. *Breast Cancer Research and Treatment*, **93**, 159–168.

3

Transforming growth factor-β receptor signalling

Gudrun Stenbeck

Biosciences, Brunel University, London

3.1 TGFβ receptors

To elicit their effect on cells, the transforming growth factor-β (TGFβ) superfamily of secreted factors binds to three different types of receptors. Type I and type II receptors are serine/threonine kinases and the type III receptor is a proteoglycan without kinase activity. Type I and type II receptors are glycoproteins of 53 and 73 kDa, respectively, that, upon ligand binding, form heterotetrameric signalling complexes, which are coordinated by the dimeric ligand. Both receptors are transmembrane proteins composed of a short *N*-terminal extracellular cysteine-rich region with a single *N*-glycosylation site, followed by a single transmembrane spanning helix and an intracellular *C*-terminal kinase domain (Hinck, 2012). The extracellular domains of both receptors contain five and six disulphide bonds, respectively, and form three-finger toxin folds, which are crucial for ligand binding. The three-finger toxin fold is a structural motif, which was first identified in neurotoxic snake venoms, where it facilitates interaction between toxin and target, that is, between African mamba toxin and the muscarinic receptor (Karlsson *et al.*, 2000). In the type I and type II receptors these modules facilitate the interaction between ligand and receptor. Upon ligand binding, the type I and type II receptors establish extensive contact points, which constrain the complex and facilitate phosphorylation of the type I receptor by the type II receptor (Groppe *et al.*, 2008). Phosphorylation of the type I receptor takes place at a glycine–serine rich region between the transmembrane domain and the kinase domain, also known as the GS box (Hinck, 2012). This phosphorylation of the GS box activates the adjacent kinase domain of the type I receptor, so that phosphorylation of Smad transcription factors can occur, which propagates the TGFβ signal to the cell interior (see Figure 3.1). The type II receptor is constitutively

Cancer Cell Signalling, First Edition. Edited by Amanda Harvey.
© 2013 John Wiley & Sons, Ltd. Published 2013 by John Wiley & Sons, Ltd.

active and does not contain a GS box (Lin *et al.*, 1992). Autophosphorylation of the type II receptor at several serine residues just outside the kinase domain is necessary for activity and is enhanced by receptor dimerisation (Luo and Lodish, 1997). In addition to phosphorylation at these serine residues, the TGFβ receptor II is also autophosphorylated at three tyrosine residues (Luo and Lodish, 1997).

The type III receptor, also known as betaglycan, has a molecular weight of 250–350 kDa and is an integral membrane protein with a large extracellular domain containing multiple glycan modifications (Lopez-Casillas *et al.*, 1991). The core protein has a molecular weight of 100 kDa but the glycan modifications increase the apparent molecular weight. The protein has a short intracellular domain, which contains a phosphorylation side but is itself without kinase activity. In addition to the phosphorylation side, the cytoplasmic domain contains a

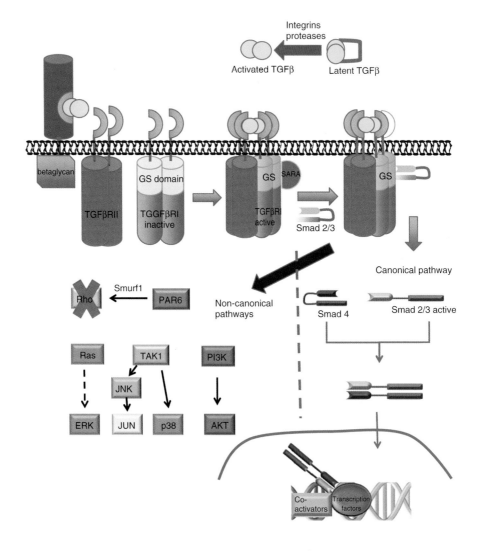

Figure 3.1 **TGFβ activated signalling pathways.** TGFβ is synthesised as precursor molecule, which is cleaved before secretion. The pro-peptide stays associated with TGFβ after cleavage (latency-associated peptide, LAP), and together with the latent TGFβ binding proteins (LTBP) forms the latent complex, which is stored in the matrix. Activation of TGFβ requires its release from LAP, which is accomplished by the action of proteases or integrins.

On the cell membrane TGFβ binds to the type III receptor, betaglycan, which presents it to the type II receptor. After binding of TGFβ, a heterotetrameric complex between the type II and the type I receptor is formed. The type II receptor phosphorylates the type I receptor at its GS domain (dark green), which activates the kinase domain of the type I receptor. The activated type I receptor phosphorylates Smad2 and 3 (R-Smads), which form a complex with Smad4 and translocate to the nucleus where they bind DNA and, together with co-factors and other transcriptions factors, activate target gene expression. Membrane recruitment of R-Smads is mediated by Smad anchor for activation (SARA).

In addition to the Smad signalling pathway, several other signalling pathways, so called non-canonical signalling pathways, are activated by TGFβ receptors. These involve amongst others mitogen activated kinases (MAPK, Erk, JNK, p38) and their activators (TAK1), phosphoinositide-3 kinase (PI3K) and its target AKT, as well as small GTPases, such as Ras and Rho. Activation of these pathways fine-tunes cellular responses. One example of this fine-tuning is the dissolution of junctional complexes and the induction of a migratory phenotype in epithelia cells. Here, the tight junction associated protein Par6 is phosphorylated by the activated TGFβ receptor complex, which triggers recruitment of ubiquitin ligase Smurf1 and subsequent ubiquitination and degradation of RhoA.

β-arrestin 2 interacting motif as well as a class I PDZ binding motif (Bilandzic and Stenvers, 2011).

Betaglycan binds and presents TGFβ to the type II receptor (Cheifetz and Massague, 1989) (see Figure 3.1). Interaction of the betaglycan with the type II receptor leads to phosphorylation of the cytoplasmic tail of betaglycan, which stimulates binding of beta-arrestin 2 and subsequent endocytosis of the beta-arrestin 2/type III/type II receptor complex via the clathrin dependent pathway (Chen *et al.*, 2003). This co-internalisation leads to down-regulation of the TGFβ signalling. The PDZ motif is important for interaction of betaglycan with GIPC, another PDZ domain containing protein, which regulates cell surface expression of betaglycan. Matrix metalloproteinases (MMPs), such as MMP1 and plasmin, cleave betaglycan close to its transmembrane domain and release it in soluble form from cells (Bilandzic and Stenvers, 2011). Recombinant soluble betaglycan acts as an inhibitor of TGFβ signalling by preventing its binding to the type II receptor. Betaglycan thus has a dual role both as enhancer and repressor of TGFβ signalling depending on its localisation (Lopez-Casillas *et al.*, 1994).

Endoglin is another type III receptor with wider ligand specificity than betaglycan that is abundantly expressed on endothelial cells and mutated in patients with haemorrhagic telangiectasia (Fernandez *et al.*, 2006). Endoglin forms a homodimer and interacts with TGFβ1 and TGFβ3, but only when it is associated with a type II receptor (Bertolino *et al.*, 2005). This is contrary to the direct interaction of endoglin with bone morphogenic proteins (BMPs).

3.2   Ligands

TGFβ belongs to a large family of dimeric growth factors with over 30 members including, amongst others, bone morphogenic proteins and activins; members have similar protein structure and downstream signalling components. The TGFβ sub-family is composed of at least five members, TGFβ1, TGFβ2, TGFβ3, TGFβ4 and TGFβ5, which are each encoded by distinct genes. TGFβ4 and TGFβ5 are only found in chicken and frog (*Xenopus laevis*), respectively, whereas TGFβ1–3 are expressed in both embryonic and adult mammalian tissues (for a review see Massague (1990) and references therein). The five isoforms show 64–82% identity at the amino acid level. However, individual isoforms have higher homologies demonstrating conservation between species (e.g. 97% identity between TGFβ1 sequences from mammalian and avian species). At the genomic level, *TGFβ* genes have similar structure and are composed of seven exons (Derynck *et al.*, 1987). Isoform genes localise to different chromosomes.

TGFβ proteins are characterised by a conserved cysteine-rich region that forms a so-called cysteine knot. This structure is important for receptor binding. Three intra-molecular disulphide bonds stabilise it and a seventh conserved cysteine is involved in homodimer formation of the mature cytokine.

All isoforms are synthesised from a large precursor containing a pro-peptide region with a hydrophobic signal sequence and several glycosylation sites. The *C*-terminal region of the precursor contains the TGFβ polypeptide of 112 amino acids (Harrison *et al.*, 2011). During processing in the endoplasmic reticulum, TGFβ precursor monomers form homodimers linked by disulphide bonds (one in the TGFβ region, and at least two in the pro-peptide domain). After transport to the Golgi apparatus and glycosylation, the pro-peptide is cleaved by furin at the pro-protein convertase cleavage site. The pro-protein, also called latency-associated peptide (LAP), remains associated with TGFβ forming the small latent complex. This complex can either be secreted directly or after binding to one of the latent TGFβ binding proteins (LTBPs). LTBPs tether the small latent complex to the extracellular matrix. Several isoforms of LTBP are expressed, LTBP1–4, with different substrate specificities (Sinha *et al.*, 1998). LTBP4 only binds TGFβ1 while LTBP1 and 3 can bind all TGFβ isoforms, LTBP2 does not bind TGFβ but competes with LTBP1 for binding to fibrillin-1, an extracellular microfibrillar protein (Hyytiainen *et al.*, 2004). Association with LAP as well as binding to LTBP segregates TGFβ and regulates its activity. Activation of TGFβ requires its release from the complexes. Several factors have been identified that are capable of releasing TGFβ including the matrix glycoprotein thromospondin-1, plasmins, matrix metalloproteinases, as well as integrins that bind LAPs via their RGD motifs localised close to their *C*-termini (LAP1 binds $\alpha v\beta 1$, $\alpha v\beta 3$, $\alpha v\beta 5$, $\alpha v\beta 6$, $\alpha v\beta 8$ and $\alpha 8\beta 1$, and LAP3 binds $\alpha v\beta 6$ and $\alpha v\beta 8$) (see Munger and Sheppard (2011) and references therein).

Virtually all cell types express TGFβ and have receptors for it. The most ubiquitous isoform is TGFβ1 while TGFβ2 and 3 are expressed in a more tissue specific/developmental dependent fashion (Wilcox and Derynck, 1988). At the mRNA level, *TGFβ1* is expressed in endothelial, hematopetic and connective tissue cells; *TGFβ2* is expressed in epithelial and neuronal cells and *TGFβ3* is primarily expressed in mesenchymal cells (Thompson *et al.*, 1989). There is discrepancy between protein and mRNA expression for the different isoforms, which could result from diffusion and accumulation of the cytokine away from the site of synthesis (Thompson *et al.*, 1989). In bone both TGFβ1 and 2 are expressed and co-purify together. Tissue culture cells respond to TGFβ1–3 equally but during development, TGFβ1 and TGFβ3 are expressed early in all structures undergoing morphogenesis, whereas TGFβ2 is expressed later in mature and differentiating epithelium. Furthermore, studies of knockout animals have shown clear distinctions between the isoforms. Depending on the genetic background, all targeted ablations of *TGFβ1–3* genes show either embryonic or postnatal lethality. Only 50% of mice with a *TGFβ1* ablation are born, the other half die *in utero*. The pups born are initially healthy but succumb within four weeks to multifocal inflammatory disease, with lesions resembling those found in autoimmune disorders (Shull *et al.*, 1992), clearly demonstrating the important role TGFβ1 plays in the regulation of the immune system. The *TGFβ2* knockdown mice die either *in utero* or shortly after birth because of multiple developmental defects, including amongst others heart, lung and craniofacial malformations (Sanford *et al.*, 1997). *TGFβ3* knockout mice have defective palatogenesis and delayed pulmonary development and die shortly after birth (Kaartinen *et al.*, 1995).

There is further distinction between the different isoforms concerning binding to the TGFβ receptors. TGFβ2 requires the type III receptor betaglycan for binding to the type II receptor because it only weakly binds to it on its own. Thus cells that do not express betaglcan are insensitive to TGFβ2. However, an alternatively spliced type II receptor binds TGFβ2 without the aid of betaglycan so renders cells responsive to TGFβ2 in the absence of betaglycan (Rotzer *et al.*, 2001). This type II receptor splice variant is ubiquitously expressed in cell lines but with prevalence in cell types from tissues where the TGFβ2 is the main isoform, such as bone cells (Hirai and Fijita, 1996).

3.3   Downstream signalling molecules and events

TGFβ has wide-ranging effects in vertebrate development as well as on homeostasis of adult tissues, especially the adaptive immune systems and wound healing. Lymphocytes, macrophages and dendritic cells all produce TGFβ1. As in other cell systems, its expression controls differentiation, proliferation and state of activation of these immune cells. TGFβ controls the inflammatory response through regulation of chemotaxis and inhibition of activated cells (Letterio and Roberts, 1998). TGFβ is thus an important factor in establishing immune tolerance and its dysregulation has been linked to malignancy, autoimmune disorders, susceptibility to opportunistic infection and to the fibrotic complications associated with chronic inflammatory conditions. During wound healing, TGFβ stimulates fibroblasts to produce extracellular-matrix proteins such as collagen and fibronectin and to up-regulate cell-adhesion integrins (Roberts *et al*., 1986). Concomitant, TGFβ decreases expression of matrix metalloproteases, such as collagenase and stromelysin, which degrade the extracellular matrix, and increases the production of proteins that inhibit matrix degradation, such plasminogen-activator inhibitor type 1 and tissue inhibitor of metalloprotease (TIMP) (Schultz and Wysocki, 2009). Furthermore, TGFβ induces the trans-differentiation of fibroblasts and epithelia cells into myofibroblasts, which actively contract the extracellular matrix, an important step in wound healing. Myofibroblasts are also important mediators of inflammation and extracellular matrix formation through the secretion of inflammatory and anti-inflammatory cytokines, chemokines, growth factors, as well as extracellular matrix proteins and proteases (Powell *et al*., 1999). In epithelia and endothelia cells, TGFβ signalling controls cell proliferation, differentiation and apoptosis.

3.3.1   Smads

Binding of TGFβ to its cognate receptors and assembly of the heterotetrameric receptor complex triggers a signalling cascade that directly activates the Smad transcription factors, which translocate to the nucleus and together with accessory proteins regulate transcriptional responses (see Figure 3.1). The name Smad is derived from the *Sma* and *Mad* gene homologues identified in nematodes (*Caenorhabiditis elegans*) and fruit fly, respectively (Derynck *et al*., 1996). In vertebrates there are eight Smads, which can be categorised into three functional classes. The R-type Smads are directly activated by the type I receptor, Smads 1, 2, 3, 5 and 8 belong to this group (Derynck *et al*., 1998). After activation they bind the common partner Smad (Co-Smad), Smad4, and translocate to the nucleus. The I-type Smads, Smads 6 and 7, inhibit TGFβ responses by competing with R-Smads for binding to the TGFβ receptor and Smad4, which reduces the amount of Smad4 available for R-Smad signalling. In addition, I-Smads induce ubiquitination of the TGFβ receptor complex targeting it for degradation (Shi and Massague, 2003).

R-Smads and Co-Smad are composed of three domains, two conserved domains with high sequence similarity, termed Mad-homology region 1 (MH1), located at the *N*-terminus, and Mad-homology region 2 (MH2), located at the *C*-terminus of the protein and a central proline-rich linker region (ten Dijke *et al*., 2000). The MH1 domains of Smad4 and Smad3 have DNA binding activity and are also important for association with other transcription factors (Shi *et al*., 1998). The MH2 domain is important for receptor interaction, dimerisation and assembly of transcriptional complexes and conserved in I-Smads. However, I-Smads contain only partial elements of the MH1 domain so are not activating transcription, but rather provide a negative feedback-loop for TGFβ signalling. In R-Smads the MH2 domain is phosphorylated at a specific serine motif close to the *C*-terminus of the protein (SSXS motif). This phosphorylation disrupts the autoinhibitory interaction between MH1 and MH2 domains and activates the R-Smad, which dissociates from the receptor and forms a heteromeric complex with Smad4 (ten Dijke *et al.*, 2000).

The activated TGFβ type I receptor phosphorylates Smads 2 and 3, Smads 1, 5 and 8 mediate signalling of other TGFβ superfamily members. Smads shuttle between the cytoplasm and the nucleus (Inman *et al.*, 2002). Non-phosphorylated Smads 2 and 3 are retained in the cytoplasm by interaction with accessory proteins that also mediate Smad membrane recruitment to the activated receptor complex. For Smads 2 and 3 membrane recruitment is controlled by a membrane-associated protein, termed Smad anchor for activation (SARA) (Cheifetz and Massague, 1989) (Figure 3.1).

3.3.2 SARA

Smad anchor for activation (SARA) contains a phospholipid binding FYVE-domain and presents Smad2 and Smad3 to the activated type I receptor by binding to both non-phosphorylated Smads and the TGFβ receptor complex. This interaction requires the presence of the cytoplasmic isoform of promyelocytic leukaemia (cPML) protein, a tumour suppressor that is required for binding of Smad2 and Smad3 to SARA (Lin *et al.*, 2004). After phosphorylation of Smad2/Smad3 and subsequent binding to Smad4, SARA is released and can recruit another set of non-activated Smad2/Smad3 for receptor presentation (Xu *et al.*, 2000).

3.3.3 Nuclear events

The Smad complex translocates to the nucleus by binding to the nuclear import machinery. In the case of Smad3 this is mediated by a lysine-rich nuclear localisation sequence (NLS) in the MH1 domain that is conserved in all R-Smads. However, the MH2 domain can directly interact with nucleoporins that regulate entry into and exit from the nucleus (Xu *et al.*, 2002). This binding is mediated by the so-called hydrophobic corridor, a region in the MH2 domain, which is also the site of interaction with SARA and nuclear transcription factors that contain a Smad interacting motif (SIM) (Randall *et al.*, 2002). R-Smad phosphorylation exposes the nuclear import signal and facilitates transport into the nucleus (Tsukazaki *et al.*, 1998). Shuttling of Smad4 is mediated by a constitutively active NLS combined with a nuclear export signal in the linker region, which is masked by interaction with the R-Smad, thus leading to accumulation of Smad4 in the nucleus (Watanabe *et al.*, 2000).

Smad transcriptional complexes activate a large array of genes by binding to target sequences and assembling transcriptional complexes. The Smad MH1 domains of all R-Smads except Smad2 recognise sequence specific DNA elements. The minimal Smad binding element (SBE) is composed of only four base pairs 5'-CAGA-3' or its complement 5'-GTCT-3' (Shi et al., 1998). MH1 domains bind only weakly to DNA but association with additional DNA-binding co-factors increases DNA affinity. Smad binding partners include forkhead, homeobox, zinc-finger, bHLH and AP1 families of transcription factors (for review see Feng and Derynck (2005) and references therein). In addition to these DNA-binding co-factors, co-activators, such as CREB-binding protein (CBP) or p300 (Moustakas et al., 2001), as well as repressors and chromatin remodeling factors, such as histone deacetylases, are recruited to the regulatory regions of target genes, which together mediate the highly specific transcriptional control of TGFβ target genes (Massague, 2012). Further factors in this regulation are epigenetic changes that render TGFβ target genes active or inactive by either opening or closing the chromatin structure, which controls access of the transcriptional machinery (Xi et al., 2011).

The main outcome of TGFβ signalling in epithelial, endothelial, hematopoietic, neural and some mesenchymal cells is cell cycle inhibition. This is achieved by activating gene responses that inhibit cyclin-dependent kinases (CDKs) and down regulate c-Myc (Frederick et al., 2004), ID1 and ID2 (Kang et al., 2003a), three transcription factors that promote cell growth and proliferation. This arrest is usually reversible but depending on cell type can lead to terminal differentiation and apoptosis.

CDKs are important for progression through the cell cycle and TGFβ arrests cells at the G1 stage of the cell cycle by depriving the cell of G1 CDKs through inducing the rapid expression of p15Ink4b and p21Cip1, inhibitors of cyclin D dependent kinases CDK4 and 6 (Ravitz and Wenner, 1997). Inhibition of CDKs prevents phosphorylation of the retinoblastoma (Rb) protein, which is required for S phase progression.

Furthermore, TGFβ induces expression of interfering miRNAs, which regulate gene translation post-transcriptionally. In general, control of miRNAs can be either achieved at the transcriptional level or at the different processing steps during their biogenesis. miRNAs are transcribed as primary transcripts (pri-miRNAs) that are processed to precursors (pre-miRNAs) in the nucleus before cytoplasmic cleavage into mature miRNAs by Dicer. A majority of TGFβ regulated miRNAs contain a consensus sequence within their stem region, similar to the SBE that is found in the promoter region of TGFβ regulated genes. Smads bind directly to this motif and induce processing of the miRNA by a nuclear miRNA processor complex composed of the RNase III enzyme Drosha and its cofactor DGCR8 (Davis et al., 2010). Thus, Smads modulate gene expression both at the transcription level through DNA binding and post-transcriptionally through miRNA binding and processing.

3.3.4   Other pathways

In addition to the Smad signalling pathway, several other signalling pathways, involving amongst others mitogen activated kinases (MAPK) and small GTPases are activated by TGFβ receptors (for review see Zhang (2009) and see also Figure 3.1). These pathways fine-tune cellular responses either by regulating Smad signalling through direct phosphorylation of the linker domain of R-Smads or through effects on the cytoskeleton and intercellular junctions. Of note in the context of cancer is the fact that in polarised epithelia the type I receptor is associated with the tight junction protein occludin and Par6 (partitioning-defective protein 6), a member of the conserved tripartite complex formed between Par3, Par6 and atypical protein kinase C (aPKC). The Par complex is important to establish and maintain adherence and tight junctions within the epithelia cell layer (Aranda *et al.*, 2008). After ligand binding the type II receptor is recruited to the complex formed between Par6 and the type I receptor and phosphorylates both proteins. For Par6 this phosphorylation event is enhanced by aPKC (Gunaratne *et al.*, 2013) and triggers recruitment of ubiquitin ligase Smurf1 to the tight junction and subsequent ubiquitination and degradation of RhoA (see Figure 3.1), which results in dissolution of junctional complexes and the induction of a migratory phenotype in epithelia cells (epithelial–mesenchymal transition (EMT)). The concomitant activation of Smad2/3 represses E-cadherin gene (*CDH1*) expression by activating a set of transcription factors (Twist, Snail, Slug, ZEB1 and ZEB2) that together negatively regulate *CDH1* expression, which leads to the dissolution of adherence junctions, completing the EMT process (Heldin *et al.*, 2012). EMT is a biological process in which polarised epithelia cells lose their contact to neighbouring cells and the basement membrane and assume a migratory phenotype (i.e. a more mesenchymal cell phenotype), which includes enhanced invasiveness, resistance to apoptosis and production of ECM components (Thiery *et al.*, 2009). EMT also induces expression and secretion of cytokines that promote cell migration such as: TGFβ; Wnt; Notch ligands; HGF (hepatocyte growth factor or scatter factor); EGF (epidermal growth factor) and PDF (platelet-derived growth factor). These changes are necessary during development but also during wound healing and are altered in cancer metastasis.

3.4   Signalling regulation

Regulation of TGFβ signalling is achieved at several steps of the pathway: ligand activation and availability, receptor and Smad activity and availability, transcriptional control through co-activators/repressors and induction of negative feedback loops. Furthermore, there is extensive cross-talk between the TGFβ pathway and several other important signalling pathways such as MAPK, Ras and Wnt pathways, which leads to phosphorylation of Smads and sharing of components (in the case of Wnt signalling) (Moustakas and Heldin, 2009).

TGFβ is secreted as an inactive small latency complex together with LAP and is stored in the matrix by association with LTBPs. Activation of TGFβ requires its release from these latency complexes, which is controlled by hydrolysis of LAP through proteinases, such as thrombospondin, MMPs and plasmin (see Figure 3.1). However, binding of integrins to LAP can also release TGFβ. As integrins are mediating the interaction of the cell with the extracellular matrix, mechanical signals such as stretch can release TGFβ (Munger and Sheppard, 2011). This is an important step in wound healing where TGFβ controls extracellular matrix formation.

The type I receptor binds the immunophilin FKBP12 at its GS domain, which prevents phosphorylation and activation by the type II receptor. FKBP12 is a peptidyl-prolyl *cis/trans* isomerase, which is inhibited by immunosuppressive drugs such as FK506 and rapamycin. By binding to the type I receptor, FKBP12 does not inhibit the interaction between type I and type II receptors but prevents activation of the type I receptor in the absence of ligand (Chen *et al.*, 1997).

I-Smad7 expression is stimulated by TGFβ and association of Smad7 with the type I receptor recruits the E3 ubiquitin ligase Smurf2 leading to ubiquitination and degradation of the receptor in the proteasome (Kavsak *et al.*, 2000). Furthermore, Smad7 masks the binding site for Smad2/3 and prevents their interaction with the receptor (see Figure 3.2).

R-Smads themselves are substrates for ubiquitination mediated by the E3 ubiquitin ligase Nedd4L and subsequent degradation by the 26S proteasome, which controls their basal levels (Gao *et al.*, 2009). Smad basal levels in turn determine the responsiveness of a cell to the incoming TGFβ signal. Smad ubiquitination is triggered by phosphorylation of the linker region by glycogen synthase kinase 3 (GSK3) (Fuentealba *et al.*, 2007). However, in the nucleus this phosphorylation is preceded by phosphorylation of other serine/threonine residues in the linker region by cyclin-dependent kinase 8 and 9 (CDK8 and CDK9), which is necessary to assemble transcriptional complexes (Alarcon *et al.*, 2009). Thus phosphorylation of the Smad linker region first enhances transcriptional activity before turning off the signal by limiting the half-life of the activated Smad (Aragon *et al.*, 2011). Furthermore, phosphorylation of the linker region by MAPK also inhibits Smad activity providing a link between TGFβ signalling and other growth factors that signal through MAPK.

Activated receptors are endocytosed via the clathrin-mediated pathway reaching endosomes where they can remain active for several hours before being routed to lysosomes for degradation (Figure 3.2). Endosomes are rich in the phospholipid phosphatidylinositol 3-phosphate, which is specifically recognised by FYVE-domain containing proteins (Kutateladze, 2006). Therefore, SARA preferentially binds to endosomes and can present Smad2/3 there to the activated receptor complex (see Figure 3.2). In the nucleus R-Smads are dephosphorylated by PPM1A (protein phosphatase 1A), which is a magnesium-dependent enzyme that belongs to the protein phosphatase 2C (PP2C) family of phosphatases (Lin *et al.*, 2006). Dephosphorylated R-Smads shuttle back to the cytoplasm where they can be

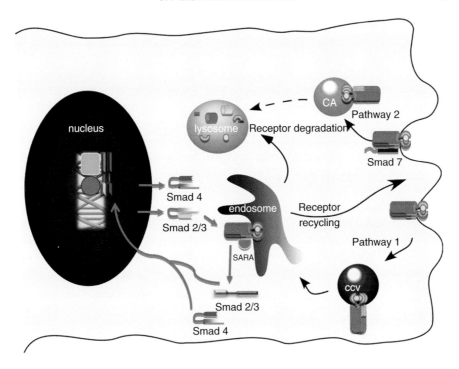

Figure 3.2 **Regulation of TGFβ signalling.** Activated receptors are endocytosed via clathrin-coated pits (pathway 1) or caveolin positive lipid rafts (pathway 2). After endocytosis, clathrin-coated vesicles (CCV) reach the endosome where TGFβ receptors can remain active for several hours before being routed to lysosomes for degradation. Endosomes are rich in the phospholipid phosphatidylinositol 3-phosphate, which is specifically recognised by FYVE-domain containing proteins such as SARA. SARA preferentially binds to endosomes and can present Smad2/3 there to the activated receptor complex, activating them. The R-Smad together with Smad4 translocates into the nucleus where they activate transcriptional responses. R-Smad and co-Smad are dephosphorylated in the nucleus and shuttle back to the cytoplasm where they can be activated again as long as the receptor is active.

Endocytosis via lipid rafts and association of Smad7 with the type I receptor stimulates degradation of the receptor by enhancing ubiquitination in caveolin-positive vesicles (CA) (pathway 2).

activated again as long as the receptor is active (Figure 3.2). Thus this phosphorylation and dephosphorylation of Smads and shuttling between nucleus and cytoplasm fine-tune the transcriptional response to TGFβ.

Receptors are also endocytosed via caveolin positive lipid rafts. However, endocytosis via lipid rafts leads directly to receptor down-regulation and degradation by enhancing ubiquitination in caveolin-positive vesicles (Di Guglielmo *et al.*, 2003) (Figure 3.2). It is not yet clear how routing to the different endocytosis pathways is achieved but recent evidence points to a regulatory function of neddylation of the type II receptor by the proto-oncogene c-Cbl, which prevents ubiquitin mediated receptor down-regulation (Zuo *et al.*, 2013). Neddylation is a post-translational modification similar to ubiquitination but with the small protein NEDD8 (neural precursor cell-expressed, developmentally down-regulated 8) instead of ubiquitin (Kamitani *et al.*, 1997).

As described in Section 3.1, the type III receptor betaglycan binds and presents TGFβ to the type II receptor (Cheifetz and Massague, 1989). The constitutive active type II receptor phosphorylates betaglycan, which stimulates binding of beta-arrestin 2 and subsequent endocytosis of the beta-arrestin 2/type III/type II complex via the clathrin dependent pathway. This endocytosis down-regulates receptors thus decreasing the response to TGFβ (Chen *et al.*, 2003). Furthermore, the extracellular domain of betaglycan can be cleaved by MMPs, which liberates a soluble TGFβ receptor preventing TGFβ from binding to the type I/type II receptor complex (Velasco-Loyden *et al.*, 2004).

In the nucleus, the Smad2/3–Smad4 complex assembles the factors necessary for transcriptional activation/repression of specific target genes. This highly selective process depends on the precise configuration of the target gene promoter, which must present the cognate sequences at the correct distance and in proper orientation. Furthermore, assembly of the transcriptional complexes is dependent on expression and availability of the required co-factors, which is cell-type dependent. For example, c-Ski and SnoN, two transcriptional repressors that activate p53 and induce apoptosis, are expressed in all mammalian tissues (Luo, 2004). However, during mammary gland development and lactation an increased expression of SnoN promotes lobular-alveolar proliferation by increasing epithelial proliferation, counteracting the anti-proliferative function of TGFβ (Jahchan *et al.*, 2010). Thus the TGFβ response is cell type and context dependent despite the relatively simple general signal transduction mechanism.

3.5   Dysregulation of signalling in cancer

Cancer is a multistep disease and requires premalignant cells to acquire several mutations in cellular pathways regulating cell proliferation and apoptosis before the disease progresses to the active stage. Given the importance and multitude of effects that TGFβ exerts in the body, key components of the pathway have been found mutated in cancer; 90% of tumours over-express TGFβ, which contributes to metastasis, angiogenesis as well as immunosuppression (Levy and Hill, 2006). Interestingly, TGFβ has a biphasic activity in cancer. During the early stages of cancer, TGFβ has a tumour suppressor function whereas at later stages it has tumour progressing activity. As described earlier, TGFβ induces EMT, which stimulates the release of cytokines and growth factors that are important mediators of metastasis. IL11 (interleukin 11) and PTHrP (parathyroid hormone related peptide) stimulate osteolysis in bone metastasis (Kang *et al.*, 2003b). VEGF (vascular endothelia growth factor) and CTGF (connective tissue growth factor) stimulate angiogenesis (Chen and Lau, 2009). TGFβ stimulates recruitment of macrophages and neutrophils to the tumour but suppresses T cell proliferation and differentiation of antigen-presenting dendritic cells effectively dampening immune responses to the tumour (for review see Flavell *et al.* (2010) and reference therein).

3.5.1 Receptor mutations

Type II receptor mutations

At the early stages of cancer the growth inhibitory effect of TGFβ prevails; however, once cancer cells acquire mutations inactivating key signalling components, such as the type II receptor, they are refractory to this growth inhibitory signal. Accordingly, inactivating mutations in the type II receptor have been found in a large number of gastrointestinal cancers, including colorectal (30%) and gastric (15%) (Levy and Hill, 2006). The sequence of the type II receptor gene (*TGFBR2*) contains a 10-bp polyadenine track, which is a common site for insertion mutations in cancers with microsatellite instability (Markowitz *et al.*, 1995). Microsatellite instability is caused by mutations in the mismatch repair system that during DNA replication repairs base pair mismatches, which are frequently observed in DNA stretches of tandem repeat nucleotides. Insertions or deletions in the 10-bp polyadenine track of the *TGFBR2* lead to expression of a truncated, inactive receptor (Markowitz *et al.*, 1995).

Intragenic mutations in the *TGFBR2* are also observed and frequently lead to expression of kinase dead receptor products (Wang *et al.*, 1997). Additionally, a large number of tumors show loss of expression of *TGFBR2* indicating that cancer cells, which loose the growth inhibitory effect of TGFβ gain survival advantage. Loss of *TGFBR2* expression is frequently linked to inhibition of expression either through promoter methylation or histone deacetylation (Zhang *et al.*, 2004).

Type I receptor mutations

Mutations in type I receptor genes (*TGFBR1*) are less frequent but are observed in ovarian, breast and pancreatic cancers. These mutations are mostly intragenic but loss of expression through promoter methylation has been observed in up to 50% of gastric cancers (Pinto *et al.*, 2003), again highlighting the fact that down-regulation of the TGFβ pathway is advantageous to tumour cells.

3.5.2 Inactivation of Smads

Inactivation of Smad genes has been identified particularly in pancreatic cancers and gliomas. Intragenic mutations and homozygous deletions as well as loss of expression have been observed. *Smad4* and *Smad2* are located on chromosome 18q21 (Thiagalingam *et al.*, 1996), which is frequently deleted or shows loss of heterozygosity, especially in colorectal cancers and *Smad4* mutations can account for about 50–60% of the 18q21 allele loss in these cancers (Miyaki and Kuroki, 2003). *Smad3* mutations have not been described but in gastric cancers loss of expression either through receptor methylation or epigenetic changes has been identified (Han *et al.*, 2004).

TGFβ signalling can also be down regulated through the over-expression of antagonists such as Smad7, Smurf2, Nedd4L and transcriptional repressors Ski and SnoN (Levy and Hill, 2006). Interestingly, *Smad7* is located on the same chromosome arm as *Smad 2* and *4*, between the two R-Smads. However, deletions of the *Smad7* locus are less frequent than in the *Smad2/4* loci and the *Smad7* locus also appears to be more frequently amplified in colorectal cancer (Boulay *et al.*, 2001), indicating a growth advantage for tumour cells in retaining activity of the I-Smad.

3.5.3   Mutations in transcriptional targets

A different scenario to the inhibition of TGFβ signalling described earlier results from mutations in TGFβ transcriptional targets such as *c-Myc*, *p15* or *p21*. When two or more of these downstream effectors are mutated, TGFβ signalling is intact but has lost its growth inhibitory function. Cancer cells with these mutations respond to TGFβ with increased EMT, cell motility and production and release of pro-angiogenic cytokines. These events enhance tumour invasiveness and metastasis.

3.6   Therapeutic opportunities

Given the important role TGFβ plays during carcinogenesis and other diseases such as fibrosis, strategies to control TGFβ signalling therapeutically have been developed, some of which are currently in Phase II/III clinical trials (for review see Nagaraj and Datta, 2010 and Akhurst and Hata, 2012).

Three strategies are used to target TGFβ signalling: interference with ligand levels/availability; ligand/receptor interaction; and targeting the intracellular signalling pathways. Drug design can be further divided into large-molecule inhibitors such as antibodies, anti-sense oligonucleotides or ligand traps and small-molecule inhibitors, that is, chemical inhibitors of receptor kinases. Several companies have developed and are still developing these molecules.

3.6.1   Ligand-targeted therapies

Several humanised antibodies directed against TGFβ1, TGFβ2 and a panTGFβ antibody recognising all three isoforms have been developed. Several of these antibodies have entered Phase I/II clinical trials. For Lerdelimumab, an anti-TGFβ2 antibody, a Phase III clinical trial was recently completed showing no efficacy over placebo in the treatment of scaring after glaucoma surgery (Trabeculectomy Study Group, 2007; Khaw *et al.*, 2007). Similarly, treatment with Metelimumab, an anti-TGFβ1 antibody, showed no efficacy in the treatment of systemic sclerosis in a Phase II clinical trial (Denton *et al.*, 2007). Only Fresolimumab, a pan-TGFβ antibody, is currently under investigation for treatment of cancer (www.clinicaltrials.gov identifier: NCT00356460, NCT01401062 and NCT01112293).

No results have been published using recombinant soluble betaglycan, the type III TGFβ receptor, in a clinical setting. However, an antibody directed against αvβ6 integrin, which is involved in the activation of latent TGFβ, has shown promising results in pre-clinical studies of fibrosis and is now in Phase II to establish safety, tolerability, pharmacokinetics, immunogenicity of the antibody in patients with idiopathic pulmonary fibrosis (NCT01371305).

3.6.2 Anti-sense oligonucleotides

Anti-sense oligonculeotides targeting *TGFβ1* and 2 have been developed but only AP-12009, also known as Trabedersen, has continued to Phase III clinical trials where it has shown promising results in the treatment of glioblastoma. However, owing to recruitment issues because of changes in the initial treatment of glioblastoma patients, the trial was recently terminated (February 2012 – see www.clinicaltrials.gov identifier: NCT00761280). The drug was also tested in patients with advanced pancreatic cancer or metastatic colorectal cancer known to overproduce TGFβ2 and showed promising results (NCT00844064) (Akhurst and Hata, 2012). Another approach has been pursued by NovaRx who used anti-sense oligonucleotides against *TGFβ2* to specifically down-regulate its expression in cells derived from patients with non-small-cell lung cancer (NSCLC). These engineered cells were then used as a cancer vaccine to boost antitumour immune responses in patients with NSCLC in a Phase III clinical trial (NCT00676507) (Nemunaitis *et al.*, 2009).

3.6.3 Small molecule inhibitors

Interestingly, there are two small molecule inhibitors (Yingling *et al.*, 2004) originally developed to target other molecules undergoing Phase II trials or having been approved for the treatment of fibrosis: Losartan, an angiotensin II type 1 receptor inhibitor (Holm *et al.*, 2011) and Pirfenidone, of unknown target specificity (Azuma *et al.*, 2005), which both have been shown to reduce TGFβ expression (Choi *et al.*, 2012). No results have been published about use of these molecules for cancer treatment. Cancer specific small molecule inhibitors are being developed that target the kinase domain of the type I receptor. LY2157299 (NCT01220271 and NCT01246986) and LY573636 (NCT00383292) are in Phase

II clinical trials for treatment of glioblastoma, melanoma and pancreatic carcinoma. Other molecules have shown promising results in pre-clinical studies (Melisi *et al.*, 2008; Ganapathy *et al.*, 2010). Furthermore, there is scope for the development of combined therapies through the discovery of cross-talk between different signalling pathways that antagonise Smad signalling, such as peroxisome proliferator-activated receptor gamma (PPARγ) (Reka *et al.*, 2010).

3.6.4   Signalling pathway inhibitors

Antibodies directed against type II receptor, or recombinant T cells expressing a dominant negative type II receptor to improve tumour detection and killing by these cytotoxic T-cells, are in Phase I clinical trials for lung cancer and EBV-positive lymphoma (NCT00889954 and NCT00368082). Furthermore, small molecule inhibitors targeting specific Smad protein–protein interactions have been developed and shown specificity in a reporter gene expression assay (Cui *et al.*, 2005). However, no further development of these molecules for clinical use has been reported. Other small molecule inhibitors targeting mainly the kinase domain of the type I receptor are in the pre-clinical stage. Some of these molecules have shown promising results at nanomolar concentrations in cell-based assays or mouse models of cancer (Halder *et al.*, 2005; Uhl *et al.*, 2004). However, some of the inhibitors show pharmacokinetic instability *in vivo* (Akhurst and Hata, 2012).

Development of anti-TGFβ drugs for cancer treatment has been hampered by the cell specific effect of this cytokine. In particular, the tumour stage and the microenvironment play an important role in determining the usefulness of using anti-TGFβ drugs. Interesting results have been obtained by using combined therapy in a mouse model of breast cancer where an anti-TGFβ antibody blocked the adverse effects of ionising radiation and doxorubicin, both of which enhance secretion of TGFβ (Biswas *et al.*, 2007). As complete ablation of TGFβ is not recommend because of the multitude of effects that the cytokine has, careful consideration has to be given to when and who to treat with these emerging drugs.

References

Akhurst, R.J. and Hata, A. (2012) Targeting the TGFbeta signalling pathway in disease. Nature reviews. *Drug Discovery*, **11** (10), 790–811.

Alarcon, C., Zaromytidou, A.I., Xi, Q. *et al.* (2009) Nuclear CDKs drive Smad transcriptional activation and turnover in BMP and TGF-beta pathways. *Cell*, **139** (4), 757–769.

Aragon, E., Goerner, N., Zaromytidou, A.I. *et al.* (2011) A Smad action turnover switch operated by WW domain readers of a phosphoserine code. *Genes and Development*, **25** (12), 1275–1288.

Aranda, V., Nolan, M.E. and Muthuswamy, S.K. (2008) Par complex in cancer: a regulator of normal cell polarity joins the dark side. *Oncogene* **27** (55), 6878–6887.

Azuma, A., Nukiwa, T., Tsubio, E. *et al.* (2005) Double-blind, placebo-controlled trial of pirfenidone in patients with idiopathic pulmonary fibrosis. *American Journal of Respiratory and Critical Care Medicine*, **171** (9), 1040–1047.

Bertolino, P., Deckers, M., Lebrin, F. *et al.* (2005) Transforming growth factor-beta signal transduction in angiogenesis and vascular disorders. *Chest*, **128** (6 Suppl), 585S–590S.

Bilandzic, M. and Stenvers, K.L. (2011) Betaglycan: a multifunctional accessory. *Molecular and Cellular Endocrinology*, **339** (1-2), 180–189.

Biswas, S., Guix, M., Rinehart, C. *et al.* (2007) Inhibition of TGF-beta with neutralizing antibodies prevents radiation-induced acceleration of metastatic cancer progression. *Journal of Clinical Investigation*, **117** (5), 1305–1313.

Boulay, J.L., Mild, G., Reuter, J. *et al.* (2001) Combined copy status of 18q21 genes in colorectal cancer shows frequent retention of SMAD7. *Genes, Chromosomes and Cancer*, **31** (3), 240–247.

Cheifetz, S. and Massague J. (1989) Transforming growth factor-beta (TGF-beta) receptor proteoglycan. Cell surface expression and ligand binding in the absence of glycosaminoglycan chains. *Journal of Biological Chemistry*, **264** (20), 12025–12028.

Chen, C.C. and Lau, L.F. (2009) Functions and mechanisms of action of CCN matricellular proteins. *International Journal of Biochemistry and Cell Biology*, **41** (4), 771–783.

Chen, W., Kirkbride, K.C., How, T. *et al.* (2003) Beta-arrestin 2 mediates endocytosis of type III TGF-beta receptor and down-regulation of its signaling. *Science*, **301** (5638), 1394–1397.

Chen, Y.G., Liu, F., Massague, J. *et al.* (1997) Mechanism of TGFbeta receptor inhibition by FKBP12. *EMBO Journal*, **16** (13), 3866–3876.

Choi, K., Lee, K., Ryu, S.W. *et al.* (2012) Pirfenidone inhibits transforming growth factor-beta1-induced fibrogenesis by blocking nuclear translocation of Smads in human retinal pigment epithelial cell line ARPE-19. *Molecular Vision*, **18**, 1010–1020.

Cui, Q., Lim, S.K., Zhao, B. *et al.* (2005) Selective inhibition of TGF-beta responsive genes by Smad-interacting peptide aptamers from FoxH1, Lef1 and CBP. *Oncogene*, **24** (24), 3864–3874.

Davis, B.N., Hilyard, A.C., Nguyen, P.H. *et al.* (2010) Smad proteins bind a conserved RNA sequence to promote microRNA maturation by Drosha. *Molecular Cell*, **39** (3), 373–384.

Denton, C.P., Merkel, P.A., Furst, D.E. *et al.* (2007) Recombinant human anti-transforming growth factor beta1 antibody therapy in systemic sclerosis: a multicenter, randomized, placebo-controlled phase I/II trial of CAT-192. *Arthritis and Rheumatism*, **56** (1), 323–333.

Derynck, R., Gelbart, W.M., Harland, R.M. *et al.* (1996) Nomenclature: vertebrate mediators of TGFbeta family signals. *Cell*, **87** (2), 173.

Derynck, R., Rhee, L., Chen, E.Y. *et al.* (1987) Intron-exon structure of the human transforming growth factor-beta precursor gene. *Nucleic Acids Research*, **15** (7), 3188–3189.

Derynck, R., Zhang, Y., Feng, X.H. *et al.* (1998) Smads: transcriptional activators of TGF-beta responses. *Cell*, **95** (6), 737–740.

Di Guglielmo, G.M., Le Roy, C., Goodfellow, A.F. *et al.* (2003) Distinct endocytic pathways regulate TGF-beta receptor signalling and turnover. *Nature Cell Biology*, **5** (5), 410–421.

Feng, X.H. and Derynck, D. (2005) Specificity and versatility in tgf-beta signaling through Smads. *Annual Review of Cell and Developmental Biology*, **21**, 659–693.

Fernandez, L.A., Sanz-Rodriguez, F., Blanco, F.J. *et al.* (2006) Hereditary hemorrhagic telangiectasia, a vascular dysplasia affecting the TGF-beta signaling pathway. *Clinical Medicine and Research*, **4** (1), 66–78.

Flavell, R.A., Sanjabi, S., Wrzesinski, S.H. *et al.* (2010) The polarization of immune cells in the tumour environment by TGFbeta. *Nature Reviews. Immunology*, **10** (8), 554–567.

Frederick, J.P., Liberati, N.T., Waddell, D.S. *et al.* (2004) Transforming growth factor beta-mediated transcriptional repression of c-myc is dependent on direct binding of Smad3 to a novel repressive Smad binding element. *Molecular and Cellular Biology*, **24** (6), 2546–2559.

Fuentealba, L.C., Eivers, E., Ikeda, A. *et al.* (2007) Integrating patterning signals: Wnt/GSK3 regulates the duration of the BMP/Smad1 signal. *Cell*, **131** (5), 980–993.

Ganapathy, V., Ge, R., Grazioli, A. *et al.* (2010) Targeting the transforming growth factor-beta pathway inhibits human basal-like breast cancer metastasis. *Molecular Cancer*, **9**, 122.

Gao, S., Alarcon, C., Sapkota, G. *et al.* (2009) Ubiquitin ligase Nedd4L targets activated Smad2/3 to limit TGF-beta signaling. *Molecular Cell*, **36** (3), 457–468.

Groppe, J., Hinck, C.S., Samavarchi-Tehrani, P. *et al.* (2008) Cooperative assembly of TGF-beta superfamily signaling complexes is mediated by two disparate mechanisms and distinct modes of receptor binding. *Molecular Cell*, **29** (2), 157–168.

Gunaratne, A., Thai, B.L. and Di Guglielmo, G.M. (2013) Atypical protein kinase C phosphorylates Par6 and facilitates transforming growth factor beta-induced epithelial-to-mesenchymal transition. *Molecular and Cellular Biology*, **33** (5), 874–886.

Halder, S.K., Beauchamp, R.D. and Datta, P.K. (2005) A specific inhibitor of TGF-beta receptor kinase, SB-431542, as a potent antitumor agent for human cancers. *Neoplasia*, **7**(5), 509–521.

Han, S.U., Kim, H.T., Seong, D.H. *et al.* (2004) Loss of the Smad3 expression increases susceptibility to tumorigenicity in human gastric cancer. *Oncogene*, **23** (7), 1333–1341.

Harrison, C.A., Al-Musawi, S.L. and Walton, K.L. (2011) Prodomains regulate the synthesis, extracellular localisation and activity of TGF-beta superfamily ligands. *Growth Factors*, **29** (5), 174–186.

Heldin, C.H., Vanlandewijck, M. and Moustakas, A. (2012) Regulation of EMT by TGFbeta in cancer. *FEBS Letters*, **586** (14), 1959–1970.

Hinck, A.P. (2012) Structural studies of the TGF-betas and their receptors – insights into evolution of the TGF-beta superfamily. *FEBS Letters*, **586** (14), 1860–1870.

Hirai, R. and Fijita, T. (1996) A human transforming growth factor-beta type II receptor that contains an insertion in the extracellular domain. *Experimental Cell Research*, **223** (1), 135–141.

Holm, T.M., Habashi, J.P., Doyle, J.J. *et al.* (2011) Noncanonical TGFbeta signaling contributes to aortic aneurysm progression in Marfan syndrome mice. *Science*, **332** (6027), 358–361.

Hyytiainen, M., Penttinen, C. and Keski-Oja, J. (2004) Latent TGF-beta binding proteins: extracellular matrix association and roles in TGF-beta activation. *Critical Reviews in Clinical Laboratory Sciences*, **41** (3), 233–264.

Inman, G.J., Nicolas, F.J. and Hill, C.S. (2002) Nucleocytoplasmic shuttling of Smads 2, 3, and 4 permits sensing of TGF-beta receptor activity. *Molecular Cell*, **10** (2), 283–294.

Jahchan, N.S., You, Y.H., Muller, W.J. *et al.* (2010) Transforming growth factor-beta regulator SnoN modulates mammary gland branching morphogenesis, post-lactational involution, and mammary tumorigenesis. *Cancer Research*, **70** (10), 4204–4213.

Kaartinen, V., Voncken, J.W., Shuler, C. *et al.* (1995) Abnormal lung development and cleft palate in mice lacking TGF-beta 3 indicates defects of epithelial-mesenchymal interaction. *Nature Genetics*, **11** (4), 415–421.

Kamitani, T., Kito, K., Nguyen, H.P. *et al.* (1997) Characterization of NEDD8, a developmentally down-regulated ubiquitin-like protein. *Journal of Biological Chemistry*, **272** (45), 28557–28562.

Kang, Y., Chen, C.R. and Massague, J. (2003a) A self-enabling TGFbeta response coupled to stress signaling: Smad engages stress response factor ATF3 for Id1 repression in epithelial cells. *Molecular Cell*, **11** (4), 915–926.

Kang, Y., Siegel, P.M., Shu, W. *et al.* (2003b) A multigenic program mediating breast cancer metastasis to bone. *Cancer Cell*, **3** (6), 537–549.

Karlsson, E., Jolkkonen, M., Mulugeta, E. *et al.* (2000) Snake toxins with high selectivity for subtypes of muscarinic acetylcholine receptors. *Biochimie*, **82** (9-10), 793–806.

Kavsak, P., Rasmussen, R.K., Causing, C.G. *et al.* (2000) Smad7 binds to Smurf2 to form an E3 ubiquitin ligase that targets the TGF beta receptor for degradation. *Molecular Cell*, **6** (6), 1365–1375.

Khaw, P., Grehn, F., Hollo, G. *et al.* (2007) A phase III study of subconjunctival human anti-transforming growth factor beta(2) monoclonal antibody (CAT-152) to prevent scarring after first-time trabeculectomy. *Ophthalmology*, **114** (10), 1822–1830.

Kutateladze, T.G. (2006) Phosphatidylinositol 3-phosphate recognition and membrane docking by the FYVE domain. *Biochimica et Biophysica Acta*, **1761** (8), 868–877.

Letterio, J.J. and Roberts, A.B. (1998) Regulation of immune responses by TGF-beta. *Annual Review of Immunology*, **16**, 137–161.

Levy, L. and Hill, C.S. (2006) Alterations in components of the TGF-beta superfamily signaling pathways in human cancer. *Cytokine and Growth Factor Reviews*, **17** (1-2), 41–58.

Lin, H.K., Bergmann, S. and Pandolfi, P.P. (2004) Cytoplasmic PML function in TGF-beta signalling. *Nature*, **431** (7005), 205–211.

Lin, H.Y., Wang, X.F., Ng-Eaton, E. *et al.* (1992) Expression cloning of the TGF-beta type II receptor, a functional transmembrane serine/threonine kinase. *Cell*, **68** (4), 775–785.

Lin, X., Duan, X., Liang, Y.Y. *et al.* (2006) PPM1A functions as a Smad phosphatase to terminate TGFbeta signaling. *Cell*, **125** (5), 915–928.

Lopez-Casillas, F., Cheifetz, S., Doody, J. *et al.* (1991) Structure and expression of the membrane proteoglycan betaglycan, a component of the TGF-beta receptor system. *Cell*, **67** (4), 785–795.

Lopez-Casillas, F., Payne, H.M., Andres, J.L. *et al.* (1994) Betaglycan can act as a dual modulator of TGF-beta access to signaling receptors: mapping of ligand binding and GAG attachment sites. *Journal of Cell Biology*, **124** (4), 557–568.

Luo, K. (2004) Ski and SnoN: negative regulators of TGF-beta signaling. *Current Opinion in Genetics and Development*, **14** (1), 65–70.

Luo, K. and Lodish, H.F. (1997) Positive and negative regulation of type II TGF-beta receptor signal transduction by autophosphorylation on multiple serine residues. *EMBO Journal*, **16** (8), 1970–1981.

Markowitz, S., Wang, J., Myeroff, L. *et al.* (1995) Inactivation of the type II TGF-beta receptor in colon cancer cells with microsatellite instability. *Science*, **268** (5215), 1336–1338.

Massague, J. (1990) The transforming growth factor-beta family. *Annual Review of Cell Biology*, **6**, 597–641.

Massague, J. (2012) TGFbeta signalling in context. *Nature Reviews. Molecular Cell Biology*, **13** (10), 616–630.

Melisi, D., Ishiyama, S., Sclabas, G.M. *et al.* (2008) LY2109761, a novel transforming growth factor beta receptor type I and type II dual inhibitor, as a therapeutic approach to suppressing pancreatic cancer metastasis. *Molecular Cancer Therapeutics*, **7** (4), 829–840.

Miyaki, M. and Kuroki, T. (2003) Role of Smad4 (DPC4) inactivation in human cancer. *Biochemical and Biophysical Research Communications*, **306** (4), 799–804.

Moustakas, A. and Heldin, C.H. (2009) The regulation of TGFbeta signal transduction. *Development*, **136** (22), 3699–3714.

Moustakas, A., Souchelnytskyi, S. and Heldin, C.H. (2001) Smad regulation in TGF-beta signal transduction. *Journal of Cell Science*, **114** (Pt 24), 4359–4369.

Munger, J.S. and Sheppard, D. (2011) Cross talk among TGF-beta signaling pathways, integrins, and the extracellular matrix. *Cold Spring Harbor Perspectives in Biology*, **3** (11), a005017.

Nagaraj, N.S. and Datta, P.K. (2010) Targeting the transforming growth factor-beta signaling pathway in human cancer. *Expert Opinion on Investigational Drugs*, **19** (1), 77–91.

Nemunaitis, J., Nemunaitis, M., Senzer, N. *et al.* (2009) Phase II trial of Belagenpumatucel-L, a TGF-beta2 antisense gene modified allogeneic tumor vaccine in advanced non small cell lung cancer (NSCLC) patients. *Cancer Gene Therapy*, **16** (8), 620–624.

Pinto, M., Oliveira, C., Cirnes, L. *et al.* (2003) Promoter methylation of TGFbeta receptor I and mutation of TGFbeta receptor II are frequent events in MSI sporadic gastric carcinomas. *Journal of Pathology*, **200** (1), 32–38.

Powell, D.W., Mifflin, R.C., Valentich, J.D. *et al.* (1999) Myofibroblasts. I. Paracrine cells important in health and disease. *American Journal of Physiology*, **277** (1 Pt 1), C1–C9.

Randall, R.A., Germain, S., Inman, G.J. *et al.* (2002) Different Smad2 partners bind a common hydrophobic pocket in Smad2 via a defined proline-rich motif. *EMBO Journal*, **21** (1-2), 145–156.

Ravitz, M.J. and Wenner, C.E. (1997) Cyclin-dependent kinase regulation during G1 phase and cell cycle regulation by TGF-beta. *Advances in Cancer Research*, **71**, 165–207.

Reka, A.K., Kurapati, H., Narala, V.R. *et al.* (2010) Peroxisome proliferator-activated receptor-gamma activation inhibits tumor metastasis by antagonizing Smad3-mediated epithelial-mesenchymal transition. *Molecular Cancer Therapeutics*, **9** (12), 3221–3232.

Roberts, A.B., Sporn, M.B., Assoian, R.K. *et al.* (1986) Transforming growth factor type beta: rapid induction of fibrosis and angiogenesis in vivo and stimulation of collagen formation in vitro. *Proceedings of the National Academy of Sciences, USA*, **83** (12), 4167–4171.

Rotzer, D., Roth, M., Lutz, M. *et al.* (2001) Type III TGF-beta receptor-independent signalling of TGF-beta2 via TbetaRII-B, an alternatively spliced TGF-beta type II receptor. *EMBO Journal*, **20** (3), 480–490.

Sanford, L.P., Ormsby, I., Gittenberger-De Groot, A.C. *et al.* (1997) TGFbeta2 knockout mice have multiple developmental defects that are non-overlapping with other TGFbeta knockout phenotypes. *Development*, **124** (13), 2659–2670.

Schultz, G.S. and Wysocki, A. (2009) Interactions between extracellular matrix and growth factors in wound healing. *Wound Repair and Regeneration: Official Publication of the Wound Healing Society [and] the European Tissue Repair Society*, **17** (2), 153–162.

Shi, Y. and Massague, J. (2003) Mechanisms of TGF-beta signaling from cell membrane to the nucleus. *Cell*, **113** (6), 685–700.

Shi, Y., Wang, Y.F., Jayaraman, L. *et al.* (1998) Crystal structure of a Smad MH1 domain bound to DNA: insights on DNA binding in TGF-beta signaling. *Cell*, **94** (5), 585–594.

Shull, M.M., Ormsby, I., Kier, A.B. *et al.* (1992) Targeted disruption of the mouse transforming growth factor-beta 1 gene results in multifocal inflammatory disease. *Nature*, **359** (6397), 693–699.

Sinha, S., Nevett, C., Shuttleworth, C.A. *et al.* (1998) Cellular and extracellular biology of the latent transforming growth factor-beta binding proteins. *Matrix Biology: Journal of the International Society for Matrix Biology*, **17** (8-9), 529–545.

ten Dijke, P., Miyazono, K. and Heldin, C.H. (2000) Signaling inputs converge on nuclear effectors in TGF-beta signaling. *Trends in Biochemical Sciences*, **25** (2), 64–70.

Thiagalingam, S., Lengauer, C., Leach, F.S. *et al.* (1996) Evaluation of candidate tumour suppressor genes on chromosome 18 in colorectal cancers. *Nature Genetics*, **13** (3), 343–346.

Thiery, J.P., Acloque, H., Huang, R.Y. *et al.* (2009) Epithelial-mesenchymal transitions in development and disease. *Cell*, **139** (5), 871–890.

Thompson, N.L., Flanders, K.C., Smith, J.M. *et al.* (1989) Expression of transforming growth factor-beta 1 in specific cells and tissues of adult and neonatal mice. *Journal of Cell Biology*, **108** (2), 661–669.

Trabeculectomy Study Group (2007) CAT-152 Trabeculectomy Study. *Ophthalmology*, **114** (10), 1950.

Tsukazaki, T., Chiang, T.A., Davison, A.F. *et al.* (1998) SARA, a FYVE domain protein that recruits Smad2 to the TGFbeta receptor. *Cell*, **95** (6), 779–791.

Uhl, M., Aulwurm, S., Wischhusen, J. *et al.* (2004) SD-208, a novel transforming growth factor beta receptor I kinase inhibitor, inhibits growth and invasiveness and enhances immunogenicity of murine and human glioma cells in vitro and in vivo. *Cancer Research*, **64** (21), 7954–7961.

Velasco-Loyden, G., Arribas, J. and Lopez-Cassillas, F. (2004) The shedding of betaglycan is regulated by pervanadate and mediated by membrane type matrix metalloprotease-1. *Journal of Biological Chemistry*, **279** (9), 7721–7733.

Wang, D., Song, H., Evans, J.A. *et al.* (1997) Mutation and downregulation of the transforming growth factor beta type II receptor gene in primary squamous cell carcinomas of the head and neck. *Carcinogenesis*, **18** (11), 2285–2290.

Watanabe, M., Masuyama, N., Fukuda, M. *et al.* (2000) Regulation of intracellular dynamics of Smad4 by its leucine-rich nuclear export signal. *EMBO Reports*, **1** (2), 176–182.

Wilcox, J.N. and Derynck, R. (1988) Developmental expression of transforming growth factors alpha and beta in mouse fetus. *Molecular and Cellular Biology*, **8** (8), 3415–3422.

Xi, Q., Wang, Z., Zaromytidou, A.I. *et al.* (2011) A poised chromatin platform for TGF-beta access to master regulators. *Cell*, **147** (7), 1511–1524.

Xu, L., Chen, Y.G. *et al.* (2000) The nuclear import function of Smad2 is masked by SARA and unmasked by TGFbeta-dependent phosphorylation. *Nature Cell Biology*, **2**(8), 559–562.

Xu, L., Kang, Y., Col, S. *et al.* (2002) Smad2 nucleocytoplasmic shuttling by nucleoporins CAN/Nup214 and Nup153 feeds TGFbeta signaling complexes in the cytoplasm and nucleus. *Molecular Cell*, **10** (2), 271–282.

Yingling, J.M., Blanchard, K.L. and Sawyer, J.S. (2004) Development of TGF-beta signalling inhibitors for cancer therapy. *Nature Reviews. Drug Discovery*, **3** (12), 1011–1022.

Zhang, H.T., Chen, X.F., Wang, M.H. *et al.* (2004) Defective expression of transforming growth factor beta receptor type II is associated with CpG methylated promoter in primary non-small cell lung cancer. *Clinical Cancer Research: An Official Journal of the American Association for Cancer Research*, **10** (7), 2359–2367.

Zhang, Y.E. (2009) Non-Smad pathways in TGF-beta signaling. *Cell Research*, **19** (1), 128–139.

Zuo, W., Huang, F., Chiang, Y.J. *et al.* (2013) c-Cbl-Mediated neddylation antagonizes ubiquitination and degradation of the TGF-beta type II receptor. *Molecular Cell*, **49** (3), 499–510.

4
Wnt signalling

David Tree

Biosciences, Brunel University, London

4.1 Introduction and overview

The cell-signalling pathway activated by the ligands of the Wnt class of proteins is an essential and widely conserved mechanism. Wnt signalling directs cell proliferation, cell polarity and cell identity both during embryonic development and during the homeostasis of many adult tissues. Reflecting its ubiquity and importance, the mis-regulation of Wnt signalling is causal in human birth defects, cancer and an increasingly wide and diverse array of disorders. This chapter focuses on our current knowledge of the best-understood cell-signalling pathway regulated by Wnt proteins, the canonical Wnt/β-catenin pathway. β-Catenin is a key cytoplasmic and nuclear mediator of signalling whose levels are key in the regulation of signalling. Other cell signalling pathways, so-called 'non-canonical' Wnt signalling pathways activated by Wnt proteins will be mentioned in passing but are beyond the scope of this work. These non-canonical pathways are extensively reviewed elsewhere (Peng and Axelrod, 2012; Vladar *et al.*, 2009).

The first *Wnt* gene to be cloned was identified in 1982 by Roel Nusse in Harold Varmus's laboratory. It was cloned by virtue of the fact that it was the gene transcriptionally unregulated by the insertion of mouse mammary tumour virus MMV-1 (Nusse and Vamus, 1982) and was named *Int-1* for integration-1. It encodes a characteristically cysteine-rich secreted protein, which can act as a morphogenetic ligand in some circumstances. Subsequently the gene affected by the *Drosophila* mutant wingless (*Wg*) was identified and the family of genes were renamed *Wnt* (Rijsewijk *et al.*, 1987). A combination of genetic, cell biological and biochemical studies in a variety of model systems have led to a detailed understanding of a highly conserved signalling pathway, although many aspects of it are less well understood and challenges in order to do so continue to lie ahead. The importance of Wnt signalling in mediating various human health problems have led to it being targeted by therapy in a variety of ways to combat these problems.

Cancer Cell Signalling, First Edition. Edited by Amanda Harvey.
© 2013 John Wiley & Sons, Ltd. Published 2013 by John Wiley & Sons, Ltd.

Comprehensive information including a considerable historical perspective can be found at the Wnt homepage (www/Stanford.edu/russe/wntwindow.html).

There are 12 conserved subfamilies of Wnt proteins and most mammalian genomes contain 19 *Wnt* genes. Wnt proteins are around 40 kDa and lipid modification of the proteins is important for their function (Willert *et al.*, 2003). The consensus view of the cytoplasmic regulation of Wnt signalling is often described as the 'two-state' model and refers to the interactions and actions of molecules when Wnt signalling is active and when Wnt signalling is inactive. While clearly not perfect, the two-state model is an attractive framework in which to understand both how signalling is regulated during normal signalling and the way in which signalling is disrupted in various mutant situations. The two-state model will be reviewed briefly here and then the various aspects of cellular regulation of signalling will be discussed (Figure 4.1).

In the 'off' state, when Wnt ligands are not present, the free cytoplasmic levels of the key mediator of signalling, β-catenin, are kept at a low level by the action of a complex of proteins referred to as the destruction complex, though it is sometimes referred to as the APC or Axin complex after the key components. The basic elements of the destruction complex are Axin, a large scaffolding protein containing an RGS (regulator of G-protein signalling) and a DIX domain, and APC (adenomatous polyposis coli) a multi-domain tumour suppressor protein that also has scaffolding properties, along with the kinases casein kinase 1 (CK1) and glycogen synthase kinase 3 (GSK3). CK1 and GSK3 sequentially phosphorylate the amino terminal end of β-catenin on conserved serine and threonine residues. This results in β-catenin being recognised by the E3 ubiquitin ligase β-Trcp, which leads to its degradation by the proteosome. Low levels of free cytoplasmic β-catenin result in very low levels of β-catenin in the nucleus and the repression of Wnt target genes by T cell factor/lymphoid enhancer factor (TCF/LEF) family proteins in concert with other transcriptional repressors, most notably Groucho. When Wnt ligands are present in the extracellular space they are able to activate the Wnt/β-catenin pathway by binding to two classes of receptor: the Frizzled (Fz) family of receptors (of which there are ten members in mammals) are seven pass transmembrane proteins and the low-density lipoprotein receptor related protein (LRP) class of receptors (consisting of LRP5 and 6) are single pass transmembrane proteins. The formation of a tripartite complex containing a member of each receptor class plus a ligand leads to the recruitment of the cytoplasmic protein Dishevelled (Dsh) to the cytoplasmic face of the membrane. This results in the phosphorylation of the cytoplasmic tail of LRP and the recruitment of at least some members of the destruction complex to the membrane. The subsequent inhibition of the destruction complex means that β-catenin is no longer phosphorylated and thus not degraded. Free β-catenin thus builds up in the cytoplasm, is transported to the nucleus, displaces Groucho from its inhibitory complexes with TCF/LEF and activates transcription of Wnt target genes (Figure 4.1).

This is an accurate if somewhat simplistic view of how Wnt signalling is regulated. The cellular organisation of signalling is discussed in more detail in the following sections.

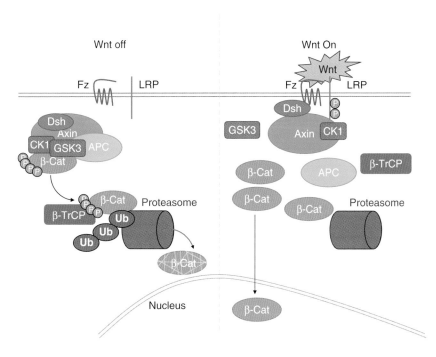

Figure 4.1 **The classic two-state model for the regulation of Wnt signalling.** The classic two-state model was developed in the mid-1990s from a combination of results from *Drosophila* and mouse genetics, *Xenopus* embryological work and *Drosophila* and mammalian cell culture experiments. In the 'off' state in the absence of a Wnt ligand, the destruction complex, containing APC, Axin, GSK3 and CK1 resides in the cytoplasm where it binds to and leads to the phosphorylation of β-catenin. Phosphorylated β-catenin exits the destruction complex and is ubiquitinated by β-TrCP that binds to phosphorylated β-catenin, which is subsequently degraded by the proteasome. In the 'on' state when Wnt binds to its receptors Frizzled and LRP a tripartite complex is formed, which induces the binding of Axin to the phosphorylated cytoplasmic tail of LRP. This induces the disassociation of the destruction complex, which leads to the accumulation of un-phosphorylated free β-catenin, which is able to enter the nucleus and direct transcription of Wnt target genes.

4.2 The ligands: Wnt proteins, their modification and secretion

Despite the central importance and numerous functions of Wnt proteins in development and disease, little was known about their biochemical nature for 30 years after the first cloning of the disease due to the technical difficulties surrounding purifying them. The biochemical purification of Wnts, first performed by Carl Willert in Roel Nusse's lab, has allowed a characterisation of their post-translational modifications and a rich understanding of their mode of biological action. Wnt proteins are lipid modified (Willert *et al.*, 2003) by a monounsaturated fatty acid, palmitoleic acid, attached to a conserved serine residue (Takada *et al.*, 2006). Wnt proteins lacking this serine are unable to activate Wnt/β-catenin signalling (Willert *et al.*, 2003; Galli *et al.*, 2007; Komekado *et al.*, 2007). The central importance of lipid modification of Wnts is underlined by the importance of the Porcupine (Porc) molecule, first identified as a mutation in *Drosophila*, the wild-type product of which is required cell-autonomously for Wnt signalling to be active and, crucially, for Wnts to be secreted (van den Heuval *et al.*, 1993; Hausmann *et al.*, 2007). Porc encodes a transmembrane endoplasmic reticulum protein with an *O*-acyl transferase domain (Hausmann *et al.*, 2007). In Porc mutants Wnts have reduced palmitoleoylation at serine 209 and the under-modified protein accumulates in the endoplasmic reticulum, unable to activate signalling (Hausmann *et al.*, 2007).

Two other systems are known to be required for the correct and efficient secretion of Wnt proteins in different model systems: the Wntless (Wls)/Eveness interrupted (Evi)/Sprinter (Srt) system, characterised in *Drosophila* and the retromer complex, characterised in *C. elegans*. Wls is a seven-pass transmembrane protein that can bind Wnts and which is found in the Golgi apparatus, endosomes and plasma membrane (Banziger *et al.*, 2006; Bartscherer *et al.*, 2006; Goodman *et al.*, 2006). In Wls mutant cells Wnts accumulate in the Golgi apparatus (Port *et al.*, 2008) and it has been suggested that Wls functions as a sorting molecule, chaperoning Wnt from the Golgi apparatus to the cell surface. The retromer complex in nematodes has been shown to be an intracellular trafficking complex, which transports endocytosed transmembrane proteins back to the Golgi body (McGough and Cullen, 2011). It has been suggested that the retromer complex may traffic endosomal Wls back to the Golgi network by retrograde transport, preventing it from being degraded in lysosomes (Port *et al.*, 2008; Belenkaya *et al.*, 2008; Franch-Marro *et al.*, 2008; Yang *et al.*, 2008). It is important to note that not all Wnt molecules will be modified in the same fashion and care should be taken applying conclusions to different gingival Wnt molecules. For example, it has been shown that the consequence of changing the two lipid-molecule amino acids on Wg secretion and function are different from changing those for Wnt3a (Franch-Marro *et al.*, 2008). Additionally, there are differences in the order in which modifications occur between Wg and Wnt3a (Komekado *et al.*, 2007; Tanak *et al.*, 2002; Zhai *et al.*, 2004). It is likely therefore that the overall level of lipid modification may be more important for the ligand activity rather than the precise location of the lipidation on the molecule.

4.3   The receptors: Frizzleds and LRPs, multiple receptors and combinations

Two fairly different receptor types are absolutely required for canonical Wnt signalling: those of the Frizzled (Fz or Fzd) (Bhanot *et al.*, 1996) are seven-pass transmembrane receptors, which may be associated with a G-protein

(Katanaev, 2010) and those of the LDL receptor-related proteins 5 and 6 (LRP5/6) (Pinson *et al.*, 2000; Tamai *et al.*, 2000). In *Drosophila* Wg shows an absolute but redundant requirement for either Fz1, which was first identified by its role in the non-canonical planar cell polarity (PCP) pathway (Adler *et al.*, 1990; Park *et al.*, 1994), or Fz2 (Bhanot *et al.*, 1999) along with the fly LRP homologue, Arrow (Arr) (Wehrli *et al.*, 2000). Much work has been done on the specificity of individual Wnts and their receptors (see, for example, Wu and Nusse, 2002; Rulifson *et al.*, 2000; Boutros *et al.*, 2000). Mammalian genomes contain 19 *Wnt* genes, ten *Fz* genes and two *LRP* genes. LRP6 is essential for embryogenesis for which LRP5 is dispensable. LRP5 shows essential roles in adult bone homeostasis (Leucht *et al.*, 2008). Each Wnt protein can bind multiple Fz molecules and each Wnt can bind multiple Fzs, each with varying degrees of affinity, and different Fz molecules have different abilities to activate β-catenin when over-expressed with various Wnt and LRP molecules (e.g. Binnerts *et al.*, 2007), there is almost certainly a large amount of functional redundancy within Fz and Wnt family members (Logan and Nusse, 2004).

We will confine our attention to the current best understanding of how canonical Wnt/β-catenin is regulated by a stereotypical Wnt, Fz and LRP. Most data support a model in which a Wnt molecule binds its receptors and induces the formation of a tertiary Wnt-Fz-LRP5/6 complex (He *et al.*, 2004). An unambiguous demonstration of such a receptor complex *in vivo* remains lacking, but there is strong evidence for its existence. Wnt binding to LRP5/6 and the formation of a Wnt1-Fz8-LRP6 complex has been shown *in vitro* and the sufficiency of a chimeric Fz-LRP5/6 to activate signalling in multiple systems support such a model (Cong *et al.*, 2004; Holmen *et al.*, 2005; Tolwinski *et al.*, 2003). We will thus follow the assumption that one Fz and one LRP receptor seem to be required for Wnt binding and signalling. Other receptors for Wnt exist, including Ryk and ROR2 (reviewed in Gordon and Nusse, 2006) but are not required for canonical Wnt/β-catenin signalling and in some cases may antagonise signalling (van Amerongen *et al.*, 2008).

4.4 Regulation of signalling

4.4.1 Extracellular Wnt antagonists: turning the signalling off at the source

In the extracellular space the cell can secrete numerous proteins that affect the ability of Wnts to interact with their receptors thus modulating signalling. The first identified, by virtue of their sharing a protein domain with Fzs, were the secreted FZ related proteins (sFRPs) (Bovolenta *et al.*, 2008). sFRPs can bind to Wnts and also to Fz molecules to down-regulate signalling. A second class of Wnt-binding extracellular antagonists are the Wnt inhibitory proteins (WIF), which act in a similar manner and are also able to modulate the non-canonical PCP pathway (Bovolenta *et al.*, 2008). Dickkopf (Dkk1) proteins repress Wnt signalling by binding to and antagonising LRP5/6. There exists some disagreement in the literature over the mode of action of Dkk1, with some groups reporting that they inhibit signalling through mediating internalisation and degradation of LRP in concert with a transmemebrane protein Kremen (Mao and Niehrs, 2003; Mao *et al.*, 2002) and others suggesting that they disrupt the formation of the tripartite Wnt–Fz–LRP complex (Ellwanger *et al.*, 2008; Semenov *et al.*, 2008; Wang *et al.*, 2008). Finally, Wise and SOST comprise another family of proteins that antagonise signalling via LRP5/6 (Itasaki *et al.*, 2003; Semenov *et al.*, 2005). SOST acts in a fashion similar to Dkk and is able to disrupt the Wnt-induced formation of Fz-LRP6 complexes *in vitro* (Semenov *et al.*, 2005) and, like Dkk, is strongly linked to human diseases.

4.4.2 Intracellular regulation

In the cytoplasm: the two-state model when off

The central mode of regulation of Wnt signalling is in the modulation of the free cytoplasmic levels of β-catenin (Aberle *et al.*, 1997). Key to this is the protein Axin, which holds together the destruction complex, using its various protein domains to bring into proximity GSK3, CK1 and β-catenin, leading to the phosphorylation of β-catenin at serine 45 by CK1a then at threonine 41 and serines 37 and 33 by GSK3 (Kimelman and Xu, 2006). These phospho-serines act as a docking site for β-TRCP, an E3 ubiquitin ligase, which tags the protein for proteolytic destruction (Maniatis, 1999). The importance of these phosphorylation events in the destruction of β-catenin and the regulation of Wnt signalling is underlined by the fact that mutations of these amino acids and those surrounding them are often found in cancers and lead to a β-catenin molecule which is refractory to phosphorylation and thus constitutively activates Wnt signalling (Polakis, 2000). Beyond the phosphorylation of β-catenin, the phosphorylation states of most of the destruction complex members are regulated to modulate the level of Wnt signalling in the cell. GSK3 and CK1 phosphorylate APC and Axin (Kimelman and Xu, 2006; Huang and He, 2008) increasing the avidity of binding within the destruction complex, thus increasing the overall level of β-catenin phosphorylation and reducing the level of signalling output. Conversely, the phosphatases PP1 and PP2A dephosphorylate Axin and APC, reducing the stability of the destruction complex and up-regulating signalling output. PP1 dephosphorylates Axin, causing the destruction complex to fall apart (Luo *et al.*, 2007) and PP2A can act to remove phosphate groups from β-catenin (Su *et al.*, 2008), leading to increased signalling output due to increased stability of β-catenin.

A key molecule in the destruction, Axin, shows numerous interesting properties. Peterson-Nedry *et al.* (2008) found that in Axin null mutant flies expression of moderate levels of Axin molecules which lack the domains responsible for binding APC, GSK3 or β-catenin led to considerable levels of rescue of the mutant phenotypes, implying that the assembly of the destruction is surprisingly robust and may result from Axin forming dimers or multimers. Luo and colleagues (2005) showed that Axin has multiple dimerisation domains that mediate homo- and heterodimeric interactions and Schwarz-Romond *et al.* (2007) found that the Axin DIX domain can form multimeric polymers in conjunction with Dishevelled (Dsh). When the levels of Wnt signalling components were determined in *Xenopus* oocytes, it was found that Axin exists in extremely low levels in the cell, orders of magnitude below the lowest of the other components (Lee *et al.*, 2003). This may indicate that the levels of Axin are limiting for destruction complex formation. The stability and cellular levels of Axin are also modulated by Wnt signalling. An Axin-centric view of the regulation of Wnt signalling regulation has been presented (Tolwinski and Wieschaus, 2004) as an alternative to the β-catenin-centric view of the regulation of Wnt signalling described by the two-state model.

In the cytoplasm: the two-state model when on

Both a Fz and an LRP molecule are required for Wnt signalling activation through the formation of a Wnt–Fz–LRP complex. A key event in activation of the pathway is the Wnt-induced phosphorylation of the cytoplasmic tail of LRP (Tamia *et al.*, 2004). The intracellular portion of LRP molecules have five conserved repeats of the amino acid sequence PPPSPxS that are key to their function. This motif is phosphorylated twice on signalling and serves as a binding site for Axin, recruiting destruction complex members to the plasma membrane (Tamia *et al.*, 2004; Davidson *et al.*, 2005; Zeng *et al.*, 2005). The importance of these residues is underlined by the fact that they can be added to a heterologous receptor to form a chimeric receptor that can constitutively activate β-catenin signalling (Tamia *et al.*, 2004; Zeng *et al.*, 2005; MacDonald *et al.*, 2008). The phosphorylation of the PPPSPxS is achieved by kinases already familiar to Wnt signalling and associated with the destruction complex: GSK3 and CK1 (Davidson *et al.*, 2005; Zeng *et al.*, 2005). Thus these kinases have dual roles in Wnt/β-catenin signalling, both as negative and positive regulators of the signalling output of the pathway. Although some reports differ (Davidson *et al.*, 2005) the majority of studies point to a model in which Wnt induces GSK3 to perform a priming phosphorylation of PPPSPxS (Binnerts *et al.*, 2007; Khan *et al.*, 2007; Pan *et al.*, 2008), which is followed by a further phosphorylation event carried out by CK1 resulting in a Wnt-induced dual phosphorylation (Zeng *et al.*, 2005). It is thought that the majority of PPPSP phosphorylation requires GSK3 as in cells null for both alpha and beta isoforms of GSK3 little phosphorylation of LRP5/6 is seen and signalling cannot be activated. Interestingly the phosphorylation of LRP5/6 by GSK3 requires and is mediated by Axin-bound GSK3 (Zeng *et al.*, 2008). Thus Wnt signalling can be viewed as being regulated by activating opposing activities of an Axin–GSK3 complex on either β-catenin to turn off signalling or on LRP to activate signalling.

Critical to and necessary for the phosphorylation of LRP is the Wnt-binding induced physical interaction between the Fz receptor and the cytoplasmic scaffolding phospho-protein Dsh (Zeng *et al.*, 2008; Wallingford and Habas, 2005; Wong *et al.*, 2003; Bilic *et al.*, 2007). Dsh binds to Axin (Wallingford and Habas, 2005) and this is a prerequisite for Axin recruitment to the plasma membrane on activation of Wnt signalling (Cliffe *et al.*, 2003). It is thus likely that the Fz–Dsh complex dependent recruitment of an Axin-GSK3 complex to the membrane is a key step in initiating LRP phosphorylation (Zeng *et al.*, 2008). Two important regulatory mechanisms of the activation of Wnt signalling by Wnt-binding and the recruitment of Dsh and Axin have been described. It has been reported that binding Axin is a prerequisite for LRP6 phosphorylation and that the phosphorylated PPPSPxS motifs act as a binding site for further Axin recruitment, which would lead to further phosphorylation of the PPPSPxP repeats. This can be thought of as a feed-forward amplification loop amplifying signalling after a priming initiation step (Baig-Lewis *et al.*, 2007), which is in agreement with the report that the phosphorylation of the PPPSPxS motifs are dependent on each other and that LRP6 activity is sensitive to copy number of these repeats (MacDonald *et al.*, 2008; Wolf *et al.*, 2008). Activated Wnt–Fz–LRP receptor complexes are also thought to cluster at the membrane in a Dsh, Axin and GSK3 dependent fashion and form 'signalosomes' in which the signal initiation and amplification can occur (Schwarz-Romond *et al.*, 2007; Bilic *et al.*, 2007). The stability of these signalosomes seems to be relatively low with the Fz–Dsh and Dsh–Axin interactions being relatively weak, with the latter being mediated by both proteins DIX domains (Schwarz-Romond *et al.*, 2007). It is thought this allows the Dsh-Axin aggregates to be dynamic in the regulation of signalling at the cytoplasmic face of the cell membrane.

It is possible that there is also a link between the Dsh-mediated activation of Wnt signalling at the membrane and phosphatidylinositol lipids. Dsh has been shown to stimulate the production of phosphatidylinositol 4,5-bisphosphate (PIP_2) by phosphatidylinositol 4-kinase type II (PI4KIIalpha) and phosphatidylinositol 4-phosphate 5-kinase type I kinase (PIP5KI) (Pan *et al.*, 2008). The DIX domain of Dsh binds to and activates PIP5K on Wnt stimulation, which leads to the production and accumulation of PIP_2 and this is thought to lead to LRP6 clustering and phosphorylation (Pan *et al.*, 2008).

A closer look at the destruction complex

A recent paper marked a considerable step forward in our understanding of how β-catenin is regulated by the endogenous destruction complex (Li *et al.*, 2012). Many of the experiments that form our view of the regulation of Wnt signalling are based on over-expression experiments and *in vitro* biochemical techniques that may not fully replicate the *in vivo* situation. The experiments reported by Li *et al.* (2012) were all performed on *in vivo* tissues and the results are summarised in Figure 4.2. These workers showed that on activation by Wnt the composition of

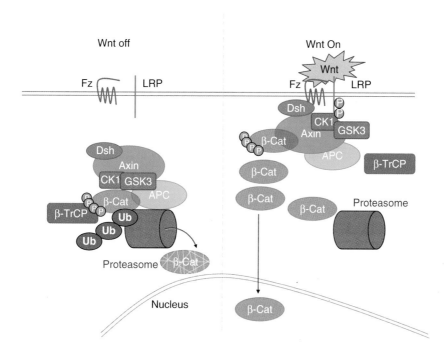

Figure 4.2 **A modern model of the cytoplasmic regulation of Wnt signalling.** This model is based on biochemical study of endogenous components of the destruction complex (Li, *et al.*, 2012). In the absence of Wnt ligands, the destruction complex in the cytoplasm binds to and leads to the phosphorylation of β-catenin that is subsequently ubiquitinated by β-TrCP and destroyed by the proteasome. The proteasome recycles the destruction complex at the end of this process. On binding of Wnt to its receptors, the intact destruction complex binds to the phosphorylated tail of LRP. After this binding the destruction complex still binds and phosphorylates β-catenin, but β-TrCP is unable to ubiquitinate it. Newly synthesised β-catenin is able to accumulate un-phosphorylated, enter the nucleus and direct transcription of Wnt target genes.

the destruction complex is not changed in terms of any of the molecules that they studied and that the activities of GSK3 or CKI are not inhibited. They showed that when signalling is inactive, phosphorylated β-catenin accumulates in the destruction complex and it is within the destruction complex that the B3 ligase β-TrCP is actively ubiquitinating β-catenin, rather than this being a downstream, distal event separate from phosphorylation of β-catenin. Ubiquitinated β-catenin is removed from the destruction complex by directly being proteolytically degraded by the proteosome within the destruction complex. This also acts to reset the destruction complex for a further round of β-catenin processing.

On activation of Wnt signalling, phosphorylated β-catenin builds up and saturates the destruction complex so that the destruction complex function is inactivated. This fits with previous observations by same the group which had previously showed that only β-catenin that has been newly synthesised after signalling activation is able to activate signalling (Staal *et al.*, 2002). Additionally, the work shows that in APC deficient colorectal cancer the destruction complex remains intact and that it is the fact that β-catenin ubiquitination is deficient in these cells that leads to increased Wnt signalling rather than the destruction complex merely falling apart. This study is in contrast to much of the literature, which has assumed that the destruction complex simply falls apart and disassembles when Wnt signalling is activated. Li and colleagues showed that the destruction complex is compositionally unchanged by the activation state of Wnt signalling. Additionally, they showed that the destruction complex is intact in colorectal cancer caused by loss of APC.

In the nucleus: β-catenin and its many friends

That the level of β-catenin is the central point of control of the level of output of Wnt signalling is clear, how the levels of β-catenin in the nucleus are regulated is much less clear (Henderson and Fagotto, 2002; Stadeli *et al.*, 2006). It is clear that the levels of β-catenin increase in the cell on Wnt signalling but it is unlikely that the levels of β-catenin in the nucleus is simply a passive product of this increased level of protein free in the cytoplasm. The levels of β-catenin in the cytoplasm and nucleus are a product of both shuttling between the two compartments and retention within them, both of which are achieved by multiple mechanisms. β-Catenin has a nuclear localisation signal (NLS) and is transported into the nucleus via the nuclear pore complex in an importin-dependent fashion (Henderson and Fagotto, 2002). Molecules of the destruction complex, APC (Henderson and Fagotto, 2002) and Axin (Cong *et al.*, 2004) along with RanBP3 (Hendriksen *et al.*, 2005) are involved in the nuclear export of β-catenin. The study of the rate of import and export of β-catenin into and out of the nucleus has found that although Axin and APC enrich it in the cytoplasm and TCF, BCL8 and Pygopus increase the levels of β-catenin in the nucleus, the actual rates of their transport is not affected, implying that these molecules act to sequester β-catenin in one compartment or another rather than being involved in its actual transport (Krieghoff *et al.*, 2006). Additionally, it has been shown the Wnt activation of Rac1, a small GTPase, is required for nuclear accumulation of β-catenin. It was found that Rac1, Jun *N*-terminal kinase 2 (JNK2) and β-catenin form a cytoplasmic complex in which JNK2 phosphorylates β-catenin on serines 191 and 605 (Wu *et al.*, 2008). This modification has been proposed to mediate the nuclear translocation of β-catenin. Rac1 has also been shown to play a role as part of the β-catenin transcription regulating complex (Esufali and Bapat, 2004) and to antagonise the destruction complex (Schlessinger *et al.*, 2009). Rac1 has long been known to play a role in non-canonical PCP signalling and its role in Wnt/β-catenin signalling remains to be elucidated further.

The major and best-understood co-activator of gene expression, which regulates Wnt signalling in the nucleus along with β-catenin, are the proteins of the TCF/LEF transcription factors. *Drosophila* and *C. elegans* only have one *TCF* gene, whereas there are four in mammals, although these undergo extensive alternative splicing and use multiple promotors to produce a vast array of proteins with different functions, some of which act as negative regulators of Wnt signalling (Arce *et al.*, 2006; Hoppler *et al.*, 2007). TCF proteins are high mobility group (HMG) DNA binding proteins. They bind to a consensus Wnt responsive element (WRE), which results in bending of the DNA and cause changes in the conformation of chromatin. In the absence of Wnt signalling, TCF represses Wnt target gene transcription by binding to WREs and interacting with the repressor protein Groucho/TLE1 by promoting histone deacetylation and chromatin compaction (Daniels and Weiss, 2005). On activation of signalling, β-catenin displaces Groucho from WREs and recruits other co-activators, such as BCL9 and Pygopus (Pygo). BCL9 binds to β-catenin via its amino-terminal Arm repeats (Parker *et al.*, 2008) and this binding recruits Pygo (Hoffman *et al.*, 2005), which also interacts with Mediator (Carrera *et al.*, 2008), which is required for transcription initiation. Pygo shows constitutive nuclear localisation and may function to recruit and retain β-catenin and BCL9 in the nucleus on signalling activation (Brembeck *et al.*, 2004; Townsley *et al.*, 2004). When Wnt signalling is inactive Pygo is found localised with, although not physically binding to, TCF at the same sites and is thought to help recruit β-catenin and BCL9 to TCF on signalling activation (de la Roche and Bienz, 2007). However these studies are mostly confined to observations in *Drosophila* and in mice Pygo function is not absolutely required for Wnt signalling, with double mutants for the two murine *Pygo* genes showing milder Wnt signalling phenotypes than would be expected if the pathways were totally inactivated by their loss (Schwab *et al.*, 2007). These and other observations imply more is to be discovered on the function of Pygo and BCL9.

Wnt signalling target genes, the ultimate target

The ultimate output of Wnt signalling is a change in the level of target genes. TCF binds to its consensus sequence the WRE that consists of: CCTTTGWW, with W representing either T or A. When complexes containing TCF and β-catenin bind DNA they cause considerable bending and alteration of chromatin structure. The promotors of Wnt responsive genes are enriched with multiple WREs, which are often found extremely distal to the AUG start codon of the open reading, frame (Hatxis *et al.*, 2008). Direct Wnt signalling target genes are usually defined as those that have been proved to have a TCF binding site, and that those sites are important for their transcriptional regulation. The Wnt homepage lists 164 proven Wnt target genes, which have been identified, in a number of different situations from the model organisms *Drosophila*, *Xenopus* and mouse and from human cancers and human cell culture. Numerous studies have been performed to identify Wnt target genes through gene expression profiling using microarrays and other genomic approaches. These have used human embryonic stem cells (Willert *et al.*, 2002), various cancer cell lines (Ziegler *et al.*, 2005; Klapholz-Bown *et al.*, 2007) and various model organisms (Morkel *et al.*, 2003). Many candidate Wnt target genes have been identified in this fashion and require validation.

Table 4.1 Feedback inhibitors of Wnt.

Target gene	Effect of Wnt signal on target gene expression	Effect of changes on Wnt pathway output	Target interacts with:	Reference
Fz	Down	Inactivate	Wnt	Muller *et al.*, 1999
Dfz2	Down	Inactivate	Wnt	Cadigan *et al.*,1998
Dfz3	Up	Activate	Wnt	Sato *et al.*, 1999
Fz7	Up	–	Wnt	Willert *et al.*, 2002
Arrow/LRP	Down	Inactivate	Wnt	Wehrli *et al.*, 2000
Dickkopf	Up	Inactivate	LRP	Niida *et al.*, 2004
				Gonzalez-Sancho *et al.*, 2004
				Chamorro *et al.*, 2004
Dally (HSPG)	Down	–	Wnt	Baeg and Perrimon, 2000
Wingful/notum	Up	Inactivate	HSPG	Giraldez *et al.*, 2002
Nemo	Up	Inactivate	TCF	Zeng and Verheyen, 2004
Naked	Up	Inactivate	Dsh	Rousset *et al.*, 2001
Axin2	Up	Inactivate	β-catenin	Yan *et al.*, 2001
				Lustig *et al.*, 2002
				Jho *et al.*, 2002
b-TCRP	Up	Inactivate	β-catenin	Spiegelman *et al.*, 2000
TCF1 (a dominant negative)	Up	Inactivate	TCF	Roose and Clevers, 1999
LEF1	Down	Activate	β-catenin	Hovanes *et al.*, 2001

It is also clear that many components of the Wnt pathways are themselves targets of Wnt signalling allowing a level of feedback control of the signalling output of the pathway (Table 4.1). These include the receptors (Wehrli *et al.*, 2000; Muller *et al.*, 1999; Cadigan *et al.*, 1998) and LEF1 (Hovanes *et al.*, 2000), positively acting Wnt signalling molecules which are down-regulated by signalling. Conversely, many negatively acting components of signalling are up-regulated by signalling (Rousset *et al.*, 2001; Niida *et al.*, 2004; Gonzalez-Sancho *et al.*, 2005; Chamorro *et al.*, 2005; Jho *et al.*, 2002; Roose *et al.*, 1999). Clearly evolution has built in multiple steps in the regulation of Wnt signalling, which allow feedback inhibition of the level of signalling.

Another direct transcriptional target of Wnt signalling is TERT, a component of telomerase, the enzyme that lengthens telomeres (Blackburn and Collins, 2011). Telomerase is necessary for stem cell renewal and its activity is required in cancer cells to maintain their telomere length (Buseman *et al.*, 2012). Wnt signalling is known to activate telomerase (Broccoli *et al.*, 1996) and mutations in the negative signalling components APC (Mizumoto *et al.*, 2001) and GSK3 (Bilsland *et al.*, 2009) lead to increased telomerase activity. One study showed that β-catenin directly regulates *TERT* expression by binding to the TERT promoter in conjunction with Klf4 rather than a TCF protein (Hoffmeyer *et al.*, 2012).

4.5 When good signalling goes bad: Wnt signalling in diseases

Given the central role of Wnt signalling in embryonic development and the homeostasis of many adult organs and the myriad levels of control of the signalling output of the pathway, it is no surprise that defects in Wnt signalling have been implicated in many hereditary disorders, diseases and carcinogenesis; see Table 4.2 for a summary. Here, the main focus is on the mis-regulation of Wnt in inherited bone mass disorders and in carcinogenesis.

Osteoporosis pseudoglioma syndrome (OPPG) is a recessive loss bone mass disorder, sufferers of which also show abnormal eye vasculature. In 2001 LRP5 loss-of-function mutations were found in sufferers of OPPG (Gong *et al.*, 2001). Around the same time gain of function mutations of LRP5 were found in individuals with high bone mass disorders (Boyden *et al.*, 2002; Little *et al.*, 2002a; Little *et al.*, 2002b). These missense mutations in LRP5 are found in its extracellular domain and prevent the binding of the Wnt signalling antagonists Dkk1 (Ai *et al.*, 2005) and SOST (Ellies *et al.*, 2006; Semenov and He, 2006). So the activation

Table 4.2 Human health conditions caused by mutated or aberrant Wnt signalling.

Gene	Disease	Reference
WNT3	Tetra-amelia	Niemann *et al.*, 2004
WNT4	Mullerian-duct regression and virilisation	Biason-Lauber *et al.*, 2004
WNT4	SERKAL syndrome	Mandel *et al.*, 2008
WNT5B	Type II diabetes	Kanazawa *et al.*, 2004
WNT7A	Fuhrmann syndrome	Woods *et al.*, 2006
WNT10A	Odonto-onycho-dermal dysplasia	Adaimy *et al.*, 2007
WNT10B	Obesity	Christodoulides *et al.*, 2006
WNT10B	Split-hand/foot malformation	Ugur and Tolun, 2008
LRP6	Late onset Alzheimer	De Ferrari *et al.*, 2007
FZD4	Familial exudative vitreoretinopathy: Retinal angiogenesis	Robitaille *et al.*, 2002 Qin *et al.*, 2005
LRP6	Late onset Alzheimer	De Ferrari *et al.*, 2007
Norrin	Familial exudative vitreoretinopathy	Xu *et al.*, 2004
APC	Polyposis coli	Kinzler *et al.*,1991; Nishisho *et al.*, 1991
AXIN1	Caudal duplication	Oates *et al.*,2006
AXIN2	Tooth agenesis	Lammli *et al.*, 2004; Marvin *et al.*, 2011
TCF7L2 (TCF4)	Type II diabetes	Grant *et al.*, 2006 Florez *et al.*, 2006
WTX	Wilms tumour	Major *et al.*, 2007; Rivera *et al.*, 2007
WTX	Skeletal dysplasia	Jenkins *et al.*, 2009
PORC1	Focal dermal hypoplasia	Grzeschik *et al.*, 2007 Wang *et al.*, 2007

status of LRP5 in Wnt signalling seems to correlate with bone mass and is thought to do so by way of the regulation of osteoblast proliferation. Interestingly, Wnt signalling is also implicated in familial exudative vitreoretinopathy (FEVR), which is also characterised by defective retinal vascularisation (Toomes *et al.*, 2004).

Wnt signalling and cancer were first linked because of the causal role of APC in early transformation during colorectal cancer (Polakis, 2007). In the gut epithelium excessive stem cell proliferation, an early step in carcinogenic transformation, is a result of a lack of control over the levels of β-catenin, from mutation of either APC or β-catenin, an essential step for intestinal neoplasia (Fuchs, 2009). Familial adenomatous polyposis (FAP) is a hereditary cancer syndrome whose sufferers carry germ-line mutations in APC and were used in its cloning and identification (Kinzler *et al.*, 1991; Nishisho *et al.*, 1991). Most cases of sporadic colorectal cancer are caused by a loss of both alleles of APC (Kinzler and Vogelstein, 1996). APC loss results in the stabilisation of β-catenin and the constitutive activation of transcription of Wnt signalling target genes. Very occasionally colorectal cancers occur without mutation of APC, but in these cases either Axin2 is lost (Liu *et al.*, 2000) or activating mutations of β-catenin are present, which remove the serine/ threonine that are phosphorylated to tag β-catenin for destruction (Polakis, 2000).

4.6 Taming the beast: drugs and small molecule inhibitors targeting Wnt signalling

Various drugs have been found to modulate Wnt signalling raising the possibility of targeting the pathway in a therapeutic environment. Nonsteroidal anti-inflammatory drugs (NSAIDs), the most well-known of which is aspirin, function by inhibiting the role of a key enzyme in the arachidonic acid cascade cyclooxy-genase (COX). A large number of studies have been conducted which show that NSAIDs are effective chemopreventative agents against colon cancer (see for example, Thun *et al.*, 2002; Thun *et al.*, 1991; Baron *et al.*, 2003) and it has been shown that they do so by acting to inhibit the Wnt signalling pathway through increasing the stability of phosphorylated β-catenin (Dihlmann *et al.*, 2001; Boon *et al.*, 2004). It is thought that increased PGE2 resulting from increases in COX suppresses β-catenin degradation, so suppression of increased COX activity in cancer cells is most likely causal in the anticancer activity of NSAIDs.

Retinoids are compounds that are naturally synthesised from vitamin A and are used in some cancer therapies and in chemoprevention. 1-α,25-Dihydroxyvitamin D3 and derivatives have shown chemopreventative properties in mouse models of breast and colorectal cancers. The mechanism by which vitamins achieve the down-regulation of Wnt signalling is not known, although a few hypotheses have been made. It has been suggested that the activated nuclear receptors for such vita-mins compete with TCF for access to β-catenin (Shah *et al.*, 2003; Palmer *et al.*, 2001). It is also possible that vitamins A and D may induce inhibitory proteins such as Disables-2 (Dab2), Dkk-1 and Dkk-2 (Jiang *et al.*, 2008; Penda-Franco *et al.*, 2008).

Polyphenols are a family of plant chemicals with the characteristic of having multiple phenol units per molecule and the polyphenols quercetin, epigallocatechin-3-gallate (EGCG), curcumin and resveratrol have been shown to inhibit Wnt signalling. It will, however, be difficult to determine their mechanism of action due to their lack of specificity and the fact that they affect numerous signalling pathways (Jaiswal *et al.*, 2002; Park *et al.*, 2005; Kim *et al.*, 2006; Roccaro *et al.*, 2008).

Owing to the large number of specific, tight physical interactions that modulate Wnt signalling, a large amount of effort has been poured into identifying small molecules that will inhibit these interactions and thus down-regulate signalling in cancer. The cytoplasmic protein Dsh is essential to Wnt signalling and acts as a scaffolding protein, with numerous binding partners having been identified. Dsh contains a PDZ domain, which is a common protein–protein interaction domain, one of whose binding partners is the COOH terminal tail of the Wnt receptor Fz (Wong *et al.*, 2003). Three small molecules have been identified through screening *in silico* and nuclear magnetic resonance spectroscopy, which have the ability to block Wnt signalling by binding the Dsh PDZ domain (Fujii *et al.*, 2007; Grandy *et al.*, 2009; Shan *et al.*, 2005). The interaction between β-catenin and TCF has been most extensively mined for small molecule inhibitors. A high-throughput screen of 6000 natural and 45 000 synthetic compounds led to the identification of eight natural molecules that interfered with the interaction between TCF and β-catenin (Lepourcelet *et al.*, 2004). Although these molecules are of limited immediate use, as they also interact with APC and thus are not sufficiently selective in their action, they suggest that such methods provide useful tools for developing small molecule inhibitors of the Wnt pathway. Another group showed that the synthetic small molecule PNU 74654 can antagonise the interaction between β-catenin and TCF using *in silico* screening, although the biological action of the inhibitor has not been shown (Trosset *et al.*, 2006).

Also of interest to those seeking to design small molecule inhibitors of Wnt signalling are the interactions between transcriptional co-activators of Wnt signalling. These include CBP, p300, BCL9 and pygopus. One group found that the small molecule ICG-001 is able to specifically inhibit the interaction between CBP and β-catenin and down-regulates a subset of Wnt signalling gene expression (Takahashi *et al.*, 2010). Finally, monoclonal antibodies developed against Wnt-1 and Wnt2 have been shown to inhibit Wnt signalling and suppress cellular growth *in vivo* (Tang *et al.*, 2009; You *et al.*, 2004; Wei *et al.*, 2009).

4.7   Conclusion and perspectives

Wnt signalling is such a fundamental and important mechanism which is reused in so many contexts in development, adult life and mis-regulated in so many human health disorders, that decades of research have led to a fairly detailed view of how the pathway is regulated; yet there remain many questions in the field that are as yet unaddressed. The cellular location of signalling events remains unknown, the transport and regulation of the levels of β-catenin in the nucleus and cytoplasm is not well understood, how much of the genome is controlled by Wnt signalling is unknown and whether Wnt signalling can really be effectively targeted in the clinic also remains unknown.

References

Aberle, H., Bauer, A., Stappert, J. *et al.* (1997) β-catenin is a target for the ubiquitin-proteasome pathway. *EMBO Journal*, **16**, 3797–3804.

Adaimy, L. Chouery, E., Megarbane, H. *et al.* (2007) Mutation in WNT10A is associated with an autosomal recessive ectodermal dysplasia: the odonto-onycho-dermal dysplasia. *American Journal of Human Genetics*, **81**, 821–828.

Adler, P.N., Vinson, C., Park, W.J. *et al.* (1990) Molecular structure of frizzled, a Drosophila tissue polarity gene. *Genetics*, **126**, 401–416.

Ai, M., Holmen, S.L., Van Hul, W., Williams, B.O. and Warman, M.L. (2005) Reduced affinity to and inhibition by DKK1 form a common mechanism by which high bone mass-associated missense mutations in LRP5 affect canonical Wnt signaling. *Molecular and Cell Biology*, **25**, 4946–4955.

Arce, L., Yokoyama, N.N. and Waterman, M.L. (2006) Diversity of LEF/TCF action in development and disease. *Oncogene*, **25**, 7492–7504.

Baeg, G.H. and Perrimon, N. (2000) Functional binding of secreted molecules to heparan sulfate proteoglycans in Drosophila. *Current Opinion in Cell Biology*, **12**, 575–580.

Baig-Lewis, S., Peterson-Nedry, W. and Wehrli, M. (2007) Wingless/Wnt signal transduction requires distinct initiation and amplification steps that both depend on Arrow/LRP. *Developmental Biology*, **306**, 94–111.

Banziger, C., Soldini, D., Schutt, C. *et al.* (2006) Wntless, a conserved membrane protein dedicated to the secretion of Wnt proteins from signaling cells. *Cell*, **125**, 509–522.

Baron, J.A., Cole, B.F., Sandler, R.S. *et al.* (2003) A randomized trial of aspirin to prevent colorectal adenomas. *New England Journal of Medicine*, **348**, 891–899.

Bartscherer, K., Pelte, N., Ingelfinger, D. and Boutros, M. (2006) Secretion of Wnt ligands requires Evi, a conserved transmembrane protein. *Cell*, **125**, 523–533.

Belenkaya, T.Y., Wu, Y., Tang, X. *et al.* (2008) The retromer complex influences Wnt secretion by recycling wntless from endosomes to the trans-Golgi network. *Developmental Cell*, **14**, 120-31.

Bhanot, P., Brink, M., Samos, C.H. *et al.* (1996) A new member of the frizzled family from Drosophila functions as a Wingless receptor. *Nature*, **382**, 225–230.

Bhanot, P., Fish, M., Jemison, J.A. *et al.* (1999) Frizzled and Dfrizzled-2 function as redundant receptors for Wingless during Drosophila embryonic development. *Development*, **126**, 4175–4186.

Biason-Lauber, A., Konrad, D., Navratil, F. and Schoenle, E.J. (2004). WNT4 mutation associated with Mullerian-duct regression and virilization in a 46,XX woman. *New England Journal of Medicine*, **351**, 792–798.

Bilic, J., Huang, Y.L., Davidson, G., *et al.* (2007) Wnt induces LRP6 signalosomes and promotes dishevelled-dependent LRP6 phosphorylation. *Science*, **316**, 1619–1622.

Bilsland, A.E., Hoare, S., Stevenson, K. *et al.* (2009) Dynamic telomerase gene suppression via network effects of GSK3 inhibition. *PLoS One*, **4**, e6459.

Binnerts, M.E., Kim, K.A., Bright, J.M. *et al.* (2007) R-Spondin1 regulates Wnt signaling by inhibiting internalization of LRP6. *Proceedings of the National Academy of Sciences, USA*, **104**, 14700–14705.

Blackburn, E.H. and Collins, K. (2011) Telomerase: an RNP enzyme synthesizes DNA. *Cold Spring Harb Perspectives in Biology*, **3**.

Boon, E.M., Keller, J.J., Wormhoudt, T.A.M. *et al.* (2004) Sulindac targets nuclear β-catenin accumulation and Wnt signalling in adenomas of patients with familial adenomatous polyposis and in human colorectal cancer cell lines. *British Journal of Cancer*, **90**, 224–229.

Boutros, M., Mihaly, J., Bouwmeester, T. and Mlodzik, M. (2000) Signaling specificity by Frizzled receptors in Drosophila. *Science*, **288**, 1825–1828.

Bovolenta, P., Esteve, P., Ruiz, J.M. *et al.* (2008) Beyond Wnt inhibition: new functions of secreted Frizzled-related proteins in development and disease. *Journal of Cell Science*, **121**, 737–746.

Boyden, L.M., Mao, J., Belsky, J. *et al.* (2002) High bone density due to a mutation in LDL-receptor-related protein 5. *New England Journal of Medicine*, **346**, 1513–1521.

Brembeck, F.H., Schwarz-Romond, T., Bakkers, J. *et al.* (2004) Essential role of BCL9-2 in the switch between β-catenin's adhesive and transcriptional functions. *Genes and Development*, **18**, 2225–2230.

Broccoli, D., Godley, L.A., Donehower, L.A. *et al.* (1996) Telomerase activation in mouse mammary tumors: lack of detectable telomere shortening and evidence for regulation of telomerase RNA with cell proliferation. *Molecular and Cell Biology*, **16**, 3765–3772.

Buseman, C.M., Wright, W.E. and Shay, J.W. (2012) Is telomerase a viable target in cancer? *Mutatation Research*, **730**, 90–97.

Cadigan, K.M., Fish, M.P., Rulifson, E.J. and Nusse, R. (1998) Wingless repression of Drosophila frizzled 2 expression shapes the Wingless morphogen gradient in the wing. *Cell*, **93**, 767–777.

Carrera, I., Janody, F., Leeds, N. *et al.* (2008) Pygopus activates Wingless target gene transcription through the mediator complex subunits Med12 and Med13. *Proceedings of the National Academy of Sciences, USA*, **105**, 6644–6649.

Chamorro, M.N., Schwartz, D.R., Vonica, A. *et al.* (2005) FGF-20 and DKK1 are transcriptional targets of β-catenin and FGF-20 is implicated in cancer and development. *EMBO Journal*, **24**, 73–84.

Christodoulides, C. Scarda, A., Granzotto, M. *et al.* (2006) WNT10B mutations in human obesity. *Diabetologia* **49**, 678–684.

Cliffe, A., Hamada, F. and Bienz, M. (2003) A role of Dishevelled in relocating Axin to the plasma membrane during wingless signaling. *Current Biology*, **13**, 960–966.

Cong, F., Schweizer, L. and Varmus, H. (2004) Wnt signals across the plasma membrane to activate the β-catenin pathway by forming oligomers containing its receptors, Frizzled and LRP. *Development*, **131**, 5103–5115.

Daniels, D.L. and Weis, W.I. (2005) β-catenin directly displaces Groucho/TLE repressors from Tcf/Lef in Wnt-mediated transcription activation. *Nature Structural and Molecular Biology*, **12**, 364–371.

Davidson, G., Wu, W., Shen, J. *et al.* (2005) Casein kinase 1 gamma couples Wnt receptor activation to cytoplasmic signal transduction. *Nature*, **438**, 867–872.

De Ferrari, G.V., Papassotiropoulos, A., Biechele, T. *et al.* (2007) Common genetic variation within the low-density lipoprotein receptor-related protein 6 and late-onset Alzheimer's disease. *Proceedings of the National Academy of Sciences, USA*, **104**, 9434–9439.

de la Roche, M. and Bienz, M. (2007) Wingless-independent association of Pygopus with dTCF target genes. *Current Biology*, **17**, 556–561.

Dihlmann, S., Siermann, A. and von Knebel Doeberitz, M. (2001) The nonsteroidal anti-inflammatory drugs aspirin and indomethacin attenuate β-catenin/TCF-4 signaling. *Oncogene*, **20**, 645–653.

Ellies, D.L., Viviano, B., McCarthy, J. *et al.* (2006) Bone density ligand, Sclerostin, directly interacts with LRP5 but not LRP5G171V to modulate Wnt activity. *Journal of Bone and Mineral Research*, **21**, 1738–1749.

Ellwanger, K., Saito, H., Clement-Lacroix, P. *et al.* (2008) Targeted disruption of the Wnt regulator Kremen induces limb defects and high bone density. *Molecular and Cell Biology*, **28**, 4875–4882.

Esufali, S. and Bapat, B. (2004) Cross-talk between Rac1 GTPase and dysregulated Wnt signaling pathway leads to cellular redistribution of β-catenin and TCF/LEF-mediated transcriptional activation. *Oncogene*, **23**, 8260–8271.

Florez, J.C., Jablonski, K.A., Bayley, N. *et al.* (2006) TCF7L2 polymorphisms and progression to diabetes in the Diabetes Prevention Program. *New England Journal of Medicine*, **355**, 241–250.

Franch-Marro, X., Wendler, F., Guidato, S. *et al.* (2008) Wingless secretion requires endosome-to-Golgi retrieval of Wntless/Evi/Sprinter by the retromer complex. *Nature Cell Biology*, **10**, 170–177.

Fuchs, E. (2009) The tortoise and the hair: slow-cycling cells in the stem cell race. *Cell*, **137**, 811–819.

Fujii, N., You, L., Xu, Z. *et al.* (2007) An antagonist of dishevelled protein-protein interaction suppresses β-catenin-dependent tumor cell growth. *Cancer Research*, **67**, 573–579.

Galli, L.M., Barnes, T.L., Secrest, S.S. *et al.* (2007) Porcupine-mediated lipid-modification regulates the activity and distribution of Wnt proteins in the chick neural tube. *Development*, **134**, 3339–3348.

Giraldez, A.J., Copley, R.R. and Cohen, S.M. (2002) HSPG modification by the secreted enzyme Notum shapes the Wingless morphogen gradient. *Developental Cell*, **2**, 667–676.

Gong, Y., Slee, R.B., Fukai, N. *et al.* (2001) LDL receptor-related protein 5 (LRP5) affects bone accrual and eye development. *Cell*, **107**, 513–523.

Gonzalez-Sancho, J.M., Aguilera, O., Garcia, J.M. *et al.* (2005) The Wnt antagonist DICKKOPF-1 gene is a downstream target of β-catenin/TCF and is downregulated in human colon cancer. *Oncogene*, **24**, 1098–1103.

Goodman, R.M., Thombre, S., Firtina, Z., *et al.* (2006) Sprinter: a novel transmembrane protein required for Wg secretion and signaling. *Development*, **133**, 4901–4911.

Gordon, M.D. and Nusse, R. (2006) Wnt signaling: multiple pathways, multiple receptors, and multiple transcription factors. *Journal of Biological Chemistry*, **281**, 22429–22433.

Grandy, D., Shan, J., Zhang, X. *et al.* (2009) Discovery and characterization of a small molecule inhibitor of the PDZ domain of dishevelled. *Journal of Biological Chemistry*, **284**, 16256–16263.

Grant, S.F., Thorleifsson, G., Reynisdottir, I., *et al.* (2006) Variant of transcription factor 7-like 2 (TCF7L2) gene confers risk of type 2 diabetes. *Nature Genetics*, **38**, 320–323.

Grzeschik, K.H., Bornholdt, D., Oeffner, F. *et al.* (2007) Deficiency of PORCN, a regulator of Wnt signaling, is associated with focal dermal hypoplasia. *Nature Genetics*, **39**, 833–835.

Hatzis, P., van der Flier, L.G., van Driel, M.A. *et al.* Genome-wide pattern of TCF7L2/TCF4 chromatin occupancy in colorectal cancer cells. *Molecular and Cell Biology*, **28**, 2732–2744.

Hausmann, G., Banziger, C. and Basler, K. (2007) Helping wingless take flight: how WNT proteins are secreted. *Nature Reviews Molecular Cell Biology*, **8**, 331–336.

He, X., Semenov, M., Tamai, K. and Zeng, X. (2004) LDL receptor-related proteins 5 and 6 in Wnt/β-catenin signaling: arrows point the way. *Development*, **131**, 1663–1677.

Henderson, B.R. and Fagotto, F. (2002) The ins and outs of APC and β-catenin nuclear transport. *EMBO Reports*, **3**, 834–839.

Hendriksen, J., Fagotto, F., van der Velde, H. *et al.* (2005) RanBP3 enhances nuclear export of active (beta)-catenin independently of CRM1. *Journal of Cell Biology*, **171**, 785–797.

Hoffmans, R., Stadeli, R. and Basler, K. (2005) Pygopus and legless provide essential transcriptional coactivator functions to armadillo/β-catenin. *Current Biology*, **15**, 1207–1211.

Hoffmeyer, K., Raggioli, A., Rudloff, S., *et al.* (2012) Wnt/β-catenin signaling regulates telomerase in stem cells and cancer cells. *Science*, **336**, 1549–1554.

Holmen, S.L., Robertson, S.A., Zylstra, C.R. and Williams, B.O. (2005) Wnt-independent activation of β-catenin mediated by a Dkk1-Fz5 fusion protein. *Biochemical and Biophysical Research Communications*, **328**, 533–539.

Hoppler, S. and Kavanagh, C.L. (2007) Wnt signalling: variety at the core. *Journal of Cell Science*, **120**, 385–393.

Hovanes, K. Li, T.W., Munguia, J.E., *et al.* (2001) Beta-catenin-sensitive isoforms of lymphoid enhancer factor-1 are selectively expressed in colon cancer. *Nature Genetics*, **28**, 53–57.

Hovanes, K., Li, T.W. and Waterman, M.L. (2000) The human LEF-1 gene contains a promoter preferentially active in lymphocytes and encodes multiple isoforms derived from alternative splicing. *Nucleic Acids Research*, **28**, 1994–2003.

Huang, H. and He, X. (2008) Wnt/β-catenin signaling: new (and old) players and new insights. *Current Opinion in Cell Biology*, **20**, 119–25.

Itasaki, N., Jones, C.M., Mercurio, S. *et al.* (2003) Wise, a context-dependent activator and inhibitor of Wnt signalling. *Development*, **130**, 4295–4305.

Jaiswal, A.S., Marlow, B.P., Gupta, N. and Narayan, S. (2002) β-Catenin-mediated transactivation and cell-cell adhesion pathways are important in curcumin (diferuylmethane)-induced growth arrest and apoptosis in colon cancer cells. *Oncogene*, **21**, 8414–8427.

Jenkins, Z.A. van Kogelenberg, M., Morgan, T. *et al.* (2009) Germline mutations in WTX cause a sclerosing skeletal dysplasia but do not predispose to tumorigenesis. *Nature Genetics*, **41**, 95–100.

Jho, E.H., Zhang, T., Domon, C. *et al.* (2002) Wnt/β-catenin/Tcf signaling induces the transcription of Axin2, a negative regulator of the signaling pathway. *Molecular and Cell Biology*, **22**, 1172–1183.

Jiang, Y., Prunier, C. and Howe, P.H. (2008) The inhibitory effects of Disabled-2 (Dab2) on Wnt signaling are mediated through Axin. *Oncogene*, **27**, 1865–1875.

Kanazawa, A., Tsukada, S., Sekine, A., *et al.* (2004) Association of the gene encoding wingless-type mammary tumor virus integration-site family member 5B (WNT5B) with type 2 diabetes. *American Journal of Human Genetics*, **75**, 832–843.

Katanaev, V.L. (2010) The Wnt/Frizzled GPCR signaling pathway. *Biochemistry (Moscow)*, **75**, 1428–1434.

Khan, Z., Vijayakumar, S., de la Torre, T.V. *et al.* (2007) Analysis of endogenous LRP6 function reveals a novel feedback mechanism by which Wnt negatively regulates its receptor. *Molecular and Cell Biology*, **27**, 7291–7301.

Kim, J., Zhang, X., Rieger-Christ, K.M. *et al.* (2006) Suppression of Wnt signaling by the green tea compound (−)-epigallocatechin 3-gallate (EGCG) in invasive breast cancer cells. Requirement of the transcriptional repressor HBP1. *Journal of Biological Chemistry*, **281**, 10865–10875.

Kimelman, D. and Xu, W. (2006) β-catenin destruction complex: insights and questions from a structural perspective. *Oncogene*, **25**, 7482–7491.

Kinzler, K.W. and Vogelstein, B. (1996) Lessons from hereditary colorectal cancer. *Cell*, **87**, 159–170.

Kinzler, K.W., Nilbert, M.C., Vogelstein, B. *et al.* (1991) Identification of a gene located at chromosome 5q21 that is mutated in colorectal cancers. *Science*, **251**, 1366–1370.

Klapholz-Brown, Z., Walmsley, G.G., Nusse, Y.M. *et al.* (2007) Transcriptional program induced by Wnt protein in human fibroblasts suggests mechanisms for cell cooperativity in defining tissue microenvironments. *PLoS One* **2**, e945.

Komekado, H., Yamamoto, H., Chiba, T. and Kikuchi, A. (2007) Glycosylation and palmitoylation of Wnt-3a are coupled to produce an active form of Wnt-3a. *Genes to Cells*, **12**, 521–534.

Krieghoff, E., Behrens, J. and Mayr, B. (2006) Nucleo-cytoplasmic distribution of β-catenin is regulated by retention. *Journal of Cell Science*, **119**, 1453–1463.

Lammi, L., Arte, S., Somer, M. *et al.* (2004) Mutations in AXIN2 cause familial tooth agenesis and predispose to colorectal cancer. *American Journal of Human Genetics*, **74** (5), 1043–1050.

Lee, E., Salic, A., Kruger, R. *et al.* (2003) The roles of APC and Axin derived from experimental and theoretical analysis of the Wnt pathway. *PLoS Biology*, **1**, E10.

Lepourcelet, M., Chen, Y.N., France, D.S. *et al.* (2004) Small-molecule antagonists of the oncogenic Tcf/β-catenin protein complex. *Cancer Cell*, **5**, 91–102.

Leucht, P., Minear, S., Ten Berge, D. *et al.* (2008) Translating insights from development into regenerative medicine: the function of Wnts in bone biology. *Seminars in Cell and Developmental Biology*, **19**, 434–443.

Li, V.S., Ng, S.S., Boersema, P.J. *et al.* (2012) Wnt signaling through inhibition of β-catenin degradation in an intact Axin1 complex. *Cell*, **149**, 1245–1256.

Little, R.D., Carulli, J.P., Del Mastro, R.G. *et al.* (2002a) A mutation in the LDL receptor-related protein 5 gene results in the autosomal dominant high-bone-mass trait. *American Journal of Human Genetics*, **70**, 11–19.

Little, R.D., Recker, R.R. and Johnson, M.L. (2002b) High bone density due to a mutation in LDL-receptor-related protein 5. *New England Journal of Medicine*, **347**, 943–944; author reply.

Liu, W., Dong, X., Mai, M. *et al.* (2000) Mutations in *AXIN2* cause colorectal cancer with defective mismatch repair by activating β-catenin/TCF signalling. *Nature Genetics*, **26**, 146–147.

Logan, C.Y. and Nusse, R. (2004) The Wnt signaling pathway in development and disease. *Annual Review of Cell and Developmental Biology*, **20**, 781–810.

Luo, W., Peterson, A., Garcia, B.A. *et al.* (2007) Protein phosphatase 1 regulates assembly and function of the β-catenin degradation complex. *EMBO Journal*, **26**, 1511–1521.

Luo, W., Zou, H., Jin, L. *et al.* (2005) Axin contains three separable domains that confer intramolecular, homodimeric, and heterodimeric interactions involved in distinct functions. *Journal of Biological Chemistry*, **280**, 5054–5060.

Lustig, B., Jerchow, B., Sachs, M., *et al.* (2002) Negative feedback loop of Wnt signaling through upregulation of conductin/axin2 in colorectal and liver tumors. *Molecular and Cellular Biology*, **22**, 1184–1193.

MacDonald, B.T., Yokota, C., Tamai, K. *et al.* (2008) Wnt signal amplification via activity, cooperativity, and regulation of multiple intracellular PPPSP motifs in the Wnt co-receptor LRP6. *Journal of Biological Chemistry*, **283**, 16115–16123.

Major, M.B., Camp, N.D., Berndt, J.D. *et al.* (2007) Wilms tumor suppressor WTX negatively regulates WNT/beta-catenin signaling. *Science* **316**, 1043–1046.

Mandel, H., Shemer, R., Borochowitz, Z.U., *et al.* (2008) ERKAL syndrome: an autosomal-recessive disorder caused by a loss-of-function mutation in WNT4. *American Journal of Human Genetics*, **82**, 39–47.

Maniatis, T. (1999) A ubiquitin ligase complex essential for the NF-kappaB, Wnt/Wingless, and Hedgehog signaling pathways. *Genes and Development*, **13**, 505–510.

Mao, B. and Niehrs, C. (2003) Kremen2 modulates Dickkopf2 activity during Wnt/LRP6 signaling. *Gene*, **302**, 179–183.

Mao, B., Wu, W., Davidson, G. *et al.* (2002) Kremen proteins are Dickkopf receptors that regulate Wnt/β-catenin signalling. *Nature*, **417**, 664–667.

Marvin, M.L. Mazzoni, S.M., Herron, C.M. *et al.* (2011) AXIN2-associated autosomal dominant ectodermal dysplasia and neoplastic syndrome. *American Journal of Human Genetics, A*, **155A**, 898–902.

McGough, I.J. and Cullen, P.J. (2011) Recent advances in retromer biology. *Traffic*, **12**, 963–971.

Mizumoto, K., Ogawa, Y., Niiyamo, H. *et al.* (2001) Possible role of telomerase activation in the multistep tumor progression of periampullary lesions in patients with familial adenomatous polyposis. *American Journal of Gastroenterology*, **96**, 1261–1265.

Morkel, M., Huelsken, J., Wakamiya, M. *et al.* (2003) β-catenin regulates Cripto- and Wnt3-dependent gene expression programs in mouse axis and mesoderm formation. *Development*, **130**, 6283–6294.

Muller, H.A., Samanta, R. and Wieschaus, E. (1999) Wingless signaling in the Drosophila embryo: zygotic requirements and the role of the frizzled genes. *Development*, **126**, 577–586.

Niemann, S., Zhao, C., Pascu, F., *et al.* (2004) Homozygous WNT3 mutation causes tetra-amelia in a large consanguineous family. *American Journal of Human Genetics*, **74**, 558–63.

Niida, A., Hiroko, T., Kasai, M. *et al.* (2004) DKK1, a negative regulator of Wnt signaling, is a target of the β-catenin/TCF pathway. *Oncogene*, **23**, 8520–8526.

Nishisho, I., Nakamura, Y., Miyoshi, Y. *et al.* (1991) Mutations of chromosome 5q21 genes in FAP and colorectal cancer patients. *Science*, **253**, 665–669.

Nusse, R. and Varmus, H.E. (1982) Many tumors induced by the mouse mammary tumor virus contain a provirus integrated in the same region of the host genome. *Cell*, **31**, 99–109.

Oates, N.A., van Vliet, J., Duffy, D.L. *et al.* (2006) Increased DNA methylation at the AXIN1 gene in a monozygotic twin from a pair discordant for a caudal duplication anomaly. *American Journal of Human Genetics*, **79**, 155–162.

Pálmer, H.G., González-Sancho, J., Espada, J. *et al.* (2001) Vitamin D(3) promotes the differentiation of colon carcinoma cells by the induction of E-cadherin and the inhibition of β-catenin signaling. *Journal of Cell Biology*, **154**, 369–387.

Pan, W., Choi, S.C., Wang, H. *et al.* (2008) Wnt3a-mediated formation of phosphatidylinositol 4,5-bisphosphate regulates LRP6 phosphorylation. *Science*, **321**, 1350–1353.

Park, C.H., Chang, J.Y., Hahm, E.R. *et al.* (2005) Quercetin, a potent inhibitor against β-catenin/Tcf signaling in SW480 colon cancer cells. *Biochemical and Biophysical Research Communications*, **328**, 227–234.

Park, W.J., Liu, J. and Adler, P.N. (1994) The frizzled gene of Drosophila encodes a membrane protein with an odd number of transmembrane domains. *Mechanisms of Development*, **45**, 127–137.

Parker, D.S., Ni, Y.Y., Chang, J.L. *et al.* (2008) Wingless signaling induces widespread chromatin remodeling of target loci. *Molecular and Cell Biology*, **28**, 1815–1828.

Pendas-Franco, N., Aguilera, O., Pereira, F. *et al.* (2008) Vitamin D and Wnt/β-catenin pathway in colon cancer: role and regulation of DICKKOPF genes. *Anticancer Research*, **28**, 2613–2623.

Peng, Y. and Axelrod, J.D. (2012) Asymmetric protein localization in planar cell polarity: mechanisms, puzzles, and challenges. *Current Topics in Developments Biology*, **101**, 33–53.

Peterson-Nedry, W., Erdeniz, N., Kremer, S. *et al.* (2008) Unexpectedly robust assembly of the Axin destruction complex regulates Wnt/Wg signaling in *Drosophila* as revealed by analysis *in vivo*. *Developmental Biology*, **320** (1), 226-241, PubMed PMID: 18561909.

Pinson, K.I., Brennan, J., Monkley, S. *et al.* (2000) An LDL-receptor-related protein mediates Wnt signalling in mice. *Nature*, **407**, 535–538.

Polakis, P. (2000) Wnt signaling and cancer. *Genes and Development*, **14**, 1837–1851.

Polakis, P. (2007) The many ways of Wnt in cancer. *Current Opinions in Genetics and Development*, **17**, 45–51.

Port, F., Kuster, M., Herr, P. *et al.* (2008) Wingless secretion promotes and requires retromer-dependent cycling of Wntless. *Nature Cell Biology*, **10**, 178–185.

Qin, M., Hayashi, H., Oshima, K., *et al.* (2005) Complexity of the genotype-phenotype correlation in familial exudative vitreoretinopathy with mutations in the LRP5 and/or FZD4 genes. *Human Mutation*, **26**, 104–112.

Rijsewijk, F., Schuermann, M., Wagenaar. E. *et al.* (1987) The Drosophila homolog of the mouse mammary oncogene int-1 is identical to the segment polarity gene wingless. *Cell*, **50**, 649–657.

Rivera, M.N., Kim, W.J., Wells, J. *et al.* (2007) An X chromosome gene, WTX, is commonly inactivated in Wilms tumor. *Science*, **315**, 642–645.

Robitaille, J., MacDonald, M.L., Kaykas, A. *et al.* (2002) Mutant frizzled-4 disrupts retinal angiogenesis in familial exudative vitreoretinopathy. *Nature Genetics*, **32**, 326–330.

Roccaro, A.M., Leleu, X., Sacco, A. *et al.* (2008) Resveratrol exerts antiproliferative activity and induces apoptosis in Waldenstrom's macroglobulinemia. *Clinical Cancer Research*, **14**, 1849–1858.

Roose, J. and Clevers, H. (1999) TCF transcription factors: molecular switches in carcinogenesis. *Biochimica et Biophysica Acta*, **1424**, M23–M37.

Rousset, R., Mack, J.A., Wharton, K.A., Jr., *et al.* (2001) Naked cuticle targets dishevelled to antagonize Wnt signal transduction. *Genes and Development*, **15**, 658–671.

Rulifson, E.J., Wu, C.H. and Nusse, R. (2000) Pathway specificity by the bifunctional receptor frizzled is determined by affinity for wingless. *Molecular Cell*, **6**, 117–126.

Sato, A., Kojima, T., Ui-Tei, K. *et al.* (1999) Dfrizzled-3, a new Drosophila Wnt receptor, acting as an attenuator of Wingless signaling in wingless hypomorphic mutants. *Development*, **126**, 4421–4430.

Schlessinger, K., Hall, A. and Tolwinski, N. (2009) Wnt signaling pathways meet Rho GTPases. *Genes and Development*, **23**, 265–277.

Schwab, K.R., Patterson, L.T., Hartman, H.A. *et al.* (2007) Pygo1 and Pygo2 roles in Wnt signaling in mammalian kidney development. *BMC Biology*, **5**, 15.

Schwarz-Romond, T., Metcalfe, C. and Bienz, M. (2007) Dynamic recruitment of axin by Dishevelled protein assemblies. *Journal of Cell Science*, **120**, 2402–2412.

Semenov, M., Tamai, K. and He, X. (2005) SOST is a ligand for LRP5/LRP6 and a Wnt signaling inhibitor. *Journal of Biological Chemistry*, **280**, 26770–26775.

Semenov, M.V. and He, X. (2006) LRP5 mutations linked to high bone mass diseases cause reduced LRP5 binding and inhibition by SOST. *Journal of Biological Chemistry*, **281**, 38276–38284.

Semenov, M.V., Zhang, X. and He, X. (2008) DKK1 antagonizes Wnt signaling without promotion of LRP6 internalization and degradation. *Journal of Biological Chemistry*, **283**, 21427–21432.

Shah, S., Hecht, A., Pestell, R. and Byers, S.W. (2003) Trans-repression of β-catenin activity by nuclear receptors. *Journal of Biological Chemistry*, **278**, 48137–48145.

Spiegelman, V.S., Slaga, T.J., Pagano, M., *et al.* (2000) Wnt/beta-catenin signaling induces the expression and activity of betaTrCP ubiquitin ligase receptor. *Molecular Cell*, **5**, 877–882.

Shan, J., Shi, D.L., Wang, J. and Zheng, J. (2005) Identification of a specific inhibitor of the dishevelled PDZ domain. *Biochemistry*, **44**, 15495–15503.

Staal, F.J., Noort Mv, M., Strous, G.J. and Clevers, H.C. (2002) Wnt signals are transmitted through N-terminally dephosphorylated β-catenin. *EMBO Reports*, **3**, 63–68.

Stadeli, R., Hoffmans, R. and Basler, K. (2006) Transcription under the control of nuclear Arm/β-catenin. *Current Biology*, **16**, R378–R385.

Su, Y., Fu, C., Ishikawa, S. *et al.* (2008) APC is essential for targeting phosphorylated β-catenin to the SCFbeta-TrCP ubiquitin ligase. *Molecular Cell*, **32**, 652–661.

Takada, R., Satomi, Y., Kurata, T. *et al.* (2006) Monounsaturated fatty acid modification of Wnt protein: its role in Wnt secretion. *Developmental Cell*, **11**, 791–801.

Takahashi-Yanaga, F. and Kahn, M. (2010) Targeting Wnt signaling: can we safely eradicate cancer stem cells? *Clinical Cancer Research*, **16**, 3153–3162.

Tamai, K., Semenov, M., Kato, Y. *et al.* (2000) LDL-receptor-related proteins in Wnt signal transduction. *Nature*, **407**, 530–535.

Tamai, K., Zeng, X., Liu, C. *et al.* (2004) A mechanism for Wnt coreceptor activation. *Molecular Cell*, **13**, 149–156.

Tanaka, K., Kitagawa, Y. and Kadowaki, T. (2002) Drosophila segment polarity gene product porcupine stimulates the posttranslational N-glycosylation of wingless in the endoplasmic reticulum. *Journal of Biological Chemistry*, **277**, 12816–12823.

Tang, Y., Simoneau, A.R., Liao, W.-X. *et al.* (2009) WIF1, a Wnt pathway inhibitor, regulates SKP2 and c-myc expression leading to G1 arrest and growth inhibition of human invasive urinary bladder cancer cells. *Molecular Cancer Therapeutics*, **8**, 458–468.

Thun, M.J., Henley, S.J. and Patrono, C. (2002) Nonsteroidal anti-inflammatory drugs as anticancer agents: mechanistic, pharmacologic, and clinical issues. *Journal of the National Cancer Instute*, **94**, 252–266.

Thun, M.J., Namboodiri, M.M. and Heath, C.W., Jr., (1991) Aspirin use and reduced risk of fatal colon cancer. *New England Journal of Medicine*, **325**, 1593–1596.

Tolwinski, N.S. and Wieschaus, E. (2004) Rethinking WNT signaling. *Trends in Genetics*, **20**, 177–181.

Tolwinski, N.S., Wehrli, M., Rives, A. *et al.* (2003) Wg/Wnt signal can be transmitted through arrow/LRP5,6 and Axin independently of Zw3/Gsk3beta activity. *Developmental Cell*, **4**, 407–418.

Toomes, C., Downey, L.M., Bottomley, H.M. *et al.* (2004) Identification of a fourth locus (EVR4) for familial exudative vitreoretinopathy (FEVR). *Molecular Vision*, **10**, 37–42.

Townsley, F.M., Cliffe, A. and Bienz, M. (2004) Pygopus and Legless target Armadillo/β-catenin to the nucleus to enable its transcriptional co-activator function. *Nature Cell Biology*, **6**, 626–633.

Trosset, J.Y., Dalvit, C., Knapp, S. *et al.* (2006) Inhibition of protein-protein interactions: the discovery of druglike β-catenin inhibitors by combining virtual and biophysical screening. *Proteins*, **64**, 60–67.

Ugur, S.A. and Tolun, A. (2008) Homozygous WNT10b mutation and complex inheritance in Split-Hand/Foot Malformation. *Human Molecular Genetics*, **17**, 2644–2653.

van Amerongen, R., Mikels, A. and Nusse, R. (2008).Alternative wnt signaling is initiated by distinct receptors. *Science Signaling*, **1**, re9.

van den Heuvel, M., Harryman-Samos, C., Klingensmith, J. *et al.* (1993) Mutations in the segment polarity genes wingless and porcupine impair secretion of the wingless protein. *EMBO Journal*, **12**, 5293–5302.

Vladar, E.K., Antic, D. and Axelrod, J.D. (2009) Planar cell polarity signaling: the developing cell's compass. *Cold Spring Harbour Perspectives in Biology*, **1**, a002964.

Wallingford, J.B. and Habas, R. (2005) The developmental biology of Dishevelled: an enigmatic protein governing cell fate and cell polarity. *Development*, **132**, 4421–4436.

Wang, K., Zhang, Y., Li, X. *et al.* (2008) Characterization of the Kremen-binding site on Dkk1 and elucidation of the role of Kremen in Dkk-mediated Wnt antagonism. *Journal of Biological Chemistry*, **283**, 23371–23375.

Wang, X. Reid Sutton, V., Omar Peraza-Llanes, J. *et al.* (2007) Mutations in X-linked PORCN, a putative regulator of Wnt signaling, cause focal dermal hypoplasia. *Nature Genetics*, **39**, 836–838.

Wehrli, M., Dougan, S.T., Caldwell, K., *et al.* (2000) Arrow encodes: an LDL-receptor-related protein essential for Wingless signalling. *Nature*, **407**, 527–530.

Wei, W., Chua, M.S., Grepper, S. and So, S.K. (2009) Blockade of Wnt-1 signaling leads to anti-tumor effects in hepatocellular carcinoma cells. *Molecular Cancer*, **8**, 76.

Willert, J., Epping, M., Pollack, J.R. *et al.* (2002) A transcriptional response to Wnt protein in human embryonic carcinoma cells. *BMC Developmental Biology*, **2**, 8.

Willert, K., Brown, J.D., Danenberg, E. *et al.* (2003) Wnt proteins are lipid-modified and can act as stem cell growth factors. *Nature*, **423**, 448–452.

Wolf, J., Palmby, T.R., Gavard, J. *et al.* (2008) Multiple PPPS/TP motifs act in a combinatorial fashion to transduce Wnt signaling through LRP6. *FEBS Letters*, **582**, 255–261.

Wong, H.C., Bourdelas, A., Krauss, A., *et al.* (2003) Direct binding of the PDZ domain of Dishevelled to a conserved internal sequence in the C-terminal region of Frizzled. *Molecular Cell*, **12**, 1251–1260.

Woods, C.G., Stricker, S., Seemann, P. *et al.* (2006) Mutations in WNT7A cause a range of limb malformations, including Fuhrmann syndrome and Al-Awadi/Raas-Rothschild/Schinzel phocomelia syndrome. *American Journal of Human Genetics*, **79**, 402–408.

Wu, C.H. and Nusse, R. (2002) Ligand receptor interactions in the Wnt signaling pathway in Drosophila. *Journal of Biological Chemistry*, **277**, 41762–41769.

Wu, X., Tu, X., Joeng, K.S. *et al.* (2008) Rac1 activation controls nuclear localization of β-catenin during canonical Wnt signaling. *Cell*, **133**, 340–353.

Xu, Q., Wang, Y., Dabdoub, A. *et al.* (2004) Vascular development in the retina and inner ear: control by Norrin and Frizzled-4, a high-affinity ligand-receptor pair. *Cell*, **116**, 883–895.

Yan, D., Wiesmann, M., Rohan, M. *et al.* (2001) Elevated expression of axin2 and hnkd mRNA provides evidence that Wnt/beta -catenin signaling is activated in human colon tumors. *Proceedings of the National Academy of Sciences, USA*, **98**, 14973–14978.

Yang, P.T., Lorenowicz, M.J., Silhankova, M. *et al.* (2008) Wnt signaling requires retromer-dependent recycling of MIG-14/Wntless in Wnt-producing cells. *Developmental Cell*, **14**, 140–147.

You, L., He, B., Xu, Z. *et al.* (2004) An anti-Wnt-2 monoclonal antibody induces apoptosis in malignant melanoma cells and inhibits tumor growth. *Cancer Research*, **64**, 5385–5389.

Zeng, X., Huang, H., Tamai, K. *et al.* (2008) Initiation of Wnt signaling: control of Wnt coreceptor Lrp6 phosphorylation/activation via frizzled, dishevelled and axin functions. *Development*, **135**, 367–375.

Zeng, X., Tamai, K., Doble, B. *et al.* (2005) A dual-kinase mechanism for Wnt co-receptor phosphorylation and activation. *Nature*, **438**, 873–877.

Zeng, Y.A. and Verheyen, E.M. (2004) Nemo is an inducible antagonist of Wingless signaling during Drosophila wing development. *Development*, **131**, 2911–2920.

Zhai, L., Chaturvedi, D. and Cumberledge, S. (2004) Drosophila wnt-1 undergoes a hydrophobic modification and is targeted to lipid rafts, a process that requires porcupine. *Journal of Biological Chemistry*, **279**, 33220–33227.

Ziegler, S., Rohrs, S., Tickenbrock, L. *et al.* (2005) Novel target genes of the Wnt pathway and statistical insights into Wnt target promoter regulation. *FEBS Journal*, **272**, 1600–1615.

5

Mammalian target of rapamycin (mTOR) signalling

Maria Thorpe and Emmanouil Karteris

Biosciences, Brunel University, London

The protein entitled mammalian target of rapamycin (mTOR) is a threonine/serine kinase present in all eukaryotic cells, which has been evolutionarily conserved (Efeyan and Sabatini, 2010; Laplante and Sabatini, 2012; Peterson *et al.*, 2009). It is considered to be the master coordinator of extracellular signals, an integration point that regulates a wide variety of processes, including cell growth, metabolism and proliferation in an appropriate and finely tuned response. Because of its essential role in directing and maintaining critical cellular processes, together with its known involvement in cancer and other human diseases (e.g. Dazert and Hall, 2011; Rosner *et al.*, 2008), mTOR has been the subject of extensive research in recent years.

5.1   Discovery of mTOR

The bacteria family of *streptomyces* produce many important secondary metabolites such as antibiotics and fungicides (Chater *et al.*, 2010). In 1975, *Streptomyces hygroscopicus* was a novel discovery, isolated from a soil sample taken from Rapa Nui, also known as Easter Island in the South Pacific (Vezina *et al.*, 1975). Rapamycin was the name given to the molecule produced by this bacterium that confers anti-fungal properties against *candida albicans, microsporum gypseum* and *trichophyton granulosum*, which are responsible for a diverse range of infections (Vezina *et al.*, 1975). Derivatives of rapamycin (also known as sirolimus) called rapalogs (e.g. temsirolimus, everolimus and ridforolimus), are also now used as immunosuppressants for grafts and organ transplants as well as promising cancer therapies (Caron *et al.*, 2010; Willems *et al.*, 2012; Zaytseva *et al.*, 2012). Using yeast, researchers identified two physical intracellular '*targets of*

Cancer Cell Signalling, First Edition. Edited by Amanda Harvey.
© 2013 John Wiley & Sons, Ltd. Published 2013 by John Wiley & Sons, Ltd.

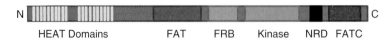

Figure 5.1   **Schematic of representation of mTOR**. The full-length protein is 289 kDa and comprises up to 20 HEAT repeat domains at the *N*-terminus plus central FAT, FRB and kinase domains with NR and FATC domains at the *C*-terminus. Adapted from Albanell *et al.*, 2007 and Bai and Jiang, 2010.

rapamycin' (TOR), named TOR1 and TOR2 (Heitman *et al.*, 1991; Kunz *et al.*, 1993). Shortly after this, the 'mammalian' TOR was described by several groups (Brown *et al.*, 1994; Chiu *et al.*, 1994; Sabatini *et al.*, 1994; Sabers *et al.*, 1995).

The mTOR gene in *homosapiens* is located on the small arm of chromosome 1 (1p36.22) (Moore *et al.*, 1996), it encodes a 2549 amino acid protein with a predicted molecular weight of 289 kDa (Chen *et al.*, 1995). It belongs to the phosphatidylinositol 3-kinase (PI3K) related family of proteins. Initially the protein was referred to as FRAP 506 binding protein 12 **r**apamycin **a**ssociated **p**rotein, rapamycin and FKBP12 target (RAFT) or rapamycin target (RAPT). More recently the 'm' for 'mammalian' has been changed to 'mechanistic' reflecting the importance given to this protein (National Centre for Biological Information (NCBI), 2012; Protein Knowledge Database (UniProtKB), 2012), and a schematic representation of the structure of this protein is shown in Figure 5.1. Albanell *et al.* (2007) and Bai and Jiang (2010) suggest that there are up to 20 **H**untingtin, **e**longation factor 3, protein phosphatase 2**A**, and the yeast PI3 kinase **T**OR1 (HEAT) repeat domains within two areas close to the *N*-terminus; however, both the NCBI (2012) and UniProtKB (2012) record the existence of just seven HEAT repeat domains located between amino acids 16 and 1186. These domains mediate protein to protein interactions. Following on from the HEAT repeat domains is the **f**ocal **a**dhesion **t**argeting (FAT) domain, which aides scaffolding, then an inhibiting section called **F**K 506 and rapamycin Binding protein (FKBP) **r**apamycin **b**inding (FRB) domain. The fourth area is its kinase domain, providing the catalytic activity, the fifth section is a putative **n**egative **r**egulatory **d**omain (NRD) and finally there is a second **FAT** before the *C*-terminus (FATC).

5.2   mTOR complexes

mTOR serves as an integration point of extracellular signalling but does not work in isolation. There are at least two distinct heteromeric complexes, referred to as mTOR complex 1 (mTORC1) and mTORC2, respectively, where mTOR provides the regulatory catalytic core. Other complexes are suspected but have yet to be elucidated (Bove *et al.*, 2011; Laplante and Sabatini, 2009). In addition to mTOR, each complex includes mammalian Lethal with Sec13 protein 8 (LST8) (also referred to as mammalian Lethal with Sec13 protein 8/G protein β subunit like protein – mLST8/GβL) (Kim *et al.*, 2003) and DEP (**d**ishevelled, **E**gl-10, **P**leckstrin) domain containing mTOR interacting protein (DEPTOR). mLST8 is a protein of 36 kDa, which interacts directly with mTOR enhancing the activity of mTOR kinase. DEPTOR, a 48 kDa protein, is a more recent discovery and was identified as an mTOR binding protein using a variety of co-immunoprecipitation techniques. It is a negative regulator, inhibiting activity of mTOR by binding to the *C*-terminal of mTOR via its postsynaptic density 95, discs large, zonula occludens 1 (PDZ) domain (Peterson *et al.*, 2009). In response to growth signals it is necessary for both of the complexes to disassociate with DEPTOR to become active. mTOR achieves this in partnership with casein kinase 1 (CS1) to phosphorylate DEPTOR, which then allows DEPTOR to be targeted by SCF/βTrCP (Skp, Cullin, F box containing complex/β transducing repeat containing protein), which in turn triggers degradation (Gao *et al.*, 2011; Duan *et al.*, 2011; Zhao *et al.*, 2011).

5.2.1   mTORC1

In addition to mLST8 and DEPTOR, mTOR complexes with the **r**egulatory **a**ssociated **p**rotein of mTOR (RAPTOR) (Hara *et al.*, 2002; Kim *et al.*, 2002) together with **p**roline **r**ich Akt **s**ubstrate **40** kDa (PRAS40) to form mTORC1 (Oshiro *et al.*, 2007; Wang *et al.*, 2007). RAPTOR is approximately 149 kDa and is a scaffold protein which links mTOR kinase with mTOR substrates and therefore actively promotes mTORC1 signalling. It is the involvement of RAPTOR with mTORC1 that has attributed this complex the additional title of '*rapamycin sensitive*'. Until recently the full function of PRAS40 (40 kDa) protein had yet to be understood, however, Wang with his collaborators proposed a dual function for PRAS40. Their research supported the earlier suggestion that PRAS40 is a physical inhibitor of mTORC1 (Wang *et al.*, 2007; Sancak *et al.*, 2007), where mTORC1 is released from this inhibition by the phosphorylation of PRAS40 by Akt (also known as protein kinase B, PKB). However, a distinctly different role for PRAS40 as a downstream substrate for mTORC1 is also suggested. It is proposed that PRAS40 directly effects the regulation of both S6 kinase 1 (S6K1) and an initiating factor 4E binding protein 1 (4E-BP1) (Wang *et al.*, 2012).

5.2.2   mTORC2

The second complex, mTORC2, comprises mTOR, DEPTOR and mLST8 associating with **r**apamycin **i**nsensitive **c**ompanion of m**TOR** (RICTOR) (Sarbassov *et al.*, 2004), **m**ammalian **s**tress activated protein kinase **in**teracting protein **1** (mSIN1), and **pro**tein observed with RIC**TOR** (PROTOR) (Pearce *et al.*, 2007). RICTOR is approximately 200 kDa and led to the term '*rapamycin insensitive*' (Sarbassov *et al.*, 2004) to define mTORC2. However, Sarbassov and colleagues have now shown this to be incorrect. They found that mTORC2 is indeed sensitive to rapamycin but needed a far longer exposure time to react to the drug in comparison with mTORC1 (Sarbassov *et al.*, 2006). mSIN1 is approximately 60 kDa with at least six known isoforms (UniProtKB, 2012; NCBI, 2012). It is understood that mSIN1 interacts directly with RICTOR to provide the physical organisation for the mTORC2 structure (Laplante and Sabatini, 2009). The last component to create mTORC2 is PROTOR. This also interacts directly with RICTOR (Chen and Sarbassov, 2011) and has a weight of approximately 43 kDa with at least four known splice isoforms (UniProtKB, 2012).

5.2.3   Complexes Upstream of mTOR

Figure 5.2 details a highly simplified view of the upstream activation and downstream effectors of both mTORC1 and mTORC2 as currently understood (Wang and Proud, 2011). Activation and inhibition of mTORC1 is achieved through its interaction with multiple signalling pathways. By comparison with what is known about mTORC1, very little is known about the signalling pathways in relation to mTORC2. However, based on the results of research conducted to date, the pathways affecting the mTOR complexes are very complicated with a high level of dynamic cross-talk combined with various feedback loops (Bai and Jiang, 2010; Galluzzi *et al.*, 2010; Wang and Proud, 2011; Willems *et al.*, 2012).

The following description of the upstream pathways affecting the mTOR complexes is only a brief overview of our present understanding of these systems.

Growth factor receptors

On the extracellular surface of the cell, a growth factor (e.g. insulin-like growth factor or epidermal growth factor) activates a tyrosine kinase receptor (RTK), which results in a conformational change on the intracellular section of the receptor. This allows the recruitment of scaffolding protein/s such as insulin receptor substrates (IRS) or perhaps the activation of growth factor receptor bound proteins (Grb). At this time three different pathways are understood to be networked to the TOR complexes from these receptors.

The first is one of two known signal transduction pathways involving phosphatidylinositol 3-kinase (PI3K). Here, via the p110 domain of PI3K, phosphatidylinositol 4,5-bisphosphate (PIP_2) is converted into phosphatidylinositol (3,4,5)-trisphosphate (PIP_3), which recruits phosphatidylinositol dependent protein kinase 1 (PDK1) with Akt to the plasma membrane. PDK1 uses the pleckstrin homology domain of PIP_3 as a docking site and activates Akt through phosphorylation. Akt then inhibits the tuberous sclerosis complexes (TSC1 and TSC2) releasing their inhibition on **r**at sarcoma **h**omolog **e**nriched in **b**rain (Rheb) allowing activation of mTORC1. A negative feedback loop is created to the PI3K/Akt pathway and is induced by the targeting of IRS directly by mTORC1. This leads to the proteasomal degradation of IRS, which produces deactivation of the pathway (Li *et al.*, 1999; Ozes *et al.*, 2001).

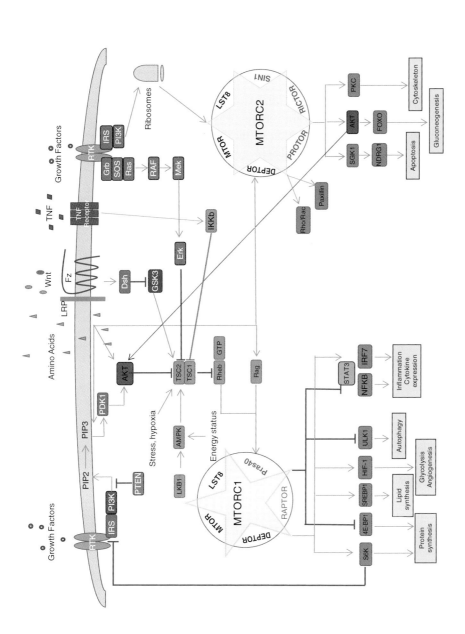

Figure 5.2 **Overview of mTOR signalling.** A schematic representation of key intracellular interactions for mTOR. Both mTORC1 and mTORC2 are activated in response to growth factor and amino acid signalling. Regulation of signalling via negative feedback loops is complex, with Akt activation via mTORC2 activating mTORC1.

The second route involving growth factors is via mTORC2. Although not completely understood, PI3K becomes activated by RTKs that ultimately signal to the ribosomes via activation of mTORC2. As a result mTORC2 achieves full phosphorylation of Akt maximising its activity and fully stimulating mTORC1 via the same TSC1 and TSC2 pathway as summarised earlier (Xie and Guan, 2011; Zinzalla et al., 2011). This discovery suggests that Akt does not need to be fully phosphorylated to activate mTORC1, and proposes mTORC2 lies upstream of mTORC1.

The third route involves the Sons of Sevenless (SOS) being recruited by Grb on the activated RTK which in turn recruits Ras. This signal is then transduced and amplified through phosphorylation of the Raf/Mek/Erk pathway, which also supresses the action of TSC1 and TSC2 as described previoulsy, allowing the activation of mTORC1 via Rheb (Lee et al., 2007).

Wingless and integrin 1 (Wnt)

Using transgenic mice, Inoki and colleagues established that the mTOR pathway was regulated by Wnt signalling via glycogen synthase kinase 3 (GSK3). In the presence of Wnt signalling, the glycolipoprotein causes the Frizzled receptor to associate with LPR5/6. The resulting intracellular signalling pathway leads to the activation of Dishevelled (DVL), which inhibits the ability of GSK3 to phosphorylate TSC2. The consequence of this is the inability of the TSC1/2 complex to inhibit Rheb leading to activation of mTORC1 (Inoki et al., 2006; Rosner et al., 2008).

Amino acids

Amino acids such as leucine, arginine and glutamine are transported into the cytoplasm in partnership with a variety of solute carrier family proteins and positively regulate mTORC1. It is now understood, although further elucidation is still required, that when amino acids are present Rag GTPases dimerise, and mediate relocation of mTORC1 to lysosomes where Rag works in conjunction with Rheb to activate mTORC1 (Laplante and Sabatini, 2009; Efeyan and Sabatini 2010; Russell et al., 2011; Yan and Lamb, 2012). More recently amino acids have also been implicated in activation of mTORC2 through the PI3K/Akt pathway. In this study this novel connection was demonstrated using a variety of cell lines which resulted in the rapid phosphorylation of Akt by both P13K and then by amino acid activated mTORC2 (Tato et al., 2011; Yan and Lamb, 2012).

Tumour necrosis factor (TNF) receptor

Cytokines such as tumour necrosis factor (TNF) activate the trimeric TNF receptor. A major kinase downstream of this receptor is IkappaB kinase beta (IKKβ). In a panel of different cancer cell lines, IKKβ was found to be responsible for the suppression of TSC1 activity by a dual phosphorylation event resulting in the activation of mTORC1 (Lee *et al.*, 2007).

Stress, hypoxia and energy status

Oxygen is critical for the survival of a cell. When oxygen levels are reduced in a state known as hypoxia, the cell is under stress and this leads to a decrease in the cellular availability of adenosine triphosphate (ATP). The reduction of ATP stimulates adenosine monophosphate activated protein kinase (AMPK) activity enhancing TSC1/2 inhibition of mTORC1 and halting activity of the complex (Dennis *et al.*, 2001; Brugarolas, *et al.*, 2004). The TSC2 complex is also phosphorylated via the liver kinase B1 (LKB1)/AMPK pathway when the cell is subjected to nutrient and oxygen deprivation (Cam and Houghton, 2011). There are other suspected players which inhibit mTORC1 when conditions dictate, but these are yet to be fully elucidated (reviewed in Laplante and Sabatini, 2009; Cam and Houghton, 2011).

5.2.4   Downstream signalling effectors

The downstream effectors of the mTORC complexes affect a wide variety of cellular activity. Ribosomal protein S6 kinase (S6K) together with eukaryotic translation initiation factor 4E binding protein 1 (4E-BP1) have been the most intensely studied to date because of their involvement in protein synthesis. Table 5.1 summarises the known pathways suppressed or activated.

5.3   mTOR dysregulation in disease

Table 5.2 summarises how mTOR participates in a selection of inherited genetic diseases and syndromes. Although it is clear that dysregulation of mTOR is also implicated in diverse conditions such as type 2 diabetes, cardiac hypertrophy and Alzheimer's disease, extensive research is currently being conducted in all of these fields to establish if a genetic connection exists (Rosner *et al.*, 2008).

5.3.1   Dysregulation of mTOR in cancers

Dysregulation of the pathways encompassing the mTOR complexes have been identified in many human diseases (Dazert and Hall, 2011; Efeyan and Sabatini, 2010; Laplante and Sabatini, 2012; Wang and Proud, 2011).

   mTOR is rarely mutated in cancer and it is not considered an early event in tumourgenesis (Albanell *et al.*, 2007). However, there are notable exceptions, such as haematological malignancies which revolve around 1p36 breakpoints, deletions

Table 5.1   Known downstream effectors of mTORC1 and mTORC2.

Downstream effector	Action	Result (brief description)
S6K	Activation	Phosphorylation of S6K by mTORC1 promotes initiation of gene translation via multiple substrates complexing together. Active S6K creates a negative feedback mechanism of mTOR via inhibition of IRS (Efeyan and Sabatini, 2010).
4E-BP1	Inhibition	Activated mTORC1 hyper-phosphorylates 4E-BP1, which inhibits its hold on eIF4E. This is a critical component of the transcription complex that is generated via S6K above. Inactivated mTORC1 results in hypo-phosphorylation of 4E-BP1, which then tightly binds eIF4E preventing any further protein translation (Weber and Gutmann, 2012).
SREBP1	Activation	mTORC1 promotes lipid synthesis by activating SREBP1, which in turn regulates the expression of enzymes required for the biosynthesis of fatty acids and cholesterol (Porstmann et al., 2008).
HIF-1	Activation	In normal conditions mTORC1's activation of HIF1 results in transcription of several proteins including prolyl hydroxylase (PHD). This protein hydroxylates HIF1 causing immediate degradation by the tumour suppressor Von Hippel-Lindau. This feedback loop ensures that HIF1 is kept at very low levels (Demidenko and Blagosklonny, 2011).
ULK1	Inhibition	mTORC1 hyper-phosphorylates ULK1 preventing the cell entering the autophagy process and allowing cell growth (Alers et al., 2011).
STAT3	Inhibition	Activated mTORC1 maximises the phosphorylation status of STAT3 enhancing its transcription ability (Yokogami et al., 2000).
NFkB	Activation	When activated mTORC1 suppresses NFkB thereby preventing the transcription of specific interleukins (Thomson et al., 2009).
IRF7	Activation	Activated mTORC1 associates with a scaffold protein called MyD88. Together they phosphorylate IRF7, which initiates transcription of interferon proteins (Thomson et al., 2009).
SGK1	Activation	Phosphorylation of SGK1 by mTORC2 results in the formation of sodium channels in the membrane of epithelial cells (Lu et al., 2010).
AKT	Activation	Phosphorylation of AKT at serine 473 by mTORC2 maximises AKT activity (Ikenoue et al., 2008).
PKC	Activation	mTORC2 activation results in phosphorylation of PKC at the C-terminal, which is essential for stability and function of the protein (Ikenoue et al., 2008).

Table 5.2 Genetic diseases and syndromes that directly affect normal mTOR function.

Name	Birth rate	Description
Tuberous sclerosis	1:6000	Mutation of either TSC1 (9q34) and/or TSC2 (16p13.3) genes. Result – skin abnormalities, neurological problems, benign tumours on the skin, in the brain, the kidneys and other organs.
Peutz–Jeghers syndrome	1:25 000	Mutation of STK11 gene (19p13.3), which normally controls growth and proliferation of cells. Result – production of hamartomatous polyps in the gastrointestinal tract, which can develop into tumours. Additional cancers reported in the pancreas, cervix, ovaries and mammary glands.
PTEN hamartoma-tumor syndromes	1:250 000+	Mutation of PTEN gene (10q23.3). Several very rare genetic conditions have been grouped together including Cowden syndrome, Bannayan–Riley–Ruvalcaba syndrome, Proteus syndrome and Lhermitte–Ducios disease. Result – the growth of hamartomas, which can be life threatening.
Von Hippel-Lindau syndrome	1:36 000	Mutation of VHL gene (3p25.3). Result – hemangio-blastomas, which are benign tumour growths of disorganised blood vessels.
Neurofibromatosis type 1	1:3/4000	Mutation of NF1 gene (17q11.2), which normally controls nerve growth by the production of neurofibromin. This acts as an RAS-GTPase and aides in the transcription of oligodendrocytes and Schwann cells which form myelin sheaths. Result – changes in skin pigmentation and tumour growths throughout the nervous system caused by aberrant Ras activity.
Polycystic kidney disease (autosomal dominant)	1:1000	Mutation of PKD1 (16p13.3) and/or PDK2 (4q22.1), which still needs to be fully elucidated, although it has been shown that polycystin-1 transcribed by PKD interacts directly with mTOR. Result – formation of multiple cysts and eventual loss of kidney function during adulthood.

Data source: NCBI 2012 and Rosner *et al.*, 2008.

and rearrangements (Onyango *et al.*, 1998; Varga *et al.*, 2001). A dichotomy also exists with the mTOR inhibitor of both protein complexes, DEPTOR, as it has been shown to be regularly over-expressed in a number of myeloma cell lines. When investigated by Peterson and colleagues, they reported with some astonishment that whilst mTORC1 was inhibited, almost 30% of multiple myeloma cell lines demonstrated over-expression of DEPTOR, which they believed caused activation of the PI3K pathway. They suggest that the action of DEPTOR over-expression drives growth and survival of this type of cancer but the mechanism of this dichotomy remains elusive. Additionally, the research team reported that this group of cell lines also lacked mutations that could be responsible for the aberrant PI3K activation, which is apparent in other myelomas (Peterson *et al.*, 2009).

In most cancers the mTOR complexes are 'hijacked' by hyper-activation as a result of events upstream (Menon and Manning, 2008). This abnormal functioning can occur by the inactivation of tumour suppressor proteins and/or aberrant onco-genic activity of other critical proteins within the different signalling pathways. The tumour suppressor gene PTEN, essential for deactivation of the PI3K-mTOR pathways, is regularly mutated and therefore inactivated in a significant propor-tion of glioblastomas, endometrial cancers and melanomas (e.g. reviewed in Benito *et al.*, 2010; Pollock *et al.*, 2002; Terakawa *et al.*, 2003). Gene mutations resulting in oncogenic activation of receptors such as EGFR and HER2 over activate mTOR in several cancers, such as breast, lung and gastric cancers, as well as glioblas-tomas (Akhavan, *et al.*, Benito *et al.*, 2010; Sharma *et al.*, 2007). Mutated Akt, RAS and RAF have also been identified as being present in a variety of tumours such as pancreatic, thyroid and ovarian cancers causing hyperactivation of mTOR (e.g. Dazert and Hall, 2011; Garnett and Marais, 2004; Nakayama *et al.*, 2006; Xing, 2005).

Although all of the mechanisms involved in the highly complicated mTOR story are still waiting to be fully understood, what has become clear is that dysregulation of the pathways encompassing the mTOR complexes have been identified in many human diseases (Dazert and Hall, 2011; Efeyan and Sabatini, 2010; Laplante and Sabatini, 2012; Wang and Proud, 2011). The following is only a small summary of how mTOR and its known complexes are implicated in ill-health, as recent published research has suggested its direct involvement in such diverse areas as cocaine addiction (Dayas *et al.*, 2012), to an orchestrator of stem cell physiology and homeostasis (Russell *et al.*, 2011) to a mediator of immune responses (Powell *et al.*, 2012).

5.3.2   Dysregulation of mTOR signalling in gynaecological malignancies

Dysregulation of the pathways encompassing the mTOR complexes have been identified in many human diseases (Dazert and Hall, 2011; Efeyan and Sabatini, 2010; Laplante and Sabatini, 2012; Wang and Proud, 2011).

Ovarian cancer

Ovarian carcinoma is associated with the highest mortality amongst gynaeco-logical malignancies in industrialised countries, with a reported 5-year survival rate of <30% (De Cecco *et al.*, 2004). The prognosis for patients with ovarian cancer is determined by conventional factors such as surgical stage and his-tological grade and type. Nevertheless, no single molecular profile has helped identify the most aggressive tumours or aided in the guidance of suitable ther-apeutic strategies for specific patients. Many carcinomas activate growth factor receptor signalling pathways that exhibit genetic alterations involving either the receptor, or other factors that drive the proliferation. Interestingly, several pathways converge on the highly conserved serine/threonine kinase mTOR (Hay and Sonenberg, 2004).

The PI3K/Akt/mTOR pathway is activated in advanced stage disease and inhibition of this pathway with inhibitors to Akt or its downstream effector, mTOR, increases chemo-sensitivity to paclitaxel in ovarian carcinoma cell lines (Kim *et al.*, 2007). mTOR and one of its substrates, S6 kinase, have been shown to be activated in ovarian cancer cell lines (Meng *et al.*, 2006; Altomare *et al.*, 2004). Rapamycin inhibits the growth of a broad spectrum of malignancies including pancreatic cancer, leukaemia and B-cell lymphoma, (Huang *et al.*, 2002). Treatment of several ovarian cancer cell lines with the rapalogue RAD001 (everolimus; an inhibitor of mTOR) resulted in dose-dependent growth inhibition (Treeck *et al.*, 2006). Furthermore, treatment with RAD001 diminished the expression of vascular endothelial growth factor in ovarian tumour-derived cell lines and inhibited angiogenesis *in vivo* (Mabuchi *et al.*, 2007).

In terms of upstream of mTOR complexes, RTK activation plays a key role in the oncogenic progression from non-neoplastic mesothelial lining of the ovaries or epithelium of the fallopian tubes to epithelial ovarian cancer. Epidermal growth factor receptor (EGFR) is amplified in approximately 4–22% of ovarian cancer and activating EGFR mutations are rare with a frequency of 4% or less (Lassus *et al.*, 2006). EGFR up-regulation is detected in approximately 60% of ovarian cancer and is associated with increased tumour cell proliferation, advanced tumour grades and poor patient prognosis (Lassus *et al.*, 2006). EGFR inhibitors were able to inhibit EGFR-mediated MAPK and Akt phosphorylation and reduce cell proliferation in ovarian cancer cell lines and tumour xenograft models. In a recent study, inhibition of multi-RTK signalling by Hsp90 suppression results in profound pro-apoptotic and anti-proliferative effects in ovarian cancer, and is associated with the inactivation of PI3K/Akt/mTOR pathway (Jiao *et al.*, 2011). In another study, it has been suggested that the PI3K pathway plays a central role in ovarian tumourgenesis, since mutations or increase of PIK3CA expression was detected in 30.5% of ovarian cancers tested (Campbell *et al.*, 2004).

Studies from our laboratory revealed significant up-regulation of DEPTOR in two paclitaxel resistant ovarian cancer cell lines (Foster *et al.*, 2010). Collectively our data suggest that in a stage of drug-resistance, over-expression of DEPTOR could drive increased survival and subsequent tumour growth and progression. Similarly, accumulation of DEPTOR conferred resistance to rapamycin and paclitaxel (Zhao *et al.*, 2011). Studies investigating DEPTOR expression have produced conflicting results. DEPTOR is down-regulated in a number of cancers such as prostate, bladder, cervix and thyroid, whereas it is highly over-expressed in a subset of multiple myelomas harbouring cyclin D1/D3 or c-MAF/MAFB translocations (Peterson *et al.*, 2009). Paradoxically, it has been demonstrated that DEPTOR can also induce Akt signalling, thus suggesting that DEPTOR can exert a dual role as an oncogene or as a tumour suppressor gene acting in a cell- and tissue-specific manner (Wang *et al.*, 2012).

Prostate cancer

Prostate cancer is the most frequent cancer in the male population. Every year, around half a million of patients are diagnosed with this type of cancer world-wide and, in the United States alone, around 30 000 die due to this cause (Jemal *et al.*, 2010). When the disease is localised, combinatorial treatments with radical surgery and radiotherapy lead to cure of this cancer (Rai *et al.*, 2010). However, in numerous cases there is a cancer progression despite ablation of testosterone and this is referred to as androgen-independent prostate cancer (Rai *et al.*, 2010).

An increasing body of evidence points towards numerous alterations of the Akt/mTOR signalling pathway in prostate cancer. Kremer *et al.*, have shown that there was a strong association between 4E-BP1 with prostate cancer, espe-cially when combined with PTEN and mTOR expression data (Kremer *et al.*, 2006). Moreover, in the same study they demonstrated a differential distribu-tion of phosphorylated mTOR (p-mTOR) between normal and cancer cells. In normal epithelial cells, p-mTOR is localised on the cell membrane, whereas in the tumour cells it acquires a cytoplasmic distribution. These workers have also shown increases in the phosphorylation status of mTOR in prostate intra-epithelial neoplasia, suggestive of potential changes in mTOR activation in the early stages of prostate carcinogenesis (Kremer *et al.*, 2006). It has also been proposed that tumours with a PTEN deletion as well as activated mTOR signalling represent a small subset of prostate cancers that respond optimally to anti-mTOR therapies (Müller *et al.*, 2013). A study of over 600 prostate cancer patients and 708 cancer-free controls documented that genetic variations of two AKT2 and mTOR variants may influence prostate cancer susceptibility in a Chinese cohort (Chen *et al.*, 2012). Interestingly, mTORC2 might also be implicated in the pathogenesis of this cancer, since the androgen receptor can induce degradation of p27 protein *in vitro* through selective activation of the mTORC2 complex (Fang *et al.*, 2012).

5.4   Therapeutic opportunities

5.4.1   Current treatments

Over the past few years there has been much clinical evaluation of mTOR inhibitors alone or in combination with other chemotherapeutic agents (Carew *et al.*, 2011). Table 5.3 summarises the latest on-going clinical trials. Current treatments for newly diagnosed ovarian tumours centre on the use of platinum containing drugs such as cisplatin or carboplatin and often in combination therapy with paclitaxel (Taxol™). Paclitaxel promotes assembly and stabilisation of the mitotic spindle and it has also been shown to induce apoptosis (Schiff *et al.*, 1980). The treatment options for recurrent or advanced disease depend on whether tumours are resistant or refractory to any previously used platinum based drugs (Yap *et al.*, 2009). Most patients with advanced disease will be

Table 5.3 Summary of ongoing and recruiting clinical trials.

Cancer/rapalogue	Disease stage	Treatments	Phase
Temsirolimus (T)			
Ovarian	Adjuvant; stages III–IV	T+carboplatin+paclitaxel and then T maintenance	II
Ovarian and endometrial	Recurrent disease	T+pegylated liposomal doxorubicin	Ib
Ovarian and endometrial and cervical	Recurrent disease	T+AZD2171	I
Ovarian	Advanced or recurrent ovarian cancer	Pegylated liposomal doxorubicin	Recruiting
Ovarian	Newly diagnosed stage III or stage IV clear cell ovarian cancer	T+carboplatin+paclitaxel	Recruiting
Everolemus (E)			
Ovarian	Recurrent disease	E+bevacizumab	II
Ovarian	Recurrent disease	E+pegylated liposomal doxorubicin	I
Ovarian	Advanced low grade ovarian cancers	E+JI-101	Terminated
Ovarian, fallopian tube and peritoneal Cancer	Recurrent disease	E+bevacizumab	Recruiting
Ridaforolemus (R)			
Ovarian and endometrial	Recurrent disease	R+carboplatin+paclitaxel	I

Source: www.clinicaltrials.gov.
Adapted from Diaz-Padilla *et al.*, 2012.

treated with paclitaxel, or in combination with other agents, such as topotecan (Agarwal and Kaye, 2003). One of the most important factors affecting patient survival is the development of drug resistance (Orr *et al.*, 2003).

Like ovarian cancer, emerging prostate cancer studies provide a positive outlook on the usage of mTOR inhibitors, either alone or in combination with other chemotherapeutic agents. Pharmacological manipulation *in vitro* of the PI3K/Akt/mTOR signalling cascade using the dual PI3K/mTOR inhibitor, temsirolimus, or an Akt inhibitor, led to reversal of sunitinib resistance in both androgen receptor (AR)-positive and AR-negative prostate cancer cell lines (Makhov *et al.*, 2012). An alternative therapeutic intervention is that of ionising radiation, especially for locally advanced prostate cancer. When chemical castration-resistant and AR-positive tumour cells were treated with rapamycin or temsirolimus, a radiosensitisation effect was observed when the inhibitors were used in conjunction with ionising radiation. When administered alone, mTOR inhibitors also exerted a profound inhibitory effect on cell proliferation (Schiewer *et al.*, 2012).

In addition to genetic factors, diet and obesity also emerge as risk factors for the aetiopathogenesis of prostate cancer (Tewari *et al.*, 2012). Interestingly, mTOR signalling is also implicated. Fisetin (a flavonol) is an inhibitor of the

PI3K/Akt/mTOR pathways and can affect cell proliferation of prostate cancer cells. Fisetin can be found in onions, cucumbers, apples, kiwis, grapes, and strawberries (Adhami *et al.*, 2012). Similarly, analogues of resveratrol (an mTOR inhibitor) can exert anti-androgenic effects *in vitro* (Iguchi *et al.*, 2012). Resveratrol can be found in red grapes, peanuts and certain food supplements. Given that resveratrol may exert cancer chemo-preventive effects, future studies should also focus on the use of this naturally occurring compound for prostate cancer (Cimino *et al.*, 2012). This can be of importance given its low toxicity. However, it should

Table 5.4   Current clinical trials using mTOR inhibitors.

Condition	Drug treatment	Stage
Castrate resistant prostate cancer; chemotherapy naïve prostate cancer; prostate cancer	Pasireotide (SOM230) with or without everolimus in treating patients with hormone resistant, chemotherapy naïve prostate cancer	Phase II
Prostate cancer	Safety study and effectiveness of docetaxel with RAD001 and bevacizumab in men with advanced prostate cancer	Phase Ib/II
Prostate cancer	Single agent temsirolimus (Torisel®) in chemotherapy-naïve castration-resistant prostate cancer patients	Phase II
Prostate cancer; adenocarcinoma of the prostate; hormone-resistant prostate cancer; recurrent prostate cancer; stage IV prostate cancer	Temsirolimus and vorinostat in treating patients with metastatic prostate cancer	Phase I
Prostate cancer	Temsirolimus and bevacizumab in hormone-resistant metastatic prostate cancer that did not respond to chemotherapy	Phase I-II
Prostate cancer	Everolimus as first-line therapy in treating patients with prostate cancer	Phase II
Prostate cancer	Carboplatin, everolimus and prednisone in treating patients with metastatic prostate cancer that progressed after docetaxel	Phase II
Newly diagnosed localised prostate cancer	Everolimus	Phase II
Metastatic, androgen independent prostate cancer; prostate cancer	The use of RAD001 with docetaxel in the treatment of metastatic, androgen independent prostate cancer	Phase I/II
Prostate cancer	Bicalutamide with or without everolimus in treating patients with recurrent or metastatic prostate cancer	Phase II

Source: www.clinicaltrials.gov.

be noted that toxicity is only one aspect that clinical trials should be concerned with. In a recent clinical trial in men with castration-resistant prostate cancer, a combinatorial treatment with RAD001 and bicalutamide was well tolerated but also exerted low activity. As a result it did not achieve the primary endpoint of an improved response compared with the effects bicalutamide exerts alone in this cohort of patients (Nakabayashi *et al.*, 2012). Table 5.4 indicates the current recruiting for clinical trials based on mTOR inhibition.

5.4.2 Future opportunities

As shown in Tables 5.3 and 5.4, whilst many trials are either on going or recruiting suitable candidates, research into mTOR inhibitors has not come to a halt. Most recently, reports have been made of a new compound VS-5584 (also known as SB2343) which binds to the ATP site of mTOR, resulting in the blocking of both mTORC1 and mTORC2. Additionally, this novel compound specifically inhibits all PI3K isoforms, resulting in an overall anti-proliferative effect in a wide range of tumour types without affecting the activity of over 400 lipid and protein kinases tested to date (Hart *et al.*, 2013).

As the complete function of mTOR and its complexes have yet to be fully elucidated, and as there is some notable controversy in this research field, the next 5–10 years could prove to be crucial in the development of mTOR targeted therapies.

References

Adhami, V.M., Syed, D.N., Khan, N. and Mukhtar, H. (2012) Dietary flavonoid fisetin: A novel dual inhibitor of PI3K/Akt and mTOR for prostate cancer management. *Biochemical Pharmacology*, **84** (10), 1277–1281.

Agarwal, R. and Kaye, S.B. (2003) Ovarian cancer: strategies for overcoming resistance to chemotherapy. *Nature Reviews Cancer*, **3** (7), 502–516.

Akhavan, D., Cloughsey, T.F. and Mischel, P.S. (2010) mTOR signaling in glioblastoma: lessons learned from bench to bedside. *Neuro-Oncology*, **12** (8), 763–764.

Albanell, J., Dalmases, A., Rovira, A. and Rojo, F. (2007) mTOR signalling in human cancer. *Clinical and Translational Oncology*, **9** (8), 484–493.

Alers, S., Loffler, A.S., Wesselborg, S. and Stork, B. (2012) Role of AMPK-mTOR-Ulk1/2 in the regulation of autophagy: cross talk, shortcuts and feedbacks. *Molecular and Cellular Biology*, **32** (1), 2–11.

Altomare, D.A., Wang, H.Q., Skele, K.L. *et al.* (2004) AKT and mTOR phosphorylation is frequently detected in ovarian cancer and can be targeted to disrupt ovarian tumor cell growth. *Oncogene*, **23** (34), 5853–5357.

Bai, X. and Jiang, Y. (2010) Key factors in mTOR regulation. *Cellular and Molecular Life Sciences*, **67** (2), 239–253.

Benito, R., Gil-Benso, R., Quilis, V. *et al.* (2010) Primary glioblastomas with and without EGFR amplification: relationship to genetic alterations and clinicopathological features. *Neuropathology: Official Journal of the Japanese Society of Neuropathology*, **30**, 392–400, as cited in Dazert and Hall, 2011.

Bove, J., Martinez-Vicente, M. and Vila, M. (2011) Fighting neurodegeneration with rapamycin: mechanical insights. *Nature Reviews Neuroscience*, **12** (8), 437–452.

Brown, E.J., Albers, M.W., Shin, T.B. *et al.* (1994) A mammalian protein targeted by G1-arresting rapamycin-receptor complex. *Nature*, **369** (6483), 756–758.

Brugarolas, J., Lei, K., Hurley, R. L. *et al.* (2004) Regulation of mTOR function in response to hypoxia by REDD1 and the TSC1/TSC2 tumor suppressor complex. *Genes and Development*, **18** (23), 2893–2904.

Cam, H. and Houghton, P. J. (2011) Regulation of mammalian target of rapamycin complex 1 (mTORC1) by hypoxia: causes and consequences. *Targeted Oncology*, **6** (2), 95–102.

Campbell, I.G., Russell, S.E., Choong, D.Y. *et al.* (2004) Mutation of the PIK3CA gene in ovarian and breast cancer. *Cancer Research*, **64** (21), 7678–7681.

Carew, J.S., Kelly, K.R. and Nawrocki, S.T. (2011) Mechanisms of mTOR inhibitor resistance in cancer therapy. *Targeted Oncology*, **6** (1), 17–27.

Caron, E., Ghosh, S., Matsuoka, Y. *et al.* (2010) A comprehensive map of the mTOR signaling network. *Molecular Systems Biology*, **6** (453), 1–15.

Chater, K.F., Biro, S., Lee, K.J. *et al.* (2010) The complex extracellular biology of Streptomyces. *Federation of European Microbiological Societies Microbiology Reviews*, **34** (2), 171–198.

Chen, L., Zheng, X.F., Brown, E.J. and Schreiber, S.L. (1995) Identification of an 11 kDa FKBP12 rapamycin binding domain within the 289 kDa FKBP12 rapamycin associated protein and characterization of a critical serine residue. *Proceedings of the National Academy of Sciences, USA*, **92** (11), 4947–4951.

Chen, C.H. and Sarbassov dos, D. (2011) The mTOR (mammalian target of rapamycin) kinase maintains integrity of mTOR complex 2. *Journal of Biological Chemistry*, **286** (46), 40386–40394.

Chen, J., Shao, P., Cao, Q. *et al.* (2012) Genetic variations in a PTEN/AKT/mTOR axis and prostate cancer risk in a Chinese population. *PLoS One*, **7** (7), e40817.

Chiu, M.I., Katz, H. and Berlin, V. (1994) RAPT1, a mammalian homolog of yeast Tor interacts with the FKBP12/rapamycin complex. *Proceedings of the National Academy of Sciences, USA*, **91** (26), 12574–12578.

Cimino, S., Sortino, G., Favilla, V. *et al.* (2012) Polyphenols: key issues involved in chemoprevention of prostate cancer. *Oxidative Medicine and Cellular Longevity*, **2012**, 632959.

Dayas, C.V., Smith, D.W. and Dunkley, P.R. (2012) An emerging role for the Mammalian target of rapamycin in pathological protein translation: relevance to cocaine addiction. *Frontiers in Neuropharmacology*, **3** (Article 13), 1–12.

Dazert, E. and Hall, M.N. (2011) mTOR signalling in disease. *Current Opinion in Cell Biology*, **23** (6), 744–755.

De Cecco, L., Marchionni, L., Gariboldi, M. *et al.* (2004) Gene expression profiling of advanced ovarian cancer: characterization of a molecular signature involving fibroblast growth factor2. *Oncogene*, **23** (49), 8171–8183.

Demidenko, Z.N. and Blagsklonny, M.V. (2011) The purpose of the HIF-1/PHD feedback loop. *Cell Cycle*, **10** (10), 1557–1562.

Dennis, P.B., Jaeschke, A, Masao, S. *et al.* (2001) Mammalian TOR: A homeostatic ATP sensor. *Science*, **294** (5544), 1102–1105.

Diaz-Padilla, I., Razak, A.R., Minig, L. *et al.* (2012) Prognostic and predictive value of CA-125 in the primary treatment of epithelial ovarian cancer: potentials and pitfalls. *Clinical and Translational Oncology*, **14** (1), 15–20.

Duan, S., Skaar, J.R., Kuchay, S. *et al.* (2011) mTOR generates an auto-amplification loop by triggering the βTrCP- and CK1α-dependent degradation of DEPTOR. *Molecular Cell*, **44** (2), 317–324.

Efeyan, A. and Sabatini, D. M. (2010) mTOR and cancer: many loops in one pathway. *Current Opinion in Cell Biology*, **22** (2), 169–176.

Fang, Z., Zhang, T., Dizeyi, N. *et al.* (2012) Androgen receptor enhances p27 degradation in prostate cancer cells through rapid and selective TORC2 activation. *Journal of Biological Chemistry*, **287** (3), 2090–2098.

Foster, H., Coley, H. M., Goumenou, A. *et al.* (2010) Differential expression of mTOR signalling components in drug resistance in ovarian cancer. *Anticancer Research*, **30** (9), 3529–3534.

Galluzzi, L., Kepp, O. and Kroemer, G. (2010) TP53 and MTOR crosstalk to regulate cellular senescence. *Aging*, **9** (2), 535–537.

Gao, D., Inuzuka, H., Tan, M. K. M. *et al.* (2011) mTOR drives its own activation via SCF(βTrCP) dependent degradation of the mTOR inhibitor DEPTOR. *Molecular Cell*, **44** (2), 317–324.

Garnett, M.J. and Marais, R. (2004) Guilty as charged: B-RAF is a human oncogene. *Cancer Cell*, **6** (4), 313–319.

Hara, K., Maruki, Y., Long, X. *et al.* (2002) Raptor, a binding partner of target of rapamycin (TOR), mediates TOR action. *Cell*, **110** (2), 177–189.

Hart, S., Novoyny-Diermayr. V., Goh, K. C. *et al.* (2013) VS-5584, a novel and highly selective PI3K/mTOR kinase inhibitor for the treatment of Cancer. *Molecular Chemical Therapeutics*, **12** (2), 151–161.

Hay, N. and Sonenberg, N. (2004) Upstream and downstream of mTOR. *Genes and Development*, **18**, 1926–1945.

Heitman, J., Movva, N.R. and Hall, M.N. (1991) Targets for cell cycle arrest by the immunosuppressant rapamycin in yeast. *Science*, **253** (5022), 905–909.

Huang, S. and Houghton, P.J. (2002) Inhibitors of mammalian target of rapamycin as novel antitumor agents: from bench to clinic. *Current Opinion in Investigational Drugs*, **3** (2), 295–304.

Iguchi, K., Toyama, T., Ito, T. *et al.* (2012) Anti-Androgenic Activity of Resveratrol Analogs in Prostate Cancer LNCaP Cells. *Journal of Andrology*, **33** (6), 1208–1215.

Ikenoue, T., Inoki, K., Yang, Q. *et al.* (2008) Essential function of TORC2 in PKC and Akt turn motif phosphorylation, maturation and signalling. *EMBO Journal*, **27** (14), 1919–1931.

Inoki, K., Ouyang, H., Zhu, T. *et al.* (2006) TSC2 integrates Wnt and energy signals via a co-ordinated phosphorylation by AMPK and GSK3 to regulate cell growth. *Cell*, **126** (5), 955–968.

Jemal, A., Siege, l.R., Xu, J. and Ward, E. (2010) Cancer statistics, 2010. *CA: A Cancer Journal for Clinicians*, **60** (5), 277–300.

Jiao, Y., Ou, W., Meng, F. *et al.* (2011) Targeting HSP90 in ovarian cancers with multiple receptor tyrosine kinase coactivation. *Molecular Cancer*, **10**, 125.

Kim, D.H., Sarbassov, D.D., Ali, S.M. *et al.* (2002) mTOR interacts with raptor to form a nutrient sensitive complex that signals to the cell growth machinery. *Cell*, **110** (2), 163–175.

Kim, D.H., Sarbassov, D.D., Ali, S.M. *et al.* (2003) GbetaL, a positive regulator of the rapamycin sensitive pathway required for the nutrient sensitive interaction between raptor and mTOR. *Molecular Cell*, **11** (4), 895–904.

Kim, S.H., Juhnn, Y.S. and Song, Y.S. (2007) Akt involvement in paclitaxel chemoresistance of human ovarian cancer cells. *Annals of the New York Academy of Sciences*, **1095**, 82–89.

Kremer, C.L., Klein, R.R., Mendelson, J. *et al.* (2006) Expression of mTOR signaling pathway markers in prostate cancer progression. *The Prostate*, **66** (11), 1203–1212.

Kunz, J., Henriquez, R., Schneider, U. *et al.* (1993) Target of rapamycin in yeast, TOR2, is an essential phosphatidylinositol kinase homolog required for G_1 progression. *Cell*, **73** (3), 585–596.

Laplante, M. and Sabatini, D.M. (2009) mTOR signalling at a glance. *Journal of Cell Science*, **122** (20), 3589–3594.

Laplante, M. and Sabatini, D.M. (2012) mTOR signalling. *Cold Harbor Perspectives in Biology*, **4** (2), 1–3.

Lassus, H., Sihto, H., Leminen, A. *et al.* (2006) Gene amplification, mutation and protein expression of EGFR and mutations of ERBB2 in serous ovarian carcinoma. *Journal of Molecular Medicine*, **84** (8), 671–681.

Lee, D. F., Kuo, H. P., Chen, C. T. *et al.* (2007) IKKβ suppression of TSC1 links inflammation and tumor angiogenesis via the mTOR pathway. *Cell*, **130** (3), 440–456.

Li, J., DeFea, K. and Roth, R.A. (1999) Modulation of insulin receptor substrate 1 tyrosine phosphorylation by an Akt/phosphatidylinositol 3 kinase pathway. *Journal of Biological Chemistry*, **274** (14), 9351–9356.

Lu, M., Wang, J., Jones, K. T. *et al.* (2010) mTOR complex 2 activates ENaC by phosphorylating SGK1. *Journal of the American Society of Nephrology*, **21** (5), 811–818.

Mabuchi, S., Altomare, D.A., Cheung, M. *et al.* (2007) RAD001 inhibits human ovarian cancer cell proliferation, enhances cisplatin-induced apoptosis, andprolongs survival in an ovarian cancer model. *Clinical Cancer Research*, **13** (14), 4261–4270.

Makhov, P.B., Golovine, K., Kutikov, A. *et al.* (2012) Modulation of Akt/mTOR signaling overcomes sunitinib resistance in renal and prostate cancer cells. *Molecular Cancer Therapeutics*, **11** (7), 1510–1517.

Meng, Q., Xia, C., Fang, J., Rojanasakui, Y. and Jiang, B.H. (2006) *Cellular Signalling*, **18** (12), 2262–2271.

Menon, P.A. and Manning, B.D. (2008) Common corruption of the mTOR signalling network in tumours. *Oncogene*, **27** (Supplement 2), S43–S51.

Moore, P.A., Rosen, C.A. and Carter, K.C. (1996) Assignment of the human FKBP12-rapamycin-associated protein (FRAP) gene to chromosome 1p36 by fluorescence in situ hybridization. *Genomics*, **33** (2), 331–332.

Müller, J., Ehlers, A., Burkhardt, L. *et al.* (2013) Loss of p(Ser2448) -mTOR expression is linked to adverse prognosis and tumor progression in ERG-fusion-positive cancers. *International Journal of Cancer*, **132** (6), 1333–1340.

Nakabayashi, M., Werner, L., Courtney, K.D., *et al.* (2012) Phase II trial of RAD001 and bicalutamide for castration-resistant prostate cancer. *BJU International*, **110** (11), 1729–1735.

Nakayama, K., Nakayama, N., Kurman, R. J. *et al.* (2006) Sequence mutations and amplification of PIK3CA and AKT2 genes in purified ovarian serous neoplasms. *Cancer Biology and Therapy*, **5**, 779–785, as cited in Dazert and Hall (2011).

National Centre for Biological Information (NCBI) (202), http://www.ncbi.nlm.nih.gov/gene/2475#general-protein-info.

Onyango, P., Lubyova, B., Gardellin, P. *et al.* (1998) Molecular cloning and expression analysis of five novel genes in chromosome 1p36. *Genomics*, **50** (2), 187–198.

Orr, G.A., Verdier-Pinard, P., McDaid, H. and Horwitz, S B. (2003) Mechanisms of Taxol resistance related to microtubules. *Oncogene*, **22** (47), 7280–7295.

Oshiro, N., Takahashi, R. Yoshino, K. *et al.* (2007) The proline rich Akt substrate of 40kDa (PRAS40) is a physiological substrate of mammalian target of rapamycin complex1. *Journal of Biological Chemistry*, **282** (28), 20329–20339.

Ozes, O.N., Akca, H., Mayo, L.D. *et al.* (2001) A phosphatidylinositol 3 kinase/Akt/mTOR pathway mediates and PTEN antagonizes tumor necrosis factor inhibition of insulin signalling through insulin receptor substrate 1. *Proceedings of the National Academy of Sciences, USA*, **98** (8), 4640–4645.

Pearce, L.R., Huang, X., Boudeau, J. *et al.* (2007) Identification of Protor as a novel Rictor biding component of mTOR complex 2. *Biochemical Journal*, **405** (3), 513–522.

Peterson, T.R., Laplante, M., Thorsen, C.C. *et al.* (2009) DEPTOR is an mTOR inhibitor frequently overexpressed in multiple myeloma cells and required for their survival. *Cell*, **137** (5), 873–886.

Pollock, P.M., Walker, G.J., Glendening, J.M. *et al.* (2002) PTEN inactivation is rare in melanoma tumours but occurs frequently in melanoma cell lines. *Melanoma Research*, **12**, 565–575 as cited in Dazert and Hall (2011).

Porstmann, T., Santos, C.R., Griffiths, B. *et al.* (2008) SREBP activity is regulated by mTORC1 and contributes to AKT-dependent cell growth. *Cell Metabolism*, **8**, 224–236.

Powell, J.D., Pollizzi, K.N., Helkamp, E.B. and Horton, M.R. (2012) Regulation of Immune Responses by mTOR. *Annual Review of Immunology*, **30**, 39–68.

Protein Knowledge Database (UniprotKB) (2012) http://www.uniprot.org/uniprot/P42345.

PubMed (2013) http://www.ncbi.nlm.nih.gov/pubmed.

Rai, J.S., Henley, M.J. and Ratan, H.L. (2010) Mammalian target of rapamycin: a new target in prostate cancer. *Urologic Oncology*, **28** (2), 134–138.

Rosner, M., Hanneder, M., Siegel, N. *et al.* (2008) The mTOR pathway and its role in human genetic diseases. *Mutation Research/Reviews in Mutation Research*, **659** (3), 284–292.

Russell, R.C., Fang, C. and Guan, K.L. (2011) An emerging role for TOR signalling in mammalian tissue and stem cell physiology. *Development*, **138** (16), 3343–3356.

Sabatini, D.M., Erdjument-Bromage, H., Lui, M. *et al.* (1994) RAFT1: A mammalian protein that binds to FKBP12 in a rapamycin dependent fashion and homologous to yeast TORs. *Cell*, **78** (1), 35–43.

Sabers, C.J, Martin, M.M., Brunn, G.J. *et al.* (1995) Isolation of a protein target of the FKBP12-rapamycin complex in mammalian cells. *Journal of Biological Chemistry*, **270** (2), 815–822.

Sancak, Y., Thoreen, C.C., Peterson, T R. *et al.* (2007) PRAS40 is an insulin-regulated inhibitor of the mTORC1 protein kinase. *Molecular Cell*, **25** (6), 903–915.

Sarbassov, D.D., Ali, S.M., Kim, D.H. *et al.* (2004) Rictor, a novel binding partner of mTOR, defines a rapamycin insensitive and raptor independent pathway that regulates the cytoskeleton. *Current Biology*, **14** (14), 1296–1302.

Sarbassov, D.D., Ali, S.M., Sengupta, S. *et al.* (2006) Prolonged rapamycin treatment inhibits mTORC2 assembly and Akt/PKB. *Molecular Cell*, **22** (2), 159–168.

Schiewer, M.J., Den, R., Hoang, D.T. *et al.* (2012) mTOR is a selective effector of the radiation therapy response in androgen receptor-positive prostate cancer. *Endocrine Related Cancers*, **19** (1), 1–12.

Schiff, P.B. and Horwitz, S.B. (1980) Taxol stabilizes microtubules in mouse fibroblast cells. *Proceedings of the National Academy of Sciences, USA*, **77** (3), 1561–1565.

Sharma, S.V., Bell, D.W., Settleman, J. and Haber, D.A. (2007) Epidermal growth factor mutations in lung cancer. *Nature Reviews Cancer*, **7**, 169–181.

Tato, I., Bartrons, R., Ventura, F. and Rosa, J.L. (2011) Amino acids activate mammalian target of rapamycin complex 2 (mTORC2) via PI3K/Akt signalling. *Journal of Biological Chemistry*, **286** (8), 6128–6142.

Terakawa, N., Kanamori, Y. and Yoshida, S. (2003) Loss of PTEN expression followed by Akt phosphorylation is a poor prognostic factor for patients with endometrial cancer. *Endocrine-related Cancer*, **10**, 203–208 as cited in Dazert and Hall (2011).

Tewari, R., Rajender, S., Natu, S.M. *et al.* (2012) Diet, obesity, and prostate health: are we missing the link? *Journal of Andrology*, **33** (5), 763–776.

Thomson, A.W., Turnquist, H.R. and Raimondi, G. (2009) Immunoregulatory functions of mTOR inhibition. *Nature Reviews Immunology*, **9** (5), 324–337.

Treeck, O., Wackwitz, B., Haus, U. and Ortmann, O. (2006) Effects of a combined treatment with mTOR inhibitor RAD001 and tamoxifen in vitro on growth and apoptosis of human cancer cells. *Gynacologic Oncology*, **102** (2), 292–299.

Varga, A.E., Dobrovic, A., Webb, G.C. and Hutchinson, R. (2001) Clustering of 1p36 breakpoints distal to 1p36.2 in haematological malignancies. *Cancer Genetics and Cytogenetics*, **125** (1), 78–79.

Vezina, C, Kudelski, A. and Sehgal, S.N. (1975) Rapamycin (AY-22,989), a new antifungal antibiotic (Taxonomy of the producing streptomycete and isolation of the active principal). *Journal of Antibiotics*, **28** (10), 721–726.

Wang, H., Zhang, Q., Wen, Q. *et al.* (2012) Proline rich Akt substrate of 40 kDa (PRAS40), a novel downstream target of PI3K/Akt signalling pathway. *Cell Signalling*, **24** (1), 17–24.

Wang, L., Harris, T.E., Roth, R.A. and Lawrence, J.C., Jr, (2007) PRAS40 regulates mTORC1 kinase activity by functioning as a direct inhibitor of substrate binding. *Journal of Biological Chemistry*, **282** (27), 20036–20044.

Wang, X. and Proud, C.G. (2011) mTORC1 signaling: what we still don't know. *Journal of Molecular Cell Biology*, **3** (4), 206–220.

Wang, Z., Zhong, J., Inuzuka, H. *et al.* (2012) An evolving role for DEPTOR in tumor development and progression. *Neoplasia*, **14** (5), 368–375.

Weber, J.D. and Gutmann, D.H. (2012) Deconvoluting mTOR biology. *Cell Cycle*, **11** (2), 236–246.

Willems, L., Tamburini, J., Chapuis, N. *et al.* (2012) PI3K and mTOR signalling pathways in cancer: new data on target therapies. *Current Oncology Reports*, **14** (2), 129–138.

Xie, X. and Guan, K. L. (2011) The ribosome and TORC2: collaborators for cell growth. *Cell*, **144** (5), 640–642.

Xing, M (2005) BRAF mutation in thyroid cancer. *Endocrine-related Cancer*, **12**, 245–262 as cited in Dazert and Hall (2011).

Yan, L. and Lamb, R.F. (2012) Amino acid sensing and regulation of mTORC1. *Seminars in Cell and Developmental Biology*, **23** (6), 621–625.

Yap, T.A., Carden, C.P. and Kaye, S.B. (2009) Beyond chemotherapy: targeted therapies in ovarian cancer. *Nature Reviews Cancer*, **9** (3), 167–181.

Yokogami, K., Wakisaka, S., Avruch, J. and Reeves, S.A. (2000) Serine phosphorylation and maximal activation of STAT3 during CNTF signalling is mediated by the rapamycin target mTOR. *Current Biology*, **10** (1), 47–50.

Zaytseva, Y.Y., Valentino, J.D., Gulhati, P. and Evers, B.M. (2012) mTOR inhibitors in cancer therapy. *Cancer Letters*, **319** (1), 1–7.

Zhao, Y., Xiong, X. and Sun, Y. (2011) DEPTOR, an mTOR inhibitor, is a physiological substrate of SCFβTrCP E3 ubiquitin ligase and regulates survival and autophagy. *Molecular Cell*, **44** (2), 304–316.

Zinzalla, V., Stracka, D., Oppliger, W. and Hall, M.N. (2011) Activation of mTORC2 by association with the ribosome. *Cell*, **144** (5), 757–768.

6

c–Met receptor signalling

Stephen Hiscox

School of Pharmacy and Pharmaceutical Sciences, Cardiff University

c-Met is a receptor tyrosine kinase that instigates signalling programmes resulting in an array of biological responses including cell proliferation and survival, angiogenesis and migration. Whilst these c-Met-driven processes are essential for normal embryonic development, particularly of the liver and muscle, liver regeneration and wound healing, the consequences of deregulated c-Met signalling, as occurs in cancer, are tumour progression and metastasis. The important role that c-Met plays in this context has led to the development of therapeutic approaches which seek to disrupt c-Met signalling in order to improve outcome for cancer patients.

6.1 Historical context – identification of the *MET* gene

The *MET* gene was first identified in the early 1980s as an oncogene (Cooper *et al.*, 1984) DNA extracted from a human osteosarcoma (HOS) cell line treated with a methylating chemical carcinogen (MNNG) was found to be able to transform NIH 3T3 cells. This suggested that treatment of HOS cells with carcinogens had resulted in genetic alterations and that mutated genes exerted a transforming capacity. By molecular cloning, MNNG-induced transforming gene (termed '*MET*' for its role in metastasis) was mapped to chromosome 7 (7q31) and subsequent work (Park *et al.*, 1986a; Dean *et al.*, 1987) identified that MNNG-treatment promoted a DNA rearrangement where a fusion of sequences from the TPR (translocated promoter region) locus on chromosome 1 and sequences from the MET locus on chromosome 7 occurred (Park *et al.*, 1986b). Further analysis of the *MET* nucleotide sequence identified it as a member of the kinase growth factor receptor family of oncogenes, although it lacked significant sequence homology with other growth factor receptor proteins, apart from the kinase domain (Dean *et al.*, 1985; Park *et al.*, 1987).

Cancer Cell Signalling, First Edition. Edited by Amanda Harvey.
© 2013 John Wiley & Sons, Ltd. Published 2013 by John Wiley & Sons, Ltd.

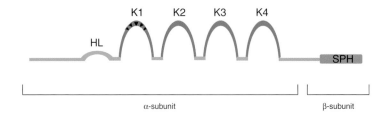

Figure 6.1   Schematic representation of HGF structure. The full-length molecule comprises a 69 kDa α-subunit and a 34 kDa β-subunit, which together represent six domains within the HGF molecule: an *N*-terminal hairpin loop (HL), four kringle domains (K1–K4) and a *C*-terminal serine protease homology (SPH) domain. The lack of proteolytic activity in the SPH domain arises from replacement of the histidine (H) and serine (S) with glutamine (Q) and tyrosine (Y), respectively. A high affinity c-Met binding site exists within K1 of the α-subunit (▼▼▼).

6.1.1   c-Met protein structure

The c-Met receptor is synthesised from the *MET* proto-oncognene as a single, 1436 amino acid polypeptide chain proteolytically processed into the mature 185 kDa transmembrane heterodimer (Migliore and Giordano, 2008). This heterodimer comprises two subunits, α and β, with the α-unit being entirely extracellular and the β-unit possessing extracellular, membrane-spanning and cytoplasmic regions (Figure 6.1).

Extracellular region

The extracellular region of Met comprises three different domains: an SEMA domain (homologous to the SEMA domain of the semaphorins and plexins) that is made up of the whole of the α-subunit and part of the β-subunit, a PSI domain (a domain also present in the **p**lexins, **s**emaphorins and **i**ntegrins), and four IPT domains (related to **i**mmunoglobulin-like domains present in **p**lexins and **t**ranscription factors), which function as general protein–protein interaction site (Comoglio *et al.*, 1993; Comoglio *et al.*, 2008. The extracellular ligand binding site in the c-Met protein is contained in regions within the *N*-terminal domain spanning the α-chain (amino acids 25–307) and the first 212 amino acids of the β-chain Gherardi *et al.*, 2003).

Intracellular region

The intracellular region of c-Met consists of three elements: a juxtamembrane sequence, important for the down-regulation of c-Met kinase activity upon phosphorylation of Ser975, a catalytic region that activates c-Met kinase activity following phosphorylation of Tyr1234 and Tyr1235, and a *C*-terminal multifunctional docking site that contains two docking tyrosine residues (Tyr1349 and Tyr1356) essential for downstream signalling (Comoglio *et al.*, 2008; Trusolino *et al.*, 2010).

6.1.2 HGF, the c-Met receptor ligand

Concurrent with the studies detailed earlier that identified the *MET* gene were other studies that ultimately revealed the ligand for the c-Met receptor: the first was concerned with the characterisation of a potent, fibroblast-derived modulator of epithelial cell motility termed 'scatter factor' (SF) (Stoker *et al.*, 1987), whilst the second study sought to understand mechanistically the remarkable ability of the liver to regenerate rapidly (for example, after removal of 60% of rodent liver mass, the remaining tissues rapidly expand to compensate for this loss in tissue, a process that takes only one week). This potent hepatocyte mitogenic factor was identified and termed 'hepatocyte growth factor' (HGF) (Nakamura *et al.*, 1986; Nakamura *et al.*, 1987). Subsequently, SF and HGF were identified as being the same molecule (Weidner *et al.*, 1991) and, importantly, the ligand for the c-Met receptor (Boaro *et al.*, 1991; Schmidt *et al.*, 1995; Bladt *et al.*, 1995).

HGF structure

HGF is a multidomain protein synthesised as a single chain inactive precursor molecule that is proteolytically converted into a functional heterodimer by extra-cellular proteases. The active HGF molecule comprises two disulphide-linked subunits of 69 kDa (α-subunit) and 34 kDa (β-subunit) in size (Nakamure *et al.*, 1989) (Figure 6.2). The complete HGF molecule consists of six domains: an *N*-terminal hairpin loop domain (HL), four kringle domains (80aa protein domains folded into loops and stabilised by disulphide bonds, which are important for protein–protein interactions) termed K1–K4, and a serine protease homology (SPH) domain, which lacks enzymatic activity. A high-affinity c-Met binding site is found within the first kringle domain of the α-chain and recognises the IPT3 and IPT4 domains of MET independently of HGF processing and maturation (Basilico *et al.*, 2008). HGF also contains a low-affinity site within its β-chain, which is only exposed after activation of HGF; this site interacts with the SEMA domain of MET (Stamos *et al.*, 2004).

HGF expression

The major sources of HGF are the mesenchymal cells of tissues – these secrete inactive HGF into the surrounding extracellular matrix (ECM) where it is sequestered by binding to heparin-like proteoglycan molecules (Lyon *et al.*, 1994; Lyon and Gallagher, 1994). HGF within the ECM is subsequently able to exert paracrine effects on surrounding epithelial cells that express the c-Met receptor.

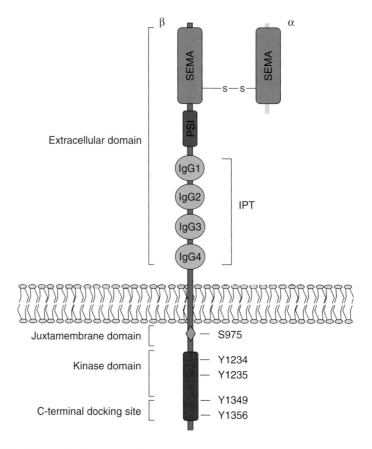

Figure 6.2 Schematic representation of the c-Met receptor structure. The mature c-Met protine is 185 kDa in size and consists of an extracellular α-subunit and a β-subunit, which spans the plasma membrane. The extracellular regions of both subunits contain SEMA domains whist the β-subunit also contains a PSI domain and four immunoglobulin repeats making up an IPT region. Several elements of the intracellular β-subunit play important roles in c-Met activation: phosphorylation of S975 in the juxtamembrane region down-regulated c-Met activity whilst ligand binding results in phosphorylation of two tyrosines (Y1234 and Y1235) in the kinase domain. Phosphorylation of two additional tyrosines (Y1349 and Y1356) downstream of the kinase domain create further docking sites for intracellular signalling proteins.

Expression of HGF in mesenchymal cells, and also c-Met in epithelial cells, can be up-regulated in response to cytokines released in response to tissue injury including TGFβ, IL-1 and IL-6 (Trusolino *et al.*, 2010; Matsumoto and Nakamura, 1996). Activation of inactive HGF through proteolytic processing also represents a further mechanism that can contribute to the process of c-Met-mediated tissue regeneration and repair, as experimental studies have shown that induction of tissue injury results in proteolytic processing of HGF exclusively within the injured tissue (Miyazawa *et al.*, 1994), a process in which the HGF-activator (HGFA) protein appears to play a central role (Miyazawwa, 2010).

6.2   c-Met expression, activation and signal transduction

The c-Met receptor is expressed in a variety of normal cell types and tissues where it mediates physiological and pathological processes (discussed in Sections 6.4 and 6.5). Activation of the c-Met receptor occurs following binding of its ligand, HGF, promoting receptor dimerisation and trans-phosphorylation of two tyrosine residues in the activation loop of the tyrosine kinase domain (Y1234 and Y1235) (Ferracini *et al.*, 1991). Subsequently, phosphorylation of two additional tyrosine residues (Y1349 and Y1356) occurs within the *C*-terminal tail, creating docking sites for recruitment of a number of kinase substrates, including phosphatidylinositol 3-kinase (PI3K)/Akt and signal transducer and activator of transcription 3 (STAT3) and also proteins with scaffolding/adaptor functions, such as growth factor receptor-bound protein 2 (Grb2), Grb2-associated adaptor protein (Gab1), Son of Sevenless (SOS) and SRC homology protein tyrosine phosphatase 3 (Shp2). The net result of these interactions is the activation of downstream signalling pathways that include the mitogen-activated protein kinase (MAPK)/extracellular signal-regulated kinase 1 (ERK1) and ERK2 pathways, JNK and p38 pathway and phosphatidylinositol 3-kinase–Akt (PI3K–Akt). Thus the downstream signalling pathways engaged as a consequence of c-Met activation include signalling modulators common to many receptor tyrosine kinases. These pathways have been reviewed in detail (Trusolini *et al.*, 2010) and are summarised here in Figure 6.3. Activation of c-Met-mediated downstream signalling results in initiation of a diverse array of biological responses encompassing cell proliferation, survival, invasion and migration.

The diversity of c-Met signalling can be further augmented through physical interactions between the c-Met receptor and a network of regulators and co-receptors. Interactions between c-Met and adaptor proteins such as GAB1 and the β4 subunit of the α6β4 integrin, which have their own specificity for distinct subsets of signalling proteins, link c-Met with additional pathways thereby broadening the consequences of cellular c-Met activation (Lai *et al.*, 2009; Furge *et al.*, 2000). The c-Met receptor may also interact with other receptors such as CD44 (Orian-Rousseau *et al.*, 2002), particularly the variant 6 and 10 isoforms. In the former case, this facilitates formation of a CD44v6/HGF/c-Met complex resulting in c-Met activation whilst also allowing the cytoplasmic domain of c-Met to be linked, via CD44-associated ERM (ezrin, radixin, moesin) proteins, to the actin cytoskeleton and resulting in Ras activation in response to HGF. Interactions between c-Met and CD44v10 have been described in endothelial cells where this results in partitioning of c-Met into caveolin-enriched membrane signalling domains along with the RAC1 exchange factor, T-lymphoma invasion and metastasis-inducing protein 1 (TIAM1), cortactin (an actin cytoskeletal regulator) and dynamin 2 (a vesicular regulator) (Singleton *et al.*, 2007). In addition, association between c-Met and members of the plexin family of receptor proteins facilitates semaphornin-dependent transactivation of c-Met and downstream signalling (Conrotto *et al.*, 2004) suggesting further mechanisms for c-Met activation

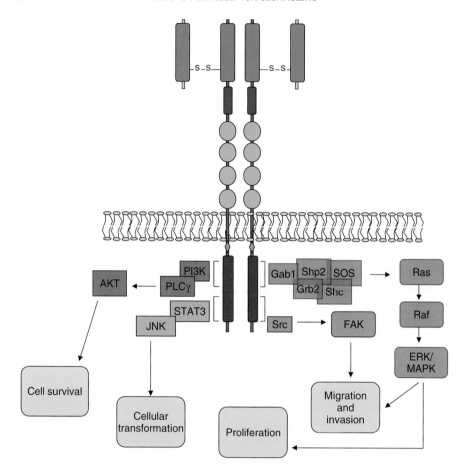

Figure 6.3　**Key intracellular binding partners for c-Met.** Binding of HGF to the c-Met receptor results in homodimerisation and receptor autophosphorylation at Y1234 and Y1235). Subsequent phosphorylation at Y1349 and Y1356 create binding sites for a variety of c-Met substrates as shown initiating intracellular signalling pathways that result in the biological responses shown. Colour has been used to highlight individual pathways, however the adaptor proteins/kinases indicated are shared between different pathways (see Chapters 1, 2, 5, 7 and 9).

independent of HGF. These instances of c-Met cross-talk with other membrane proteins points to the dynamic nature of the cellular c-Met function and demonstrates the capacity for cellular augmentation of biological responses in which c-Met is involved.

6.2.1　Regulation of Met signalling

Negative regulation of c-Met signalling is crucial to maintain its tightly-controlled cellular activity and prevent aberrant activation. Endogenous regulation of c-Met activation and signalling occur through two broad mechanisms: endocytotic trafficking/proteosomal degradation and also sequential proteolytic cleavage at juxtamembrane sites within c-Met. HGF activation of c-Met leads to receptor ubiquitination (Peschard *et al.*, 2001) and entry into early endosomes prior to sorting into multivesicular bodies. These structures ultimately fuse with lysosomes leading to receptor degradation (Kermorgant and Parker, 2008). Interestingly, internalisation of c-Met is also important for STAT3 activation, where PKCα-mediated c-Met sorting targets the receptor to a peri-nuclear location where it can interact with STAT3, promoting its nuclear translocation.

Met signalling can also be down-regulated through proteolytic cleavage, which occurs sequentially at two juxtamembrane sites within the molecule. The first cleavage, mediated by ADAM (**a d**isintegrin **a**nd **m**etalloprotease) family members, results in generation of a c-Met fragment that sequesters HGF thus antagonising receptor activity. Cleavage at a second site within the intracellular domain is mediated by a γ-secretase and results in a fragment that is proteosomally degraded (Foveau *et al.*, 2009).

6.3 Physiological roles of c-Met

c-Met is generally expressed in epithelial cells and activated by its natural ligand, HGF, in a paracrine manner when produced by surrounding mesenchymal cells, or in an endocrine fashion when present within the circulation. During embryogenesis c-Met signalling is necessary for the development of many tissues, including the placenta, liver, kidney and neuronal tissue and also for the directional migration of skeletal muscle cells. In adult tissues, c-Met signalling promotes regeneration and wound healing. Thus, through eliciting biological growth, survival and migration responses, the c-Met receptor pathway has been implicated in tissue remodelling, developmental morphogenesis, wound repair and organ homeostasis.

6.3.1 c-Met and development

HGF-induced c-Met activation is well established as an essential element of the developmental process, where it is responsible for 3D morphogenesis and organogenesis. Early studies sought to examine the physiological role of c-Met in development through generation of mouse models harbouring targeted disruption of the *MET* or *HGF* genes. Embryos from these models fail to survive due to impaired placental development and, in addition, display livers that are significantly smaller and have higher levels of apoptosis than normal embryos (Schmidt *et al.*, 1995; Uehara *et al.*, 1995).

c-Met signalling also participates in the migration of cells during development, a process required for the establishment of numerous tissues and organs. For example, expression of c-Met in myogenic precursor cells in the dermo-myotome facilitates their HGF-induced migration to the limb buds and diaphragm where they differentiate into skeletal muscle cells. Experimental ablation of the *HGF* or *MET* gene results in impairment of migratory capacity of these precursor cells and an absence of skeletal muscle in mouse embryos (Bladt *et al.*, 1995).

c-Met expression and activity is also a prerequisite for the successful development of the vertebrate nervous system. Axons within the developing nervous system are guided to their targets by chemoattractants produced by cells within the target tissues and organs. Expression of c-Met in axonal cells has been shown to facilitate their HGF-induced migration towards muscle and also their survival at later stages of development (Ebens *et al.*, 1996). c-Met is also implicated in glial as well as neuronal development since c-Met expression on oligodendrocyte progenitor cells facilitates their differentiation into oligodendrocytes (Ohya *et al.*, 2007).

6.3.2 Tissue morphogenesis and organogenesis

HGF-c-Met signalling plays an important role in the regulation of epithelial development and organ morphogenesis. c-Met is expressed in epithelial cells that are in close proximity to the neighbouring mesenchymal cells which produce HGF. This suggests a paracrine mode of regulation of the behaviour of c-Met expressing cells. Such epithelial–mesenchymal interactions mediate crucial aspects of development and affect tissue induction and epithelial morphogenesis and include stimulation of branching tubulogenesis within the kidney epithelia, mammary glands and lung and morphogenesis of tooth epithelium (Birchmeier and Gherardi, 1998).

c-Met signalling is essential for regeneration of the liver (Borowiak *et al.*, 2004) and also the skin during wound repair (Chmielowiec *et al.*, 2007). More recently, c-Met has been implicated in regeneration of heart tissue by exerting a cardioprotective role: c-Met expression and activity are usually low in adult cardiomyocytes, however, in response to heart injury, *MET* and *HGF* gene expression are up-regulated, which results in enhanced c-Met signalling ad initiation of apoptosis resistance mechanisms (Nakamura *et al.*, 2000; Ueda *et al.*, 2001) and cardiac regeneration (Urbanek *et al.*, 2005). These observations suggest that stimulation of Met activity by HGF may present a means to treat post-ischemic heart failure. However, the cardioprotective role of c-Met is not clear since, in contrast to these observations, over-activation of the Met receptor in embryonic development has been shown to result in cardiac damage, suggesting that Met may be implicated in the pathogenesis of cardiac disease (Leo *et al.*, 2011).

More recently, studies in rodents have pointed to some novel physiological roles of c-Met signalling: its role in learning and memory function has been proposed based on observations that mice, in which brain levels of HGF have been experimentally up-regulated, displayed an improved short- and long-term memory function, demonstrated by better performance in maze tests (Kato *et al.*, 2012). A role for c-Met in pregnancy, specifically maternal β-cell adaptation, may also be apparent since pregnant mice lacking pancreatic c-Met display detrimental alterations in β-cell proliferation and gestational diabetes mellitus (Demirci *et al.*, 2012). Given that gestational diabetes mellitus is one of the most common metabolic disorders during pregnancy, identification of c-Met as a potential contributor in this disorder presents a potential means of therapeutic intervention.

6.4 c-Met and cancer

c-Met signalling is fundamental to proteolytic remodelling of the extracellular matrix and promotes cell proliferation, migration and invasion. In cancer, the c-Met pathway can be deregulated leading to tumour progression and metastasis, the most important factor that determine a patient's prognosis.

Over-expression of either c-Met or HGF in cell lines prior to their implantation into nude mice provided the initial evidence that c-Met signalling can promote an invasive, metastatic phenotype (Rong *et al.*, 1994). Additionally, mice engineered to express c-Met or HGF were shown to develop metastatic tumours (Takayama *et al.*, 1997) whilst down-regulation of c-Met expression in human tumour cells is reported to be associated with a loss of tumour growth and metastatic capacity (Liang *et al.*, 2004; Abounader *et al.*, 2002; Herynk *et al.*, 2003).

Deregulated c-Met expression and/or activity plays a key role in tumour progression and may occur through a number of mechanisms including: (i) mutations within the *MET* gene leading to receptor activation, c-Met amplification, modulation of ligand binding or loss of receptor down-regulation, (ii) autocrine production of HGF and (iii) over-expression of c-Met and/or HGF.

6.4.1 Mutations

Over 20 mutations in the *MET* gene have been identified. Whilst somatic mutations on the *MET* gene are rarely found in patients with nonhereditary cancer, missense mutations have been identified in the tyrosine kinase domain, the SEMA and juxtamembrane domains (Cipriani *et al.*, 2009).

Mutations in the *MET* kinase region resulting in a constitutively active c-Met receptor have been identified in a variety of tumour types including lung cancer (NSCLC), hepatocellular carcinomas, gliomas, gastric and breast carcinomas (Stella *et al.*, 2011; Ma *et al.*, 2008; Giordano *et al.*, 2000). *MET* mutations have also been identified in renal carcinoma (Schmidt *et al.*, 2004), the functional consequence of which is to enhance both intrinsic c-Met activity and also ligand sensitivity, promoting a tumourogenic phenotype in animal models (Jeffers *et al.*, 1997).

Although relatively rare, intronic mutations of the *MET* gene have been reported in lung cancer, which result in the production of alternatively-spliced MET transcripts that encode a version of the c-Met receptor lacking in the juxtamembrane domain. This leads to loss of Cbl E3-ligase binding and enhanced receptor expression through loss of control of receptor down-regulation (Kong-Beltran *et al.*,

2006). The frequency of MET mutations in lung cancer appear to vary with ethnicity, with an N375S mutation observed to be prevalent within the East Asian population and males smokers (Krishnaswamy *et al.*, 2009). Interestingly, this particular mutation appears to confer cellular resistance to small molecule MET inhibitors, possibly through affecting HGF-c-Met binding since this mutation occurs in the semaphorin domain of the met receptor. This in turn may result in less efficient ligand-induced Met activation and thus a reduced sensitivity to the inhibitor.

MET gene amplification has been reported in lung cancers possessing EGFR mutations (Bean *et al.*, 2009) where it is associated with resistance to EGFR inhibitors (Engelman *et al.*, 2007). Furthermore, amplification of *MET* is reported in approximately 20% of tumours with acquired resistance to EGFR inhibitors compared with only 7% (maximum) of EGFR inhibitor-naïve tumour suggesting that co-targeting of MET and EGFR might offer an important therapeutic opportunity in lung cancer.

Mutations within the juxtamembrane region (T1010I and G1085X) and the SEMA domain (N375S, M431V and N454I) have been identified in mesothelioma cell lines and patient tissues (Jagadeeswaran *et al.*, 2006), which may influence receptor down-regulation and HGF binding, respectively.

6.4.2   Autocrine HGF production

Intrinsic activation of c-Met can also occur through autocrine production of HGF. This has been reported for tumours such as osteosarcomas and rabdomyosarcomas that are derived from mesenchymal, HGF-producing cells. Autocrine activation of c-Met as a consequence of intrinsic HGF production has been identified in human glioblastomas (Xie *et al.*, 2012), myeloma (Borset *et al.*, 1996) and Hodgkin lymphoma (Teofili *et al.*, 2001). Over-expression of both HGF and c-Met in breast epithelial cells leads to autocrine c-Met activation and mammary tumorigenesis and metastasis (Gallego *et al.*, 2003; Rahimi *et al.*, 1996; Tuck *et al.*, 1996), whilst co-expression of HGF and c-Met has also been reported in breast cancer, where it is associated with a mesenchyme-like invasive phenotype and a poor prognosis (Elliott *et al.*, 2002; Jin *et al.*, 1997).

6.4.3   c-Met/HGF over-expression in tumours

Over-expression of the c-Met receptor in the tumour tissue and/or its ligand in surrounding stromal cells represents the most frequent mechanism of Met deregulation found in human cancer. c-Met/HGF over-expression is reported in a wide variety of human tumours encompassing both solid malignancies including breast, colon, lung, ovary, liver, kidney, pancreatic and prostate cancers and also haematopoietic malignancies such as lymphomas (reviewed in Birchmeier *et al.*,

2003). Over-expression of c-Met and/or HGF are associated with increased tumour aggressiveness, higher stage/grade disease and are correlated with a poor clinical outcome (Birchmeier *et al.*, 2003; Kmmula *et al.*, 2007; Abounader and Laterra, 2005).

Tumours exist within a microenviroment populated by other cells including those of mesenchymal origin and of the immune system; these cell types are the major source of HGF. Biological cross-talk between tumour and stroma represents a major route to the paracrine activation of c-Met and such events are augmented in the context of increased c-Met and/or HGF expression.

6.4.4   Met and tumour progression

c-Met signalling activities have emerged as a critical feature of the majority of human cancers and is linked to a poor outcome (Knudsen *et al.*, 2008). Such clinical correlations are not surprising, given the role that c-Met has in mediating biological behaviours that are central to tumour progression and metastasis. Key pathways regulated by c-Met in this context are detailed in the following sections.

Angiogenesis

Angiogenesis represents a process fundamental to both tumour formation and dissemination. HGF-mediated activation of c-Met is known to be a potent promoter of endothelial cell growth and promotes angiogenesis and lymphamgiogenesis in cell models and *in vivo* (Abounader and Laterra, 2005; Bussolini *et al.*, 1992; Nakagawa *et al.*, 2010). Importantly, activation of the c-Met pathway can alter the balance of expression of pro/anti-angiogeneic factors in favour of the former. As such, c-Met signalling has been demonstrated to induce expression of the major angiogenic-promoting ligand, VEGFA, whilst suppressing thrombospondin 1 (TSP1), a negative regulator of angiogenesis (Zhang *et al.*, 2003). A level of synergy exists between c-Met and the VEGFR, with activation of these receptors augmenting angiogenesis *in vivo*; this level of interaction has been suggested to occur through downstream signalling elements common to both pathways including MAPK, AKT and FAK (Sulpice *et al.*, 2009).

Of particular importance to its role in angiogenesis is the fact that c-Met is a target of the HIF-1α (hypoxia-inducible factor 1α) transcription factor (Comito *et al.*, 2011; Pennacchietti *et al.*, 2003). Subsequently, hypoxia-driven c-Met expression has been described for a number of tumour types including pancreatic cancer (Kitajima *et al.*, 2008), glioma (Eckerich *et al.*, 2007), breast cancer (Chen *et al.*, 2007) and salivary gland tumours (Hara *et al.*, 2006).

Although the predominant site of c-Met expression are the epithelial cells, c-Met is also expressed on endothelial cells (Bussolino *et al.*, 1992) where it can promote endothelial proliferation and migration to form new vessels (Cantelmo *et al.*, 2010). The important role that c-Met plays in angiogenesis is further underscored by clinical studies which report that c-Met expression is associated with greater levels of tumour vascularisation and metastasis (Strohmeyer *et al.*, 2004).

Migration, invasion and metastasis

One of the central aspects of cellular behaviour controlled by c-Met is that of invasion and migration, and as such the role of c-Met signalling in tumour spread has gained wide interest over the past few decades. Indeed, the presence of activated c-Met is associated with a migratory phenotype in a wide range of tumours including prostate (Dai and Sieman, 2012), melanoma (Kwak *et al.*, 2011), gastric (Park *et al.*, 2005) and renal cancer (Nakamura *et al.*, 2001).

Mechanistically, the effects of c-Met on migratory behaviour appear to occur through activation of PI3K and subsequent PI3K-dependent cytoskeletal regulation (Nakamura *et al.*, 2001; Maulik *et al.*, 2002). However, c-Met-promoted migratory responses are not exclusive to this pathway as HGF also promotes transcription of genes involved in migratory responses through a process involving enhancement of ERK and MPK2 phosphatase activation, which then down-regulate the activity of JNK, a transcriptional inhibitor of HGF response (Paumelle *et al.*, 2000). c-Met mediated ERK activation can also result in activation of RNA modulating proteins of the Sam family and migratory responses in breast cancer (Locatelli and Lange, 2011).

c-Met mediated migratory responses can also occur through activation of focal adhesion kinase (FAK), which is localised to cellular adhesion complexes. FAK is activated downstream of c-Met through phosphorylation by members of the Src kinase family, which have been shown to associate directly with c-Met (Ponzetto *et al.*, 1994). The interaction between activated c-Met, Src and FAK results in cell migration (Hui *et al.*, 2009). One explanation for this is that activation of FAK signalling can result in integrin expression and modulate cancer cell-extracellular matrix adhesive interactions, important for migratory behaviour (Matsumoto *et al.*, 1994).

Recently, intriguing data have revealed that activation of c-Met can promote expression of the v5 isoform of CD44 in keratinocytes, a CD44 associated with cancer progression, through a mechanism involving ERK activation of the RNA processing protein Sam68 (Locatelli and Lange, 2011).

Activation of c-Met signalling can also result in increased expression and secretion of proteolytic enzymes from cancer cells including MMP2, MMP7, MMP9 and uPA that are involved in matrix and basement membrane degradation (Davies *et al.*, 2001; Dunsmore *et al.*, 1996; Rosenthal *et al.*, 1998). As such, the c-Met pathway also results in invasive cell behaviour able to support a metastatic phenotype. As a consequence, c-Met has been shown to drive invasive responses in skin (Syed *et al.*, 2011), ovarian (Zillhardt *et al.*, 2011) and bladder cancers (Yeh *et al.*, 2011) *in vitro* and *in vivo*. c-Met may additionally promote tumour cell invasion through cross-talk with other pathways. For example, interaction between c-Met and the WNT pathway which can occur at a transcriptional level is associated with breast cancer invasion (Huang *et al.*, 2012a; Previdi *et al.*, 2010).

In view of the role of c-Met on tumour cell migration and invasion, one would expect c-Met to exert some considerable influence on the metastatic capacity of tumour cells. Consequently, the ability of HGF-induced c-Met signalling to induce metastasis has been widely reported.

c-Met signalling through PI3K and PKCzeta have been shown to promote expression of the chemokine receptor, CXCR4 (Huang *et al.*, 2012b) which, when activated by its ligand, CXCL12, has been demonstrated to mediate the metastasis of many malignant tumours.

c-Met and drug resistance

One area of particular importance in which c-Met has been implicated is that of drug resistance. Acquired resistance to the BRAF inhibitor, PLX4032, in BRAF-mutant melanoma is mediated by c-Met in concert with Src kinase (Vergani *et al.*, 2011), whilst high levels of c-Met protein are reported on endothelial cells from tumours resistant to the VEGFR inhibitor, sunitinib (Shojaei *et al.*, 2010), suggesting a role for an HGF/c-Met pathway in development of resistance to anti-angiogenic therapy. Furthermore, amplification of *MET* has been implicated in driving resistance to EGFR therapies in lung cancer (Engleman *et al.*, 2007); interestingly, a number of studies have reported that a large cohort of lung cancers representing tumours that have relapsed on EGFR inhibitor treatment display *MET* amplification (Bean *et al.*, 2007; Turke *et al.*, 2010; Cappuzzo *et al.*, 2009). Given that a low incidence of *MET* amplification is reported for EGFR inhibitor-naïve tumours, these data suggest that existence of drug-resistant clones harbouring amplified *MET* may exist within the initial tumour population (Turke *et al.*, 2010).

One mechanism proposed to explain the consequence of c-Met activation for drug response and resistance is that the up-regulation of c-Met activity and signalling likely leads to the activation of downstream signalling intermediates common to a number of receptor tyrosine kinase pathways. Thus, inhibition of EGFR itself may not necessarily prevent the activation of its signalling components shared with the c-Met pathway. Cross-talk between c-Met and other receptors appears also to represent a key mechanism underlying c-Met mediated therapeutic resistance (Lai *et al.*, 2009). In such cases, transphosphorylation of other receptor tyrosine kinases such as erbB family members by c-Met can amplify the biological effects of c-Met activation.

6.4.5   Prognostic value of c-Met and HGF

A number of studies on clinical tissue have demonstrated that high levels of c-Met and/or HGF expression are associated with a poor patient outcome. For example, over-expression of c-Met and HGF are widely reported in lung adenocarcinomas where they correlate with metastasis, therapeutic resistance and represent a poor prognostic indicator (De Bacco *et al.*, 2011; Matsui *et al.*,

2010; Navab *et al.*, 2009; Masuya *et al.*, 2004). In breast cancer, high levels of c-Met/HGF are associated with advanced histological grade, high proliferation rate, metastasis and a poor prognosis (Chen *et al.*, 2007; Garcia *et al.*, 2007; Edakuni *et al.*, 2001; Yamashita *et al.*, 1994).

6.5   c-Met as a potential therapeutic target in malignancy

In light of the pro-metastatic role that it plays in cancer, c-Met represents an obvious target for the development of anti-tumour therapies (Migliore and Giordano, 2008). With this in mind, several lines of approach have been taken that seek to antagonise c-Met signalling at various levels, including peptides and antibodies that interfere with ligand binding and receptor dimerisation and the direct inhibition of c-Met activity using small molecule inhibitors.

6.5.1   c-Met peptides

c-Met peptides are large molecules derived from the carboxy-terminal tail region of the c-Met receptor. Binding of these peptides to c-Met subsequently inhibits HGF binding and migration/invasion signalling (Bardelli *et al.*, 1999).

6.5.2   c-Met antibodies

The therapeutic strategy of targeting c-Met signalling using monoclonal antibodies has displayed promising results in c-Met-over-expressing tumours or in the context of increased HGF production. Antibody-mediated inhibition of the c-Met pathway can be achieved either by targeting the c-Met directly, or through targeting HGF.

Early studies revealed that antibody-mediated targeting of HGF resulted in effective inhibition of c-Met signalling and suppression of cancer cell growth (Cao *et al.*, 2001). Subsequent development of antibody-mediated therapeutic approaches has led to the development of agents that can block binding of HGF with c-Met and thus c-Met activation. Rilotumumab (AMG102) is one such antibody (Giordano, 2009) and is currently being tested in Phase I/II clinical trials (Wen *et al.*, 2011; Schoffski *et al.*, 2011) where it has been found to suppress c-Met phosphorylation and is associated with disease stabilisation.

A number of antibodies that target the c-Met receptor have been developed. MetMAb (OA-5D5) (Jin *et al.*, 2008) is a monovalent antibody that binds to the SEMA domain of c-Met and antagonises receptor activation by HGF. MetMAb has been shown to suppress *in vivo* growth and metastasis of glioblastoma and pancreatic cancer cells (Jin *et al.*, 2008; Martens *et al.*, 2006); in Phase II clinical trials of lung cancer patients, MetMAb has been tested in combination with the EGFR inhibitor, erlotinib, and found to extend patient survival in tumours that are c-Met positive (Surati *et al.*, 2011). A further bivalent c-Met antibody, DN-30 (Petrelli *et al.*, 2006), also antagonises c-Met activity through promoting receptor down-regulation.

6.5.3 c-Met tyrosine kinase inhibitors

Small molecules designed to target the c-Met tyrosine kinase domain represent the largest class of c-Met inhibitory compounds. Targeting of receptor tyrosine kinases using small molecules has proven effective in many cases and thus taking such an approach to suppress c-Met activity may well represent a promising strategy.

Several small molecule inhibitors selective for c-Met are currently being investigated for their anti-tumour effects. SU11274 (Sugen Inc.) binds to c-Met, preventing its phosphorylation at sites that promote signalling through the PI3K, AKT and mTOR pathway (Sattler *et al.*, 2003). Interestingly, this compound has also recently been demonstrated to induce ERK-dependent Bcl2 phoshphorylation and autophagy in lung cancer cells (Liu *et al.*, 2012). *In vivo* testing of this compound demonstrated effective inhibition of melanoma growth and metastasis (Kenessey *et al.*, 2010).

PHA665752 (Pfizer, Inc.) displays efficacy in cell models of lung cancer, where it inhibits phosphorylation of c-Met and downstream activation of AKT and p70-S6K (Ma *et al.*, 2005a). Furthermore, PHA665752 displays cooperative effects when used in combination with rapamycin in NSCLC cells, resulting in inhibition of tumour migration and growth and induction of cell cycle arrest and apoptosis (Ma *et al.*, 2005b). *In vivo*, PHA665752 treatment of mouse lung cancer xenografts resulted in a significant reduction in tumour volume and angiogenesis (Puri *et al.*, 2007).

A further small molecule inhibitor of c-Met kinase activity under development by Pfizer Inc. (PF2341066) also suppresses c-Met phosphorylation in lung cancer cells and is accompanied by a reduction in HGF-mediated migration and invasion *in vitro* and a reduction in tumour volume *in vivo* (Zou *et al.*, 2007). Importantly, this compound also inhibited HGF-stimulated endothelial cell survival and invasion and serum-stimulated tubulogenesis *in vitro*, pointing to its potential anti-angiogenic properties.

ARQ197 (Tivantinib, Arqule, Inc.) has shown pre-clinical activity against a number of human xenografts, and is currently undergoing testing in Phase II clinical trials following encouraging results in Phase I trials where the compound was well tolerated with stable disease reported in 50% of patients (Rosen *et al.*, 2011).

6.6 Summary

Since its discovery over two decades ago, the c-Met pathway has emerged as a key element within physiological developmental processes but also as a central factor governing tumour progression and spread. c-Met now represents an important target for cancer therapy with several c-Met inhibitory strategies being currently investigated for their ability to suppress tumour growth, invasion and metastasis. A further benefit from targeting this pathway appears to be the opportunity to circumvent resistance to anti-EGFR therapy. Although results from early-phase clinical trials are encouraging in that they confirm the importance and effectiveness of c-Met inhibition in cancer, c-Met monotherapies will invariably be met with resistance. The challenge now is to explore and exploit biological mechanisms that may lead to resistance to further improve c-Met targeted therapies in the clinic.

References

Abounader, R. and Laterra, J. (2005) Scatter factor/hepatocyte growth factor in brain tumor growth and angiogenesis. *Neuro-Oncology*, **7** (4), 436–451.

Abounader, R., Lal, B., Luddy, C. *et al.* (2002) In vivo targeting of SF/HGF and c-met expression via U1snRNA/ribozymes inhibits glioma growth and angiogenesis and promotes apoptosis. *FASEB Journal*, **16** (1), 108–110.

Bardelli, A., Longati, P., Williams, T.A. *et al.* (1999) A peptide representing the carboxyl-terminal tail of the met receptor inhibits kinase activity and invasive growth. *Journal of Biological Chemistry*, **274** (41), 29274–29281.

Basilico, C., Arnesano, A., Galluzzo, M. *et al.* (2008) A high affinity hepatocyte growth factor-binding site in the immunoglobulin-like region of Met. *Journal of Biological Chemistry*, **283** (30), 21267–21277.

Bean, J., Brennan, C., Shih, J.Y. *et al.* (2007) MET amplification occurs with or without T790M mutations in EGFR mutant lung tumors with acquired resistance to gefitinib or erlotinib. *Proceedings of the National Academy of Sciences, USA*, **104** (52), 20932–20937.

Birchmeier, C. and Gherardi, E. (1998) Developmental roles of HGF/SF and its receptor, the c-Met tyrosine kinase. *Trends in Cell Biology*, **8** (10), 404–410.

Birchmeier, C., Birchmeier, W., Gherardi, E. and Vande Woude, G.F. (2003) Met, metastasis, motility and more. *Nature Reviews Molecular Cell Biology*, **4** (12), 915–925.

Bladt, F., Riethmacher, D., Isenmann, S. *et al.* (1995) Essential role for the c-met receptor in the migration of myogenic precursor cells into the limb bud. *Nature*, **376** (6543), 768–771.

Borowiak, M., Garratt, A.N., Wustefeld, T. (2004) Met provides essential signals for liver regeneration. *Proceedings of the National Academy of Sciences, USA*, **101** (29), 10608–10613.

Borset, M., Hjorth-Hansen, H., Seidel, C. *et al.* (1996) Hepatocyte growth factor and its receptor c-met in multiple myeloma. *Blood*, **88** (10), 3998–4004.

Bottaro, D.P., Rubin, J.S., Faletto, D.L. *et al.* (1991) Identification of the hepatocyte growth factor receptor as the c-met proto-oncogene product. *Science*, **251** (4995), 802–804.

Bussolino, F., Di Renzo, M.F., Ziche, M. *et al.* (1992) Hepatocyte growth factor is a potent angiogenic factor which stimulates endothelial cell motility and growth. *Journal of Cell Biology*, **119** (3), 629–641.

Cantelmo, A.R., Cammarota, R., Noonan, D.M. *et al.* (2010) Cell delivery of Met docking site peptides inhibit angiogenesis and vascular tumor growth. *Oncogene*, **29** (38), 5286–5298.

Cao, B., Su, Y., Oskarsson, M., Zhao, P. *et al.* (2001) Neutralizing monoclonal antibodies to hepatocyte growth factor/scatter factor (HGF/SF) display antitumor activity in animal models. *Proceedings of the National Academy of Sciences, USA*, **98** (13), 7443–7448.

Cappuzzo, F., Janne, P.A., Skokan, M. *et al.* (2009) MET increased gene copy number and primary resistance to gefitinib therapy in non-small-cell lung cancer patients. *Annals of Oncology*, **20** (2), 298–304.

Chen, H.H., Su, W.C., Lin, P.W. *et al.* (2007) Hypoxia-inducible factor-1alpha correlates with MET and metastasis in node-negative breast cancer. *Breast Cancer Research and Treatment*, **103** (2), 167–175.

Chmielowiec, J., Borowiak, M., Morkel, M. *et al.* (2007) c-Met is essential for wound healing in the skin. *Journal of Cell Biology*, **177** (1), 151–162.

Cipriani, N.A., Abidoye, O.O., Vokes, E. and Salgia R (2009) MET as a target for treatment of chest tumors. *Lung Cancer*, **63** (2), 169–179.

Comito, G., Calvani, M., Giannoni, E. *et al.* (2011) HIF-1alpha stabilization by mitochondrial ROS promotes Met-dependent invasive growth and vasculogenic mimicry in melanoma cells. *Free Radical Biology and Medicine*, **51** (4), 893–904.

Comoglio, P.M. (1993) Structure, biosynthesis and biochemical properties of the HGF receptor in normal and malignant cells. *EXS*, **65**, 131–165.

Comoglio, P.M., Giordano, S. and Trusolino, L. (2008) Drug development of MET inhibitors: targeting oncogene addiction and expedience. *Nature Reviews Drug Discovery*, **7** (6), 504–516.

Conrotto, P., Corso, S., Gamberini, S. *et al.* (2004) Interplay between scatter factor receptors and B plexins controls invasive growth. *Oncogene*, **23** (30), 5131–5137.

Cooper, C.S., Park, M., Blair, D.G., *et al.* (1984) Molecular cloning of a new transforming gene from a chemically transformed human cell line. *Nature*, **311** (5981), 29–33.

Dai, Y. and Siemann, D.W. (2012) Constitutively active c-Met kinase in PC-3 cells is autocrine-independent and can be blocked by the Met kinase inhibitor BMS-777607. *BMC Cancer*, **12** (1), 198.

Davies, G., Jiang, W.G. and Mason, M.D. (2001) Matrilysin mediates extracellular cleavage of E-cadherin from prostate cancer cells: a key mechanism in hepatocyte growth factor/scatter factor-induced cell-cell dissociation and in vitro invasion. *Clinical Cancer Research*, **7** (10), 3289–3297.

De Bacco, F., Luraghi, P., Medico, E. *et al.* (2011) Induction of MET by ionizing radiation and its role in radioresistance and invasive growth of cancer. *Journal of the National Cancer Institute*, **103** (8), 645–661.

Dean, M., Park, M., Le Beau, M.M. *et al.* (1985) The human met oncogene is related to the tyrosine kinase oncogenes. *Nature*, **318** (6044), 385–388.

Dean, M., Park, M. and Vande Woude, G.F. (1987) Characterization of the rearranged tpr-met oncogene breakpoint. *Molecular and Cellular Biology*, **7** (2), 921–924.

Demirci, C., Ernst, S., Alvarez-Perez, J.C. *et al.* (2012) Loss of HGF/c-Met signaling in pancreatic beta-cells leads to incomplete maternal beta-cell adaptation and gestational diabetes mellitus. *Diabetes*, **61** (5), 1143–1152.

Dunsmore, S.E., Rubin, J.S., Kovacs, S.O. *et al.* (1996) Mechanisms of hepatocyte growth factor stimulation of keratinocyte metalloproteinase production. *Journal of Biological Chemistry*, **271** (40), 24576–24582.

Ebens, A., Brose, K., Leonardo, E.D. *et al.* (1996) Hepatocyte growth factor/scatter factor is an axonal chemoattractant and a neurotrophic factor for spinal motor neurons. *Neuron*, **17** (6), 1157–1172.

Eckerich, C., Zapf, S., Fillbrandt, R. *et al.* (2007) Hypoxia can induce c-Met expression in glioma cells and enhance SF/HGF-induced cell migration. *International Journal of Cancer*, **121** (2), 276–283.

Edakuni, G., Sasatomi, E., Satoh, T. *et al.* (2001) Expression of the hepatocyte growth factor/c-Met pathway is increased at the cancer front in breast carcinoma. *Pathology International*, **51** (3), 172–178.

Elliott, B.E., Hung, W.L., Boag, A.H. and Tuck, A.B. (2002) The role of hepatocyte growth factor (scatter factor) in epithelial-mesenchymal transition and breast cancer. *Canadian Journal of Physiology and Pharmacology*, **80** (2), 91–102.

Engelman, J.A., Zejnullahu, K., Mitsudomi, T. *et al.* (2007) MET amplification leads to gefitinib resistance in lung cancer by activating ERBB3 signaling. *Science*, **316** (5827), 1039–1043.

Ferracini, R., Longati, P., Naldini, L. *et al.* (1991) Identification of the major autophosphorylation site of the Met/hepatocyte growth factor receptor tyrosine kinase. *Journal of Biological Chemistry*, **266** (29), 19558–19564.

Foveau, B., Ancot, F., Leroy, C. *et al.* (2009) Down-regulation of the met receptor tyrosine kinase by presenilin-dependent regulated intramembrane proteolysis. *Molecular Biology of the Cell*, **20** (9), 2495–2507.

Furge, K.A., Zhang, Y.W. and Vande Woude, G.F. (2000) Met receptor tyrosine kinase: enhanced signaling through adapter proteins. *Oncogene*, **19** (49), 5582–5589.

Gallego, M.I., Bierie, B. and Hennighausen, L. (2003) Targeted expression of HGF/SF in mouse mammary epithelium leads to metastatic adenosquamous carcinomas through the activation of multiple signal transduction pathways. *Oncogene*, **22** (52), 8498–8508.

Garcia, S., Dales, J.P., Charafe-Jauffret, E. *et al.* (2007) Poor prognosis in breast carcinomas correlates with increased expression of targetable CD146 and c-Met and with proteomic basal-like phenotype. *Human Pathology*, **38** (6), 830–841.

Gherardi, E., Youles, M.E., Miguel, R.N. *et al.* (2003) Functional map and domain structure of MET, the product of the c-met protooncogene and receptor for hepatocyte growth factor/scatter factor. *Proceedings of the National Academy of Sciences, USA*, **100** (21), 12039–12044.

Giordano, S. (2009) Rilotumumab, a mAb against human hepatocyte growth factor for the treatment of cancer. *Current Opinion in Molecular Therapeutics*, **11** (4), 448–455.

Giordano, S., Maffe, A., Williams, T.A. *et al.* (2000) Different point mutations in the met oncogene elicit distinct biological properties. *FASEB Journal*, **14** (2), 399–406.

Hara, S., Nakashiro, K., Klosek, S.K. *et al.* (2006) Hypoxia enhances c-Met/HGF receptor expression and signaling by activating HIF-1alpha in human salivary gland cancer cells. *Oral Oncology*, **42** (6), 593–598.

Herynk, M.H., Stoeltzing, O., Reinmuth, N. *et al.* (2003) Down-regulation of c-Met inhibits growth in the liver of human colorectal carcinoma cells. *Cancer Research*, **63** (11), 2990–2996.

Huang, F.I., Chen, Y.L., Chang, C.N. *et al.* (2012a) Hepatocyte growth factor activates Wnt pathway by transcriptional activation of LEF1 to facilitate tumor invasion. *Carcinogenesis*, **33** (6), 1142–1148.

Huang, S., Ouyang, N., Lin, L. *et al.* (2012b) HGF-induced PKCzeta activation increases functional CXCR4 expression in human breast cancer cells. *PLoS One*, **7** (1), e29124.

Hui, A.Y., Meens, J.A., Schick, C. *et al.* (2009) Src and FAK mediate cell-matrix adhesion-dependent activation of Met during transformation of breast epithelial cells. *Journal of Cellular Biochemistry*, **107** (6), 1168–1181.

Jagadeeswaran, R., Ma, P.C., Seiwert, T.Y. *et al.* (2006) Functional analysis of c-Met/hepatocyte growth factor pathway in malignant pleural mesothelioma. *Cancer Research*, **66** (1), 352–361.

Jeffers, M., Schmidt, L., Nakaigawa, N. *et al.* (1997) Activating mutations for the met tyrosine kinase receptor in human cancer. *Proceedings of the National Academy of Sciences, USA*, **94** (21), 11445–11450.

Jin, L., Fuchs, A., Schnitt, S.J. *et al.* (1997) Expression of scatter factor and c-met receptor in benign and malignant breast tissue. *Cancer*, **79** (4), 749–760.

Jin, H., Yang, R., Zheng, Z. R *et al.* (2008) MetMAb, the one-armed 5D5 anti-c-Met antibody, inhibits orthotopic pancreatic tumor growth and improves survival. *Cancer Research*, **68** (11), 4360–4368.

Kammula, U.S., Kuntz, E.J., Francone, T.D. *et al.* (2007) Molecular co-expression of the c-Met oncogene and hepatocyte growth factor in primary colon cancer predicts tumor stage and clinical outcome. *Cancer Letters*, **248** (2), 219–228.

Kato, T., Funakoshi, H., Kadoyama, K. *et al.* (2012) Hepatocyte growth factor over-expression in the nervous system enhances learning and memory performance in mice. *Journal of Neuroscience Research*, **90** (9), 1743–1755.

Kenessey, I., Keszthelyi, M., Kramer, Z. *et al.* (2010) Inhibition of c-Met with the specific small molecule tyrosine kinase inhibitor SU11274 decreases growth and metastasis formation of experimental human melanoma. *Current Cancer Drug Targets*, **10** (3), 332–342.

Kermorgant, S. and Parker, P.J. (2008) Receptor trafficking controls weak signal delivery: a strategy used by c-Met for STAT3 nuclear accumulation. *Journal of Cell Biology*, **182** (5), 855–863.

Kitajima, Y., Ide, T., Ohtsuka, T. and Miyazaki, K. (2008) Induction of hepatocyte growth factor activator gene expression under hypoxia activates the hepatocyte growth factor/c-Met system via hypoxia inducible factor-1 in pancreatic cancer. *Cancer Science*, **99** (7), 1341–1347.

Knudsen, B.S. and Vande Woude, G. (2008) Showering c-MET-dependent cancers with drugs. *Current Opinion in Genetics and Development*, **18** (1), 87–96.

Kong-Beltran, M., Seshagiri, S., Zha, J. *et al.* (2006) Somatic mutations lead to an oncogenic deletion of met in lung cancer. *Cancer Research*, **66** (1), 283–289.

Krishnaswamy, S., Kanteti, R., Duke-Cohan, J.S. *et al.* (2009) Ethnic differences and functional analysis of MET mutations in lung cancer. *Clinical Cancer Research*, **15** (18), 5714–5723.

Kwak, I.H., Shin, Y.H., Kim, M. *et al.* (2011) Epigallocatechin-3-gallate inhibits paracrine and autocrine hepatocyte growth factor/scatter factor-induced tumor cell migration and invasion. *Experimental and Molecular Medicine*, **43** (2), 111–120.

Lai, A.Z., Abella, J.V. and Park, M. (2009) Crosstalk in Met receptor oncogenesis. *Trends in Cell Biology*, **19** (10), 542–551.

Leo, C., Sala, V., Morello, M. *et al.* (2011) Activated Met signalling in the developing mouse heart leads to cardiac disease. *PLoS One*, **6** (2), e14675.

Liang, H., O'Reilly, S., Liu, Y. *et al.* (2004) Sp1 regulates expression of MET, and ribozyme-induced down-regulation of MET in fibrosarcoma-derived human cells reduces or eliminates their tumorigenicity. *International Journal of Oncology*, **24** (5), 1057–1067.

Liu, Y., Yang, Y., Ye, Y.C. *et al.* (2012) Activation of ERK-p53 and ERK-mediated phosphorylation of Bcl-2 are involved in autophagic cell death induced by the c-Met inhibitor SU11274 in human lung cancer A549 cells. *Journal of Pharmacological Sciences*, **118** (4), 423–432.

Locatelli, A. and Lange, C.A. (2011) Met receptors induce Sam68-dependent cell migration by activation of alternate extracellular signal-regulated kinase family members. *Journal of Biological Chemistry*, **286** (24), 21062–21072.

Lyon, M. and Gallagher, J.T. (1994) Hepatocyte growth factor/scatter factor: a heparan sulphate-binding pleiotropic growth factor. *Biochemical Society Transanctions*, **22** (2), 365–370.

Lyon, M., Deakin, J.A., Mizuno, K. *et al.* (1994) Interaction of hepatocyte growth factor with heparan sulfate. Elucidation of the major heparan sulfate structural determinants. *Journal of Biological Chemistry*, **269** (15), 11216–11223.

Ma, P.C., Jagadeeswaran, R., Jagadeesh, S. *et al.* (2005a) Functional expression and mutations of c-Met and its therapeutic inhibition with SU11274 and small interfering RNA in non-small cell lung cancer. *Cancer Research*, **65**(4), 1479–1488.

Ma, P.C., Schaefer, E., Christensen, J.G. and Salgia, R. (2005b) A selective small molecule c-MET Inhibitor, PHA665752, cooperates with rapamycin. *Clinical Cancer Research*, **11** (6), 2312–2319.

Ma, P.C., Tretiakova, M.S., MacKinnon, A.C. *et al.* (2008) Expression and mutational analysis of MET in human solid cancers. *Genes Chromosomes and Cancer*, **47** (12), 1025–1037.

Martens, T., Schmidt, N.O., Eckerich, C. *et al.* (2006) A novel one-armed anti-c-Met antibody inhibits glioblastoma growth in vivo. *Clinical Cancer Research*, **12** (20 Pt 1), 6144–6152.

Masuya, D., Huang, C., Liu, D. *et al.* (2004) The tumour-stromal interaction between intratumoral c-Met and stromal hepatocyte growth factor associated with tumour growth and prognosis in non-small-cell lung cancer patients. *British Journal of Cancer*, **90** (8), 1555–1562.

Matsui, S., Osada, S., Tomita, H. *et al.* (2010) Clinical significance of aggressive hepatectomy for colorectal liver metastasis, evaluated from the HGF/c-Met pathway. *International Journal of Oncology*, **37** (2), 289–297.

Matsumoto, K. and Nakamura, T. (1996) Emerging multipotent aspects of hepatocyte growth factor. *Journal of Biochemistry*, **119** (4), 591–600.

Matsumoto, K., Nakamura, T. and Kramer, R.H. (1994) Hepatocyte growth factor/scatter factor induces tyrosine phosphorylation of focal adhesion kinase (p125FAK) and promotes migration and invasion by oral squamous cell carcinoma cells. *Journal of Biological Chemistry*, **269** (50), 31807–31813.

Maulik, G., Madhiwala, P., Brooks, S. *et al.* (2002) Activated c-Met signals through PI3K with dramatic effects on cytoskeletal functions in small cell lung cancer. *Journal of Cellular and Molecular Medicine*, **6** (4), 539–553.

Meiners, S., Brinkmann, V., Naundorf, H. and Birchmeier, W. (1998) Role of morphogenetic factors in metastasis of mammary carcinoma cells. *Oncogene*, **16** (1), 9–20.

Migliore, C. and Giordano, S. (2008) Molecular cancer therapy: can our expectation be MET? *European Journal of Cancer*, **44** (5), 641–651.

Miyazawa, K. (2010) Hepatocyte growth factor activator (HGFA), a serine protease that links tissue injury to activation of hepatocyte growth factor. *FEBS Journal*, **277** (10), 2208–2214.

Miyazawa, K., Shimomura, T., Naka, D. and Kitamura, N. (1994) Proteolytic activation of hepatocyte growth factor in response to tissue injury. *Journal of Biological Chemistry*, **269** (12), 8966–8970.

Nakagawa, T., Tohyama, O., Yamaguchi, A. *et al.* (2010) E7050: a dual c-Met and VEGFR-2 tyrosine kinase inhibitor promotes tumor regression and prolongs survival in mouse xenograft models. *Cancer Science*, **101** (1), 210–215.

Nakamura, T., Teramoto, H and Ichihara, A. (1986) Purification and characterization of a growth factor from rat platelets for mature parenchymal hepatocytes in primary cultures. *Proceedings of the National Academy of Sciences, USA*, **83** (17), 6489–6493.

Nakamura, T., Nawa, K., Ichihara, A. *et al.* (1987) Purification and subunit structure of hepatocyte growth factor from rat platelets. *FEBS Letters*, **224** (2), 311–316.

Nakamura, T., Nishizawa, T., Hagiya, M. *et al.* (1989) Molecular cloning and expression of human hepatocyte growth factor. *Nature*, **342** (6248), 440–443.

Nakamura, T., Mizuno, S., Matsumoto, K. *et al.* (2000) Myocardial protection from ischemia/reperfusion injury by endogenous and exogenous HGF. *Journal of Clinical Investigation*, **106** (12), 1511–1519.

Nakamura, T., Kanda, S., Yamamoto, K. *et al.* (2001) Increase in hepatocyte growth factor receptor tyrosine kinase activity in renal carcinoma cells is associated with increased motility partly through phosphoinositide 3-kinase activation. *Oncogene*, **20** (52), 7610–7623.

Navab, R., Liu, J., Seiden-Long, I. *et al.* (2009) Co-overexpression of Met and hepatocyte growth factor promotes systemic metastasis in NCI-H460 non-small cell lung carcinoma cells. *Neoplasia*, **11** (12), 1292–1300.

Ohya, W., Funakoshi, H., Kurosawa, T. and Nakamura, T. (2007) Hepatocyte growth factor (HGF) promotes oligodendrocyte progenitor cell proliferation and inhibits its differentiation during postnatal development in the rat. *Brain Research*, **1147**, 51–65.

Orian-Rousseau, V., Chen, L., Sleeman, J.P. *et al.* (2002) CD44 is required for two consecutive steps in HGF/c-Met signaling. *Genes Development*, **16** (23), 3074–3086.

Park, M., Gonzatti-Haces, M., Dean, M. *et al.* (1986a) The met oncogene: a new member of the tyrosine kinase family and a marker for cystic fibrosis. *Cold Spring Harbor Symposium on Quantitative Biology*, **51** (Pt 2), 967–975.

Park, M., Dean, M., Cooper, C.S. *et al.* (1986b) Mechanism of met oncogene activation. *Cell*, **45** (6), 895–904.

Park, M., Dean, M., Kaul, K. *et al.* (1987) Sequence of MET protooncogene cDNA has features characteristic of the tyrosine kinase family of growth-factor receptors. *Proceedings of the National Academy of Sciences, USA*, **84** (18), 6379–6383.

Park, M., Park, H., Kim, W.H. *et al.* (2005) Presence of autocrine hepatocyte growth factor-Met signaling and its role in proliferation and migration of SNU-484 gastric cancer cell line. *Experimental and Molecular Medicine*, **37** (3), 213–219.

Paumelle, R., Tulasne, D., Leroy, C. *et al.* (2000) Sequential activation of ERK and repression of JNK by scatter factor/hepatocyte growth factor in madin-darby canine kidney epithelial cells. *Molecular Biology of the Cell*, **11** (11), 3751–3763.

Pennacchietti, S., Michieli, P., Galluzzo, M. *et al.* (2003) Hypoxia promotes invasive growth by transcriptional activation of the met protooncogene. *Cancer Cell*, **3** (4), 347–361.

Peschard, P., Fournier, T.M., Lamorte, L *et al*. (2001) Mutation of the c-Cbl TKB domain binding site on the Met receptor tyrosine kinase converts it into a trans-forming protein. *Molecular Cell*, **8** (5), 995–1004.

Petrelli, A., Circosta, P., Granziero, L. *et al*. (2006) Ab-induced ectodomain shedding mediates hepatocyte growth factor receptor down-regulation and hampers biolog-ical activity. *Proceedings of the National Academy of Sciences, USA*, **103** (13), 5090–5095.

Ponzetto, C., Bardelli, A., Zhen, Z. *et al*. (1994) A multifunctional docking site medi-ates signaling and transformation by the hepatocyte growth factor/scatter factor receptor family. *Cell*, **77** (2), 261–271.

Previdi, S., Maroni, P., Matteucci, E. *et al*. (2010) Interaction between human-breast cancer metastasis and bone microenvironment through activated hepatocyte growth factor/Met and beta-catenin/Wnt pathways. *European Journal of Cancer*, **46** (9), 1679–1691.

Puri, N., Khramtsov, A., Ahmed, S. *et al*. (2007) A selective small molecule inhibitor of c-Met, PHA665752, inhibits tumorigenicity and angiogenesis in mouse lung cancer xenografts. *Cancer Research*, **67** (8), 3529–3534.

Rahimi, N., Tremblay, E., McAdam, L. *et al*. (1996) Identification of a hepatocyte growth factor autocrine loop in a murine mammary carcinoma. *Cell Growth Differ-entiation*, **7** (2), 263–270.

Rong, S., Segal, S., Anver, M. *et al*. (1994) Invasiveness and metastasis of NIH 3T3 cells induced by Met-hepatocyte growth factor/scatter factor autocrine stimulation. *Proceedings of the National Academy of Sciences, USA*, **91** (11), 4731–4735.

Rosen, L.S., Senzer, N., Mekhail, T. *et al*. (2011) A phase I dose-escalation study of Tivantinib (ARQ 197) in adult patients with metastatic solid tumors. *Clinical Cancer Research*, **17** (24), 7754–7764.

Rosenthal, E.L., Johnson, T.M., Allen, E.D. (1998) Role of the plasminogen activator and matrix metalloproteinase systems in epidermal growth factor- and scatter factor-stimulated invasion of carcinoma cells. *Cancer Research*, **58** (22), 5221–5230.

Sattler, M., Pride, Y.B., Ma, P. *et al*. (2003) A novel small molecule met inhibitor induces apoptosis in cells transformed by the oncogenic TPR-MET tyrosine kinase. *Cancer Research*, **63** (17), 5462–5469.

Schmidt, C., Bladt, F., Goedecke, S. *et al*. (1995) Scatter factor/hepatocyte growth factor is essential for liver development. *Nature*, **373** (6516), 699–702.

Schmidt, L.S., Nickerson, M.L., Angeloni, D. *et al*. (2004) Early onset hereditary pap-illary renal carcinoma: germline missense mutations in the tyrosine kinase domain of the met proto-oncogene. *Journal of Urology*, **172** (4 Pt 1), 1256–1261.

Schoffski, P., Garcia, J.A., Stadler, W.M. *et al*. (2011) A phase II study of the efficacy and safety of AMG 102 in patients with metastatic renal cell carcinoma. *BJU International*, **108** (5), 679–686.

Shojaei, F., Lee, J.H., Simmons, B.H, *et al*. (2010) HGF/c-Met acts as an alterna-tive angiogenic pathway in sunitinib-resistant tumors. *Cancer Research*, **70** (24), 10090–10100.

Singleton, P.A., Salgia, R., Moreno-Vinasco, L. *et al*. (2007) CD44 regulates hep-atocyte growth factor-mediated vascular integrity. Role of c-Met, Tiam1/Rac1, dynamin 2, and cortactin. *Journal of Biological Chemistry*, **282** (42), 30643–30657.

Stamos, J., Lazarus, R.A., Yao, X. *et al*. (2004) Crystal structure of the HGF beta-chain in complex with the Sema domain of the Met receptor. *EMBO Journal*, **23** (12), 2325–2335.

Stella, G.M., Benvenuti, S., Gramaglia, D. *et al.* (2011) MET mutations in cancers of unknown primary origin (CUPs). *Human Mutation*, **32** (1), 44–50.

Stoker, M., Gherardi, E., Perryman, M. and Gray, J. (1987) Scatter factor is a fibroblast-derived modulator of epithelial cell mobility. *Nature*, **327** (6119), 239–242.

Strohmeyer, D., Strauss, F., Rossing, C. *et al.* (2004) Expression of bFGF, VEGF and c-met and their correlation with microvessel density and progression in prostate carcinoma. *Anticancer Research*, **24** (3a), 1797–1804.

Sulpice, E., Ding, S., Muscatelli-Groux, B. *et al.* (2009) Cross-talk between the VEGF-A and HGF signalling pathways in endothelial cells. *Biology of the Cell*, **101** (9), 525–539.

Surati, M., Patel, P., Peterson, A. and Salgia, R. (2011) Role of MetMAb (OA-5D5) in c-MET active lung malignancies. *Expert Opinion on Biological Therapy*, **11** (12), 1655–1662.

Syed, Z.A., Yin, W., Hughes, K. *et al.* (2011) HGF/c-met/Stat3 signaling during skin tumor cell invasion: indications for a positive feedback loop. *BMC Cancer*, **11**, 180.

Takayama, H., LaRochelle, W.J., Sharp, R. *et al.* (1997) Diverse tumorigenesis associated with aberrant development in mice overexpressing hepatocyte growth factor/scatter factor. *Proceedings of the National Academy of Sciences, USA*, **94** (2), 701–706.

Teofili, L., Di Febo, A.L., Pierconti, F. *et al.* (2001) Expression of the c-met proto-oncogene and its ligand, hepatocyte growth factor, in Hodgkin disease. *Blood*, **97** (4), 1063–1069.

Trusolino, L., Bertotti, A. and Comoglio, P.M. (2010) MET signalling: principles and functions in development, organ regeneration and cancer. *Nature Reviews Molecular Cell Biology*, **11** (12), 834–848.

Tuck, A.B., Park, M., Sterns, E.E. *et al.* (1996) Coexpression of hepatocyte growth factor and receptor (Met) in human breast carcinoma. *American Journal of Pathology*, **148** (1), 225–232.

Turke, A.B., Zejnullahu, K., Wu, Y.L. *et al.* (2010) Preexistence and clonal selection of MET amplification in EGFR mutant NSCLC. *Cancer Cell*, **17** (1), 77–88.

Ueda, H., Nakamura, T., Matsumoto, K. *et al.* (2001) A potential cardioprotective role of hepatocyte growth factor in myocardial infarction in rats. *Cardiovascular Research*, **51** (1), 41–50.

Uehara, Y., Minowa, O., Mori, C. *et al.* (1995) Placental defect and embryonic lethality in mice lacking hepatocyte growth factor/scatter factor. *Nature*, **373** (6516), 702–705.

Urbanek, K., Rota, M., Cascapera, S. *et al.* (2005) Cardiac stem cells possess growth factor-receptor systems that after activation regenerate the infarcted myocardium, improving ventricular function and long-term survival. *Circulation Research*, **97** (7), 663–673.

Vergani, E., Vallacchi, V., Frigerio, S. *et al.* (2011) Identification of MET and SRC activation in melanoma cell lines showing primary resistance to PLX4032. *Neoplasia*, **13** (12), 1132–1142.

Weidner, K.M., Arakaki, N., Hartmann, G. *et al.* (1991) Evidence for the identity of human scatter factor and human hepatocyte growth factor. *Proceedings of the National Academy of Sciences, USA*, **88** (16), 7001–7005.

Wen, P.Y., Schiff, D., Cloughesy, T.F. *et al.* (2011) A phase II study evaluating the efficacy and safety of AMG 102 (rilotumumab) in patients with recurrent glioblastoma. *Neuro-Oncology*, **13** (4), 437–446.

Xie, Q., Bradley, R., Kang, L. *et al.* (2012) Hepatocyte growth factor (HGF) autocrine activation predicts sensitivity to MET inhibition in glioblastoma. *Proceedings of the National Academy of Sciences, USA*, **109** (2), 570–575.

Yamashita, J., Ogawa, M., Yamashita, S. *et al.* (1994) Immunoreactive hepatocyte growth factor is a strong and independent predictor of recurrence and survival in human breast cancer. *Cancer Research*, **54** (7), 1630–1633.

Yeh, C.Y., Shin, S.M., Yeh, H.H. *et al.* (2011) Transcriptional activation of the Axl and PDGFR-alpha by c-Met through a ras- and Src-independent mechanism in human bladder cancer. *BMC Cancer*, **11**, 139.

Zhang, Y.W., Su, Y., Volpert, O.V. and Vande Woude, G.F. (2010) Hepatocyte growth factor/scatter factor mediates angiogenesis through positive VEGF and negative thrombospondin 1 regulation. *Proceedings of the National Academy of Sciences, USA*, **100** (22), 12718–12723.

Zillhardt, M., Park, S.M., Romero, I.L. *et al.* (2011) Foretinib (GSK1363089), an orally available multikinase inhibitor of c-Met and VEGFR-2, blocks proliferation, induces anoikis, and impairs ovarian cancer metastasis. *Clinical Cancer Research*, **17** (12), 4042–4051.

Zou, H.Y., Li, Q., Lee, J.H. *et al.* (2007) An orally available small-molecule inhibitor of c-Met, PF-2341066, exhibits cytoreductive antitumor efficacy through antiproliferative and antiangiogenic mechanisms. *Cancer Research*, **67** (9), 4408–4417.

7

Vascular endothelial growth factor and its receptor family

Katarzyna Leszczynska, Christopher Hillyar and Ester M. Hammond
The Cancer Research UK/MRC Gray Institute for Radiation Oncology and Biology, The University of Oxford, Oxford

Vascular endothelial growth factor (VEGF) is a small multifunctional cytokine that was first discovered in the late 1970s by Dvorak and colleagues (Senger *et al.*, 1983; Dvorak *et al.*, 1979). They found that tumours secreted a signalling molecule, which enhanced the permeability of blood vessels. This cytokine was originally called vascular permeability factor (VPF) and currently VEGF, which comprises several family members. VEGF molecules signal through binding to their cognate receptors (VEGFRs) and regulate many cellular processes including cell proliferation, migration and survival. The most prominent role of VEGF/VEGFR signalling is in endothelial cells where it drives the formation of blood vessels from the pre-existing ones. This process, called angiogenesis, is essential in physiological processes such as development, ovulation and wound healing, but can also be critical in the pathogenesis of many diseases, including solid tumours (Folkman *et al.*, 1989; Carmeliet *et al.*, 2011).

7.1 VEGF receptors

The family of human and mouse VEGFRs belongs to the superfamily of receptor tyrosine kinases (RTKs) and consists of VEGFR1 (alternative name Flt1, for fms-like tyrosine kinase 1), VEGFR2 (alternative names include KDR, for kinase domain receptor, and Flk1 for foetal liver kinase 1) and VEGFR3 (alternative name Flt4, for fms-related tyrosine kinase 4). VEGFR1 is mainly expressed in macrophages and monocytes, while VEGFR2 in vascular endothelial cells and VEGFR3 in lymphatic vessels. This classification however is not strict, as there are other expression sites reported for each receptor (Table 7.1) (referenced in Koch *et al.*, 2011; Olsson *et al.*, 2006).

Cancer Cell Signalling, First Edition. Edited by Amanda Harvey.
© 2013 John Wiley & Sons, Ltd. Published 2013 by John Wiley & Sons, Ltd.

Table 7.1　Expression sites reported for VEGFRs (referenced in Koch *et al.*, 2011; Olsson *et al.*, 2006).

Receptor	Expression site
VEGFR1	Monocytes, macrophages, vascular endothelial cells, trophoblasts, renal mesangial cells, vascular smooth muscle cells, dendritic cells, various cancer cells, placenta
VEGFR2	Vascular endothelial cells, pancreatic duct cells, retinal progenitor cells, megakaryocytes, haematopoietic cells, various cancer cells
VEGFR3	Lymphatic endothelial cells, vascular endothelial cells, neuronal progenitors, macrophages, some cancer cells

VEGFRs, once stimulated by their ligands, can form homo- or heterodimers (Figure 7.1). Each of the receptor monomer units is composed of an extracellular domain containing seven immunoglobulin (Ig)-like loops, a transmembrane domain, a juxtamembrane domain, a tyrosine kinase domain with a kinase insert domain, and a *C*-terminal tail. The fifth Ig-like loop in VEGFR3 is substituted by a disulphide bridge. Alternative splicing of VEGFR1-2 results in their soluble isoforms (sVEGFR1 and sVEGFR2, respectively), which contain only six *N*-terminal Ig-like loops and a unique 31 amino acid *C*-terminal domain (Kendall and Thomas, 1993; Albuquerque *et al.*, 2009; Pavlakovic *et al.*, 2010). These soluble isoforms lack the transmembrane domain and are secreted into the circulation. In humans, VEGFR3 can also be alternatively spliced leading to the expression of a truncated protein. This shorter isoform lacks 65 amino acids at the *C*-terminal end, including some of the important phosphorylation sites in the tyrosine kinase domain (Galland *et al.*, 1993).

Some of the receptors can interact with each other or form heterodimers, as in the case of VEGFR1/2 (Auerio *et al.*, 2003; Rahimi *et al.*, 2000; Huang *et al.*, 2001; Mac Gabhann and Popel, 2007; Kou *et al.*, 2005) or VEGFR2/3 (Nilsson *et al.*, 2010). VEGFRs can also function in conjunction with other cell surface molecules. These, serving as co-receptors, can influence the downstream outcome of VEGF/VEGFR signalling (Grunewald *et al.*, 2010). The VEGFR co-receptors include heparan sulphate (HS), heparin, heparan sulphate proteoglycans (HSPGs), neuropilins (NRPs) and integrins (Uniewicz *et al.*, 2008; Xu *et al.*, 2011; Stringer, 2006; Borges *et al.*, 2000; Mahabeleshwar *et al.*, 2008; Koch, 2012).

7.2　Ligands

The signal transduction of VEGFRs is mediated by their ligands, VEGFs, which comprise a family of structurally related signalling molecules including VEGFA, VEGFB, VEGFC, VEGFD and placental growth factor (PlGF). Non-mammalian structurally related VEGFs have also been characterised, including parapox

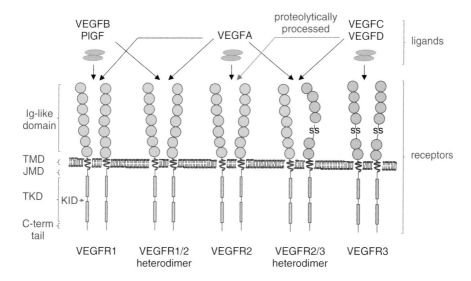

Figure 7.1 **VEGFRs and their ligands.** VEGFR1–3 can be activated by their multiple lig-ands, as indicated. VEGF ligands are comprised of covalently linked two monomer units. Receptors consist of seven immunoglobulin (Ig)-like domains, transmembrane domain (TMD); juxtamembrane domain (JMD), tyrosine kinase domain (TKD) separated by kinase insert domain (KID) and *C*-terminal tail. The fifth Ig-like domain in VEGFR3 is replaced by a disulphide bridge. VEGFRs can form homo- or heterodimers.

virus-encoded VEGFE (Ogawa *et al.*, 1998) and that present in snake venom VEGFF (Yamazaki *et al.*, 2005). VEGFs are glycopeptides and form functional homodimers covalently linked by disulphide bonds (Senger *et al.*, 1983). Some VEGFs, such as VEGFA and PlGF, can also assemble into heterodimers (DiSalvo *et al.*, 1995). Particular VEGF ligands can bind to more than one receptor (Figure 7.1). VEGFA can bind to VEGFR1 and 2 or VEGFR1/2 heterodimer, while VEGB and PlGF bind more specifically to VEGFR1 and a heterodimer VEGFR1/2. VEGFC and VEGFD are mainly ligands for VEGFR3 or VEGFR2/3 heterodimers, but after proteolytic processing they can also stimulate VEGFR2 (Olsson *et al.*, 2006).

VEGF genes are alternatively spliced, resulting in protein isoforms of various sizes (Ladomery *et al.*, 2007). This also leads to a variable affinity of particu-lar ligands to their receptors and co-receptors, and allows some of the ligands to acquire anti-angiogenic properties (Nowak *et al.*, 2008; Bates *et al.*, 2002). The *VEGF* gene is comprised of eight exons (Figure 7.2). The full-length mRNA transcript (without an alternative exon 8b) produces the VEGF ligand contain-ing 206 amino acids, hence it is denoted $VEGF_{206}$. Exons 3 and 4 encode the sequences responsible for ligand dimerisation and binding to VEGFRs. The fifth exon includes the plasmin cleavage site. The first five exons are included in all the isoforms identified. Exons 6 and 7, which are alternatively spliced, encode

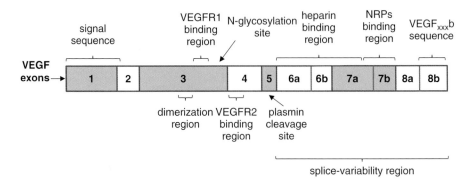

Figure 7.2 Exon structure organisation of VEGF gene. VEGF gene is comprised of eight exons, which encode various regions important for the functional VEGF protein, as indicated. The region spanning exons 6–8 is alternatively spliced in multiple VEGF isoforms (Nowak *et al.*, 2008); NRPs, neuropilins.

sequences enabling interaction with co-receptors such as heparin or NRPs. VEGF splice variants missing different regions in exons 6–8 include $VEGF_{189}$, $VEGF_{183}$, $VEGF_{165}$, $VEGF_{148}$, $VEGF_{145}$ and $VEGF_{121}$.

In addition most of the VEGF isoforms can be alternatively spliced at their 3′-untranslated regions. This generates a unique amino acid sequence at the *C*-terminus of these ligands and classifies them as anti-angiogenic isoforms, as they interfere with the pro-angiogenic properties of conventional VEGF ligands (Nowak *et al.*, 2008). The anti-angiogenic VEGF variants are denoted as $VEGF_{xxx}b$ (where 'xxx' stands for the number of amino acids in the corresponding regular isoform, and 'b' for the presence of an alternative exon 8b sequence). Moreover, as opposed to typical VEGF ligands, some $VEGF_{xxx}b$ isoforms were found to be down-regulated in many cancers (Bates *et al.*, 2002; Woolard *et al.*, 2004; Varey *et al.*, 2008; Pritchard-Jones *et al.*, 2007), which emphasises their potential anti-angiogenic and anticancer properties. The dominant and most studied isoform of the pro-angiogenic VEGFA is $VEGF_{165}$, which will be described in the subsequent sections of this chapter and denoted onwards as VEGFA.

VEGFs can bind to their receptors in a cis and a trans manner Koch *et al.*, 2011). The former occurs when diffused ligand is accessible from the extracellular space or is presented by a co-receptor expressed on the same cell. In the latter scenario, the ligand is presented by the co-receptor on the neighbouring cell. Upon binding of VEGF ligand, two monomer receptor units undergo dimerisation, which is stabilised at contact points of Ig-like loops in the extracellular domain and by transmembrane and juxtamembrane domains (Figure 7.3). Dimerisation of receptors is concomitant with conformational changes in the intracellular domains resulting in the exposure of the ATP-binding site and subsequent ATP-dependent auto- and trans-phosphorylation of tyrosine (Tyr) residues on the dimer receptor itself or on the VEGFR-interacting signalling molecules (Stuttfeld and Ballmer-Hofer, 2009).

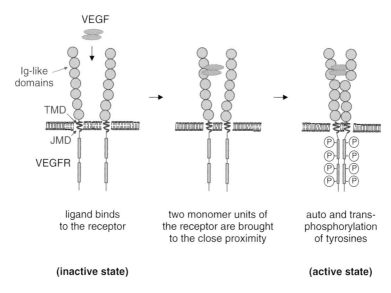

Figure 7.3 **The cascade of events during VEGFR activation.** Ig-like domains of VEGFR are recognised by appropriate VEGF ligand dimers, which brings together two monomer units of the receptor. The VEGF/VEGFR complex is then stabilised by interactions in Ig-like domains, transmembrane domain (TMD) and juxtamembrane domain (JMD). This induces conformational changes in the intracellular tyrosine kinase domain and enables auto- and transphosphorylation of various tyrosine residues (marked as circled P), leading to the activation of the receptor. The scheme of VEGFR activation is based on the one proposed in Stuttfeld and Ballmer-Hofer (2009).

Thus, upon binding by their ligands, VEGFRs undergo intra-molecular changes that lead to their reorganisation into dimers and phosphorylation of multiple tyrosine sites, and therefore their activation.

7.3 Downstream signalling molecules and events

Once activated, VEGFRs can transduce the signalling cascade inside the cell to induce or regulate specific cellular processes. The intracellular domains of active VEGFRs are phosphorylated on multiple tyrosine sites and many proteins that are recruited to these sites contain phospho-tyrosine interacting domains, such as the Src homology domain 2 (SH2). The research on VEGFRs-mediated signalling is growing very fast, and the major interactions of these receptors with downstream signalling molecules, leading to specific cellular events, will now be presented.

7.3.1 VEGFR1-mediated signalling

VEGFR1-mediated signalling regulates diverse physiological processes (Figure 7.4). This includes monocyte migration, haematopoiesis, recruitment of

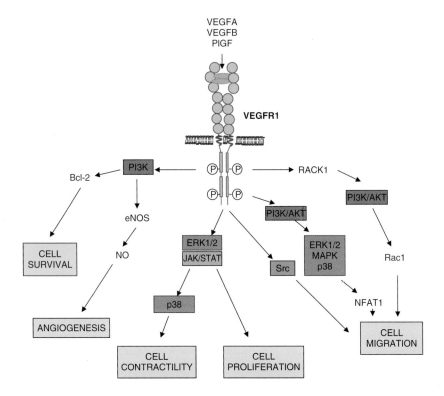

Figure 7.4   **VEGFR1-mediated signalling.** VEGFR1-mediated signalling cascades are important for many cellular processes such as proliferation, migration, survival or contractility, as indicated in the boxes at the end of each pathway. Please refer to the text for the description of summarised signalling pathways. Abbreviations: PI3K, phosphatidylinositol 3-kinase; Bcl-2, B cell lymphoma 2; eNOS, endothelial nitric oxide synthase; NO, nitric oxide; ERK1/2, extracellular signal-regulated kinase; JAK, Janus kinase; STAT, signal transducer and activator of transcription; RACK1, receptor for activated protein kinase C 1; MAPK, mitogen-activated protein kinase; NFAT1, nuclear factor of activated T-cells 1.

haematopoietic progenitor cells from the bone marrow, vascular permeability or regulation of vasculature formation during development (Koch *et al.*, 2011; Olsson *et al.*, 2006).

VEGFR1-mediated signalling is induced by VEGFA, VEGFB or PlGF ligands (Koch *et al.*, 2011). This receptor can bind VEGFA with much higher affinity than VEGFR2 (Shinkai *et al.*, 1998). However, its tyrosine kinase activity induced by VEGFA is very weak in comparison with activity of VEGFR2 (Gille *et al.*, 2000; Meyer *et al.*, 2006; Ito *et al.*, 1998; Kendall *et al.*, 1994). Consequently, VEGFR1 and its soluble isoform, sVEGFR1, have an additional function in endothelial cells, which is trapping of VEGFA ligand and limiting its availability to VEGFR2 (Kappas *et al.*, 2008; Hiratsuka *et al.*, 1998). This is supported by the finding that *Vegfr1*$^{-/-}$ mice die prematurely at embryonic day 9 due to enhanced endothelial cell proliferation and incorrect development of the vascular system (Kappas *et al.*, 2008; Hiratsuka *et al.*, 1998; Fong *et al.*, 1995). When activated by PlGF, VEGFR1 plays an important role in mobilisation of inflammatory cells during wound healing and to the pathological sites in the body, such as cancer (Carmeliet *et al.*, 2001a). PlGF signalling through VEGFR1 also significantly contributes to pathological angiogenesis and other diseases, such as atherosclerosis, obesity, or rheumatoid arthritis (De Falco, 2012). Stimulation of VEGFR1 by VEGFB has a main role in development of the cardiovascular system (Li *et al.*, 2008; Hagberg *et al.*, 2010; Aase *et al.*, 2001; Bellomo *et al.*, 1997).

The tyrosine phosphorylation sites identified on VEGFR1 include Tyr794, Tyr-1169, Tyr1213, Tyr1242, Tyr1327 and Tyr1333 (reviewed in Koch *et al.*, 2011) These create docking sites for downstream signalling molecules, such as phospholipase C (PLC) γ (Cunningham *et al.*, 1997; Swano *et al.*, 1997), growth-factor-receptor bound protein 2 (GRB2), SH2-domain-containing protein tyrosine phosphatase 2 (SHP2) and the non-catalytic region of tyrosine kinase adaptor protein (Nck) (Ito *et al.*, 1998; Igarashi *et al.*, 1998). These interactions are evidenced by *in vitro* studies; however, their significance in physiological conditions is unclear.

It has been reported that VEGF/VEGFR1-induced signalling regulates endothelial cell migration (Hiratsuka *et al.*, 1998; Kearney *et al.*, 2004). Receptor for activated protein kinase C 1 (RACK1), which is a scaffolding protein, binds directly to phosphorylated VEGFR1 and regulates cell migration via the phosphatidylinositol 3-kinase (PI3K), Akt and Rac1 signalling pathways (Wang *et al.*, 2011). Some studies indicate that VEGFR1 can directly bind the p85 subunit of PI3K (Yu *et al.*, 2001; Cunningham *et al.*, 1995). The activation of the PI3K pathway by VEGFR1 may lead to increased activity of endothelial nitric oxide (NO) synthase (eNOS) and release of NO, which promotes angiogenesis (Ahmad *et al.*, 2006). In addition, VEGFR1 can contribute to angiogenesis by promoting cell survival signalling. This is through activation of PI3K and increased expression of anti-apoptotic protein B cell lymphoma 2 (Bcl-2) (Cai *et al.*, 2003).

In vascular smooth muscle cells (VSMCs) PlGF/VEGFR1 signalling can be induced by hypoxia. This leads to activation of extracellular-signal regulated kinase (ERK1/2) and the Janus kinase (JAK)/signal transducer and activator of transcription (STAT) to induce cell proliferation. On the other hand, VEGFR1 activates the p38 kinase pathway to promote contraction of VSMCs (Bellik *et al.*, 2005). VEGF ligand can induce VEGR1 proliferative signalling in hypoxic VSMCs through an autocrine mechanism (Osada-Oka *et al.*, 2008).

In monocytes and other macrophage lineage cells VEGFR1 can mediate signalling involved in cell migration (Krysiak *et al.*, 2005; Barleon *et al.*, 1996; Kerber *et al.*, 2008; Muramatsu *et al.*, 2010). This includes activation of the nuclear factor of activated T-cells 1 (NFAT1), ERK1/2, mitogen-activated protein kinase (MAPK), p38 and PI3K/Akt (Ding *et al.*, Tchaikovski *et al.*, 2008). As an example, VEGFR1-mediated activation of NFAT is dependent on simultaneous induction of tumour necrosis factor α (TNFα), which then leads to recruitment of myelomonocytic cells to the tumour sites and contributes to the tumour inflammation (Ding *et al.*, 2010). Monocytes, which are recruited to the cancer sites via PlGF/VEGFR1 signalling can produce elevated levels of VEGF ligands and stimulate angiogenesis (Carmeliet *et al.*, 2001b).

Growing evidence suggests that VEGFR1 can drive the migratory/invasive phenotype in cancer cells, which then contributes to cancer metastases (Li, Wang, Zhang, *et al.*, 2012). As an example, migration of some colon cancer cell types is induced by VEGFR1/Src signalling (Lesslie *et al.*, 2006), while in breast cancer cells by VEGFR1-induced activation of ERK1/2 kinase (Taylor *et al.*, 2010).

7.3.2 VEGFR2-mediated signalling

Despite VEGFR2 being expressed in various cell types as indicated in Table 7.1, its role as a signalling molecule is emphasised as a stimulator of endothelial cell migration, proliferation, survival, and other pro-angiogenic processes. This is reinforced by the $Vegfr2^{-/-}$ mice phenotype, where these animals have defects in the development of haematopoietic and endothelial cells and die at embryonic day E8.5 (Shalaby *et al.*, 1995). Since this phenotype is very similar to $Vefga^{-/-}$ mice (Carmeliet *et al.*, 1996; Ferrara *et al.*, 1996), it is supposed that VEGFR2 is the main receptor for VEGFA signalling in endothelial cells.

Once activated by VEGF ligands, VEGFR2 undergoes phosphorylation at its multiple tyrosine sites in its intracellular domain. These sites then recruit and further phosphorylate various downstream molecules, as summarised in Figure 7.5. The known tyrosine phosphorylation sites on VEGFR2 include: Tyr801, Tyr951, Tyr1054, Tyr1059, Tyr1175, Tyr1214, Tyr1223, Tyr1305, Tyr1309 and Tyr1319 (reviewed in Koch *et al.*, 2011).

Src kinase is recruited to phosphorylated Tyr1059 on VEGR2 and mediates its further phosphorylation on subsequent tyrosines. This signalling event recruits other proteins, which also undergo Src-mediated phosphorylation. As an example, recruitment and activation of IQ-motif-containing GTPase-activating protein 1 (IQGAP1) regulates cell proliferation, migration and vascular endothelial (VE)-cadherin containing cell–cell junctions. In activated endothelial cells IQGAP1 contributes to the loss of cell–cell contacts in order to facilitate cell migration, while in quiescent endothelial cells it is important for the formation of these cell–cell connections (Yamaola-Tojo *et al.*, 2006; Meyer *et al.*, 2008). VEGFR2 and Src-dependent signalling can also promote endothelial cell migration through activation of focal adhesion kinase (FAK) (Le Boeuf *et al.*, 206; Abu-Ghazaleh *et al.*, 2001; Holmqvist *et al.*, 2003). Phosphorylation and activity of this protein is important for turnover of focal adhesions, the dynamic cell-to-extracellular matrix contact points that facilitate cell movement (Ilic *et al.*, 1995; Webb *et al.*, 2004). VEGF-induced activation of FAK can also stimulate vascular permeability (Chen *et al.*, 2012). In this case activated FAK localises to

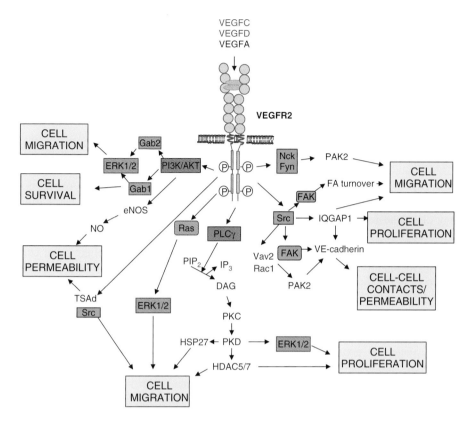

Figure 7.5   **VEGFR2-mediated signalling.** VEGFR2 is the most studied receptor in endothelial cells, which is mirrored here by the plethora of signalling pathways that it is transducing. It plays a crucial role in cellular processes including proliferation, migration, survival, regulation of cell-cell contacts, as indicated in the boxes at the end of each pathway. All these processes are critical for the formation of blood vessels. Abbreviations: PI3K, phosphatidylinositol 3-kinase; Gab1/2, GRB2-associated-binding protein 1/2; eNOS, endothelial nitric oxide synthase; NO, nitric oxide; ERK1/2, extracellular signal-regulated kinase; FA, focal adhesions; FAK, focal adhesion kinase; VE-cadherin, vascular endothelial cadherin; PAK2, p21-activated protein kinase 2; IQGPAP1, Ras GTPase-activating-like protein 1; Nck, non-catalytic region of tyrosine kinase adaptor protein 1; PLCγ, phospholipase γ; PIP$_2$, phosphatidylinositol 4,5-bisphosphate; DAG, diacylglycerol; IP$_3$, inositol 1,4,5-trisphosphate; mPKC, protein kinase C; PKD, protein kinase D; HSP27, heatshock protein 27; HDAC5/7, histone deacetylase 5/7; TSAd, T-cell-specific adapter molecule.

cell−cell junctions and leads to dissociation of VE-cadherin/β-catenin complexes and therefore enables breakdown of endothelial cell connections. T-cell-specific adapter molecule (TSAd) also promotes vascular permeability and endothelial cell migration in response to VEGF/VEGFR2 signalling by inducing Src activity. TSAd contains an SH2-domain, which directly binds to VEGFR2 Tyr951 site (Sun *et al.*, 2012; Matsumoto *et al.*, 2005).

VEGFR2 activation can drive endothelial cell proliferation by direct activation of PLCγ (Takahashi *et al.*, 1999; Xia *et al.*, 1996) or other PLC isoforms α, β and ζ (Takahashi *et al.*, 1999; Wang *et al.*, 2008; Wellner *et al.*, 1999). PLCγ catalyses the hydrolysis of phosphatidylinositol 4,5-bisphosphate (PIP$_2$) to diacylglycerol (DAG) and inositol 1,4,5-trisphosphate (IP$_3$). DAG activates protein kinase C (PKC), which in turn activates protein kinase D (PKD) and induces ERK1/2 signalling, leading to increased cell proliferation (Wong *et al.*, 2005; Qin *et al.*, 2006). VEGF-activated PKC/PKD signalling axis can also promote cellular proliferation by inducing nuclear translocation of histone deacetylases HDAC5 and HDAC7 (Wang *et al.*, 2008; Ha *et al.*, 2008). Once in the nuclei, these enzymes promote cell proliferation and migration by facilitating expression of VEGF-responsive genes such as *RCAN2* or *Nur22*. VEGF/PKC/PKD signalling may also lead to phosphorylation of heatshock protein HSP27, which promotes endothelial cell migration and tubulogenesis (Evans *et al.*, 2008).

Pro-migratory and proliferative effects of VEGF signalling in endothelial cells can be mediated by activation of small GTPase Ras (Meadows *et al.*, 2001). VEGF-induced Ras promotes cell migration by triggering actin cytoskeleton rearrangements as well as cell proliferation by activation of ERK1/2 signalling (Rak and Kerbel, 2001; Meadows *et al.*, 2004; Kranenburg *et al.*, 2004).

VEGFR2 phosphorylation at Tyr1214 recruits Nck and Fyn kinases, which then activate p21-activated protein kinase (PAK) 2 that mediates stress fibre formation and endothelial cell migration (Lamalice *et al.*, 2006). In response to VEGF treatment, VEGFR2 can also form a complex with the integrin αvβ5 and recruit filamin B, small GTPase Rac1 and its guanine nucleotide exchange factor, Vav2. Formation of this complex leads to activation of PAK4/5/6 kinases and endothelial cell migration (Dei Valle-Perez *et al.*, 2010). On the other hand, VEGF/VEGFR2-initiated and Src/Vav2/Rac1-mediated activation of PAK2 promotes vascular permeability. Active PAK2 phosphorylates VE-cadherin, which then recruits beta-arrestin 2 and is internalised into clathrin-coated vesicles, which results in disassembly of cell–cell contacts (Gavard *et al.*, 2006).

Phosphorylation of scaffolding adapter proteins Gab1 and Gab2 (GRB2-associated-binding protein 1 and 2), which also play a role in endothelial cell biology, has been attributed to VEGF/VEGFR2 signalling. Phosphorylated Gab1 can associate with PI3K and SHP2 proteins and positively regulate Akt, Src and ERK1/2-mediated endothelial cell migration and capillary formation (Larmee *et al.*, 2007) as well as cell survival (Caron *et al.*, 2009). Phosphorylated Gab2 can also interact with PI3K and SHP2 and contributes to VEGF/VEGFR2 induced cell migration but is not required for endothelial cell survival (Caron *et al.*, 2009). PI3K/Akt signalling pathway is a very important player in VEGF/VEGFR2 induced endothelial cell proliferation and survival, both of which processes contribute to angiogenesis (Fujio and Walsh, 1999; Dayanir *et al.*, 2001). Another aspect of VEGF/VEGFR2-induced Akt activity is to induce vascular permeability. This is through activation eNOS and subsequent elevation of NO levels (Dimmeler *et al.*, 1999; Fukumura *et al.*, 2001; Fulton *et al.*, 1999; Murohara *et al.*, 1998; Wu *et al.*, 1996; Thibeault *et al.*, 2010).

7.3.3   VEGFR3-mediated signalling

The ligands that activate VEGFR3 signalling include VEGFC and VEGFD and inactivation of genes that encode those cytokines leads to faulty development of lymphatic vessels (Haiko *et al.*, 2008). The expression of mutated or truncated forms of VEGFR3 also negatively impacts the development of lymphatics (Zhang *et al.*, 2010). Hence, the main function attributed to VEGFR3 is to regulate development of the lymphatic system. However, *Vegfr3*$^{-/-}$ mice die at embryonic day 10.5 due to disorganised vasculature formation and cardiovascular defects before the lymphatic system forms (Dumont *et al.*, 1998). This proves that in addition to transduction of VEGFC/VEGFD-mediated lymphatic functions, VEGFR3 also has a non-redundant role in the development of the cardiovascular system. VEGFR3 can form heterodimers with VEGFR2 (Nilsson *et al.*, 2010), and phenotype of *Vegfr3*$^{-/-}$ mice with defects in vasculature might be due to the lack of VEGFR2/3 heterodimer formation in these animals. This is supported by the fact that mice expressing kinase-dead VEGFR3 can still normally develop blood vessels (Zhang *et al.*, 2010).

Tyrosine residues that undergo phosphorylation on VEGFR3 during VEGFC/VEGFD-induced activation include Tyr1063, Tyr1068, Tyr1230, Tyr1231, Tyr-1265, Tyr1337 and Tyr1363 (Koch *et al.*, 2011). Another set of tyrosines includes Tyr830, Tyr833, Tyr853, Tyr1063, Tyr1333 and Tyr1337, which are phosphorylated by integrins in a VEGFC/VEGFD-independent manner (Koch *et al.*, 2011). Current reports indicate that VEGFR3 signalling is not as complex as VEGFR2 signalling. Nevertheless, it still influences at least several downstream signalling pathways (Figure 7.6).

Lymphatic vessels can contribute to the metastasis of various cancers (Osaki *et al.*, 2004; Roma *et al.*, 2006). Activation of VEGFR3 by VEGFC in lymphatic endothelial cells induced PI3K/Akt signalling, leading to phosphorylation of P70SRK, eNOS, PLCγ1 and ERK1/2. This can contribute to lymph node metastases in primary small lung cell carcinoma. Similarly, increased activity of VEGFR3 and PI3K was reported in metastatic lymph nodes in melanoma, colon and breast cancer tissues (Coso *et al.*, 2012). Activation of the VEGFR3/Akt/PKC/ERK1/2 signalling axis was shown to promote the growth and survival of lymphatic endothelial cells (Makinen *et al.*, 2001). The expression and activity of VEGFR3 is regulated by H-, N-, and Kras proteins, which contribute to normal development of lymphatic cells (Ichise *et al.*, 2010).

VEGFR3-dependent signalling was also shown to activate Akt and ERK1/2 kinases in vascular endothelial cells (Salameh *et al.*, 2005). This is mediated via SH2-containing transforming protein 1 (SHC) and GRB2 that directly bind to phosphorylated VEGFR3. In addition, VEGFR3 recruits C10 regulator of kinase (CRKI/II), which then activates a cascade of signals via mitogen-activated protein kinase kinase-4 (MKK4) and c-Jun *N*-terminal kinase (JNK), all of which contribute to survival, proliferation and migration of endothelial cells (Salameh *et al.*, 2005). The integrin mediated and Src-dependent phosphorylation of VEGFR3 also recruits SHC and CRKI/II and leads to activation of JNK (Galvagni *et al.*, 2010).

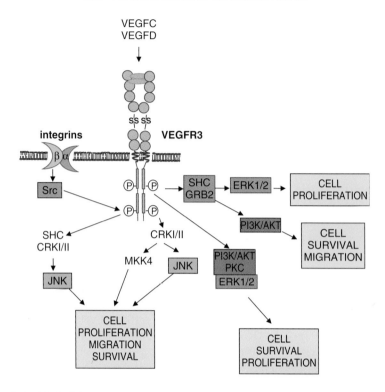

Figure 7.6 **VEGFR3-mediated signalling.** VEGFR3 is known to signal through several pathways in order to regulate mainly cell survival, proliferation and migration. This receptor is crucial for the development and signalling in the lymphatic vessels but it also plays a role in angiogenesis. Abbreviations: PI3K, phosphatidylinositol 3-kinase; GRB2, growth-factor-receptor bound protein 2; SHC, Src homology 2 domain containing transforming protein 1; CRKI/II, C10 regulator of kinase; ERK1/2, extracellular signal-regulated kinase; PKC, protein kinase C; JNK, c-Jun N-terminal kinase; MKK4, mitogen-activated protein kinase kinase-4.

7.4   Signalling regulation

There is huge complexity and multiple levels of regulation of VEGFR signalling. VEGFs can stimulate their cognate receptors expressed on these same cells or on distant/dissimilar types of cells. The first mode of signalling is called 'autocrine' and is exemplified in breast cancer cells, which express both VEGFA ligand and its receptors, VEGFR1 and 2. It was demonstrated that stimulation of VEGFR2 by VEGFA in an autocrine manner leads to an increase in ERK1/2 and Akt activity and therefore is important for proliferation and survival of breast cancer cells (Weigand *et al.*, 2005). The 'paracrine' signalling would be then mediated by VEGFA released by cancer cells, which binds to VEGFR2 on endothelial cells in order to drive the growth of blood vessels into the cancer tissue. Another example of paracrine signalling is the release of VEGF cytokines by macrophages, dendritic cells or myelomonocytic cells, which then stimulate receptors expressed on endothelial or cancer cells (David Dong *et al.*, 2009).

An additional level of regulation occurs through the cellular localisation of VEGFRs. The full-length VEGFRs localise to the plasma membrane. However, some pool of VEGFRs traffics between the plasma membrane and endosomes and may conduct signalling from both of these locations (Lampugnani *et al.*, 2006; Scott and Mellor, 2009; Lanahan *et al.*, 2010; Gampel *et al.*, 2006). Internalisation and intracellular trafficking of VEGFRs can be regulated by various molecules including caveolin-1, dynamin-2, ADP-ribosylation factor 6 (ARF6) or ephrin-B2 (Wang *et al.*, 2010; Labrecque *et al.*, 2003; Bhattacharya *et al.*, 2005; Ikeda *et al.*, 2005). The internalisation of VEGFRs, on the other hand, may regulate their surface levels and therefore the sensitivity of cells to VEGF signalling from the extracellular environment. Some proportion of VEGFRs can be sent from endosomes to lysosomes for degradation (Scott and Mellor, 2009; Kobayashi *et al.*, 2004; Ewan *et al.*, 2006).

As mentioned earlier, activation of VEGFRs and their interaction with downstream signalling molecules largely depends on the phosphorylation status of their multiple Tyr residues. Thus the obvious way to down-regulate VEGFR activity is through its de-phosphorylation. Various phosphatases have been reported to target phospho-tyrosine sites on VEGFRs, including density enhanced phosphatase 1 (DEP-1), protein tyrosine phosphatase β (PTPβ), PTP-1B, low molecular weight PTP (LMW-PTP), SHP-1 and SHP-2 (Kappart *et al.*, 2005). Although most phosphatases seem to inhibit VEGFR activity, some of them appear to actually enhance its downstream response, which emphasises how complex the regulation of VEGFR signalling is. DEP-1 is a phosphatase, which targets most of the VEGFR2 phosphorylation sites. However, it can positively regulate VEGF-induced and Src-mediated Akt activation leading to endothelial cell survival (Chabot *et al.*, 2009; Grazia Lampugnani *et al.*, 2003).

The amount of VEGF ligands available to transduce some of the VEGFRs can be often controlled through binding by their soluble forms sVEGFRs, so called 'decoy receptors'. As an example, sVEGFR1, which has a high affinity to VEGFA, can efficiently trap this ligand and limit its availability for VEGFR2 and therefore control its signalling and the subsequent formation of newly forming vessels (Kendall *et al.*, 1994; Kappas *et al.*, 2008). On the other hand, sVEGFR2 can bind VEGFC and therefore limit its availability for VEGFR3, affecting some processes important for lymphatic endothelial cells, such as their proliferation (Albuquerque *et al.*, 2009).

Signal transduction by VEGFRs might be facilitated and amplified by various co-receptors. HS, for example, when expressed on pericytes, can present the VEGFA ligand to VEGFR2 expressed on neighbouring cells in a trans manner. This significantly augments the downstream VEGFR2 signalling (Jakobsson *et al.*, 2006). In addition, HS or some other extracellular matrix molecules can bind and retain the supplies of VEGF ligands. Their release can be controlled by matrix metalloproteases, which remodel the extracellular matrix and in this way create a gradient of VEGF ligands (Small *et al.*, 2008; Liu *et al.*, 2007). This, in turn, is important for the formation of branching of the vasculature (Ruhrberg *et al.*, 2002). NRPs, which are receptors for semaphorins, can bind some of the isoforms of VEGF ligands and also heparin sulphate (Vander Kool *et al.*, 2007). These complexes are important in regulating endothelial cell migration, permeability and other processes important for angiogenesis (Favier *et al.*, 2006; Wang *et al.*, 2003; Becker *et al.*, 2005; Kawamura *et al.*, 2008). Another group of molecules bridged to VEGFRs by VEGF ligands are integrins (Mahabeleshwar *et al.*, 2006, 2008). These transmembrane proteins are responsible for cellular adhesion to extracellular matrix components. They are also important mediators of signalling between the intracellular cytoskeleton and extracellular microenvironment (Dubash *et al.*, 2009; Shattil *et al.*, 2010). As an example, in respect to VEGFR signalling, αvβ3 integrin plays an important role in VEGFR2-mediated angiogenesis in wounds and at tumour sites (Mahabeleshwar *et al.*, 2006; Miao *et al.*, 1999).

7.5   Dysregulation of signalling in cancer

Although *VEGFR3* is not widely expressed on cells other than vascular and lymphatic endothelial cells in tumour tissues (Petrova *et al.*, 2008; Wang *et al.*, 2012) there is growing evidence indicating abundant expression of *VEGFR1* and 2 genes on many cancer cell types (Kampen, 2012). These include bladder tumours (Xia *et al.*, 2006), hepatocellular carcinomas (Huang *et al.*, 2011; Li, Zhang, Tang, *et al.*, 2012), breast cancers (Guo *et al.*, 2010; Dhakal *et al.*, 2012), melanoma cancers (Graells *et al.*, 2004), ovarian cancers (Spannuth *et al.*, 2009; Trinh *et al.*, 2009), malignant pleural mesotheliomas (Loganathan *et al.*, 2011), medullary thyroid carcinomas (Rodriguez-Antona *et al.*, 2010), colorectal cancers (Giatromanolaki *et al.*, 2007), non-small-cell lung carcinomas (NSCLC) (Yang *et al.*, 2011; Pajares *et al.*, 2012), oral squamous cell carcinomas (Stinga *et al.*, 2011; Ciurea *et al.*, 2011), some types of lymphomas (Jorgensen *et al.*, 2009; Gratzinger *et al.*, 2010) or bone marrow cells from patients with multiple myeloma (Giatromanolaki *et al.*, 2010) and myeloid leukaemia (Padro *et al.*, 2002). In many of these studies it was shown that high expression of *VEGFRs* correlated with the advanced stage of cancer and its invasive phenotype, high probability of metastasis and therefore a poor prognosis for patients.

In some cases the expression of *VEGF* and *VEGFR* genes can be regulated in an epigenetic manner. The *VEGFA* promoter region can be targeted by small RNAs, which then alter histone modifications and can positively or negatively regulate the expression of this gene (Turunen *et al.*, 2009; Turunen and Yla-Herttuala, 2011). Furthermore, in high-grade transitional cell carcinoma (TCC) cells, VEGFA is expressed at higher levels than in low-grade TCCs. This is due to the hypermethylation of *VEGFA* promoter in the low-grade TCCs, which also corresponds with the less invasive phenotype of these cells in comparison to the high-grade TCCs (Ping *et al.*, 2012). Similarly, DNA methylation regulates the expression of *VEGFRs* in various cell types including some cancers with high methylation matching with a very low or no expression of these receptors (Turunen and Yla-Herttuala, 2011; Quentmeier *et al.*, 2012).

Hypoxic regions, which very often occur in solid tumours, promote angiogenesis in order to supply the extremely fast growing cancer tissues with nutrients and oxygen. Hypoxia very potently induces expression of *VEGF* and its receptors (Rankin and Giaccia, 2008). This is mainly through hypoxia-inducible factor (HIF), which is composed of α- and β-subunits, and is rapidly stabilised when tissue oxygen levels drop down below the norm (Wang *et al.*, 1995). This transcription factor can bind to the HIF response elements (HRE) located in the promoter regions of many genes, including *VEGF*, *VEGFR1* and *VEGFR2* and potently activate their expression (Rankin and Giaccia, 2008). Interestingly, hypoxic regions can also drive *VEGF* expression in normal physiological situations, such as development of organs in the embryo (Carmeliet, 2003). It is important to note that expression of *VEGF* and its receptors can also be regulated by HIF-independent pathways, for example through the reactive oxygen species (ROS) (Ushio-Fukai and Nakamura, 2008) or the family of E-twenty six (ETS) transcription factors (Randi *et al.*, 2009).

7.6 Therapeutic opportunities

In 1971, Judah Folkman proposed a mechanism, where inhibition of tumour growth might be achieved by targeting the blood vessels in order to deprive a cancer tissue of oxygen and nutrients (Folkman, 1971). Since then, anti-angiogenic therapies have emerged as very encouraging strategies for targeting cancer (Denekamp, 1990), and inhibiting VEGF/VEGFR signalling plays a crucial role in these strategies (Kerber and Folkman, 2002). Many years after Folkman pointed out the importance of angiogenesis in anticancer treatment, Rakesh Jain proposed that in some cases inhibiting angiogenesis is more suitable in combination with chemotherapy. Blood vessels that grow in the cancer are very often deformed, leaky and disorganised. Therefore, inhibiting VEGF signalling slows down the hyperactive VEGFR signalling and helps to initially normalise the vasculature. This consequently enables efficient delivery of drugs through the blood system that would eventually destroy not only the endothelial cells but also the cancer cells themselves (Jain, 2001, 2005). Various means of inhibiting VEGF/VEGFR signalling for anticancer treatment have evolved so far and these include VEGF/VEGFR neutralising antibodies, soluble VEGF receptors for trapping VEGF ligands, ribozymes specifically destroying VEGF/VEGFR mRNAs, compounds that decrease VEGF and VEGFR expression and tyrosine kinase inhibitors (TKIs), which are small molecules that directly inhibit the activity of VEGFRs (reviewed broadly in Ferrara and Kerber, 2005; Heath and Bicknell, 2009; Tugues *et al.*, 2011). These various drugs are summarised in Figure 7.7.

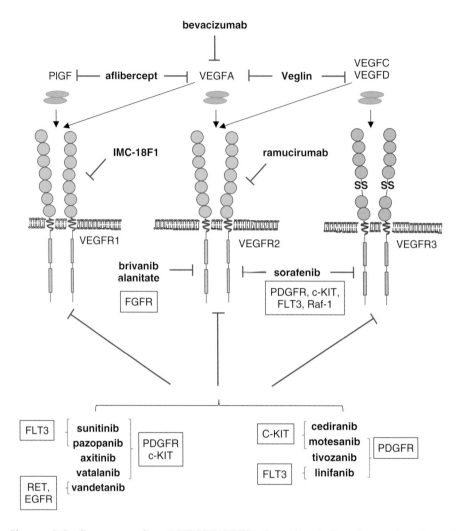

Figure 7.7 **Summary of anti-VEGF/VEGFR therapies.** Indicated are the sites of VEGF/VEGFR inhibition by various drugs. Tyrosine kinase inhibitors (TKIs), which inhibit the intracellular tyrosine kinase domain may also target other proteins, as indicated in the boxes. Ramucirumab and IMC-18F1 are monoclonal antibodies, which bind to extracellular Ig-like domains of indicated receptors. Bevacizumab, which is a also a monoclonal antibody, inhibits specifically VEGFA. Veglin oligonucleotide binds to the DNA of *VEGFA*, *VEGFC* and *VEGFD* genes, preventing their expression. Aflibercept is a soluble receptor that traps VEGFA and PlGF ligands. For the references see Tugues *et al.* (2011). Abbreviations: FGFR, fibroblast growth factor receptor; PDGFR, platelet-derived growth factor receptor; EGFR, epidermal growth factor receptor; FLT3, FMS-like tyrosine kinase 3; RET, rearranged during transfection.

7.6.1 Current therapies

Bevacizumab (also known as Avastin; from Genentech Inc.) is a humanised monoclonal antibody, which traps and neutralises VEGFA ligand, and therefore prevents its binding to VEGFRs (Van Meter and Kim, 2010). In 2004 bevacizumab was the first anti-angiogenic drug approved by the Food and Drug Administration (FDA) for clinical use in a combination with 5-fluorouracil (5-FU) to treat metastatic colorectal cancers. Subsequently, it was further approved as a drug for NSCLC, metastatic breast cancers, glioblastomas and also in combination with chemotherapy and in metastatic renal cell carcinomas as a single therapy (Van Meter and Kim, 2010). Currently bevacizumab is being tested in hundreds of various trials in combination with chemotherapy or alone, and some of the results appear to be promising. As an example, in patients with metastatic colorectal cancer, especially in the older population aged over 65 years, bevacizumab taken in combination with chemotherapy improved progression free survival, with relatively little side effects (Cassidy *et al.*, 2010). However, other studies showed that disease-free survival is not improved by bevacizumab in colorectal cancer and it is more likely to be useful as a maintenance therapy (Van Meter and Kim, 2010). In general, bevacizumab is a promising anti-angiogenic drug, especially when used in combination with chemotherapy. However, the general trend observed in many of the cancers treated is that it tends to improve progression free survival with little or no effect on overall patient survival. Thus, there is a need for more studies to optimise the doses, duration of the treatment and the chemotherapy added, in order to improve the beneficiary effects for the patients (Heath and Bicknell, 2009; Tugues *et al.*, 2011; Van Meter and Kim, 2010).

In addition to bevacizumab, which blocks VEGFA ligand, monoclonal antibodies that bind and inhibit VEGFR1 and VEGFR2 directly (IMC-18F1 and ramucirumab/IMC-1121B, respectively; from ImClone Systems) have also been developed (Wu *et al.*, 2006; Spratlin, 2011). Some promising preliminary effects of these antibodies in mouse tumour xenografts have been demonstrated (Wu *et al.*, 2006; Spratlin, 2011), and ramucirumab is being tested further in various clinical trials including breast cancers and gastric cancers (Van Meter and Kim, 2010; Spratlin, 2011).

Synthetic soluble VEGFR called VEGF-Trap (aflibercept; from Sanofi-Aventis, Regeneron), which is a decoy receptor, has been developed as another strategy to silence pro-angiogenic signalling (Teng *et al.*, 2010). Pre-clinical studies in tumour xenografts have proved that aflibercept inhibits angiogenesis and tumour growth, which was confirmed by the early phase clinical trials, where improved initial patient survival was observed. However, in the later Phase III trials the overall survival in various cancers varied a lot, with fairly promising outcomes in metastatic colorectal cancer but less good ones in lung, pancreatic and prostate cancers (Gaya and Tse, 2012). It is also currently being tested in paediatric tumours (Chau and Figg, 2012).

An alternative way to decrease the abundance of VEGF ligands is to decrease their expression. Veglin, which is an oligonucleotide (from Vasgene Therapeutics/USC) was designed to specifically bind DNA of *VEGFA*, *VEGFC* and *VEGFD* genes (Levine *et al.*, 2006). Preliminary clinical trials showed relatively good tolerance of Veglin, reduction of VEGF levels in the plasma and inhibition of various cancer types in some patients (Levine *et al.*, 2006).

The use of drugs, such as bevacizumab or aflibercept, which are directed against a narrow list of targets, may not be so efficient in inhibiting angiogenesis, as there are other signalling pathways that drive the growth of blood vessels into the tumour, for example the fibroblast growth factor (FGF) and its receptors (FGFRs) (Claesson-Welch, 2012). Therefore, another strategy is to design small molecule inhibitors that would target not only VEGFR signalling but also a broader selection of proteins. Hence, many TKIs have been developed that in addition to VEGFR1-3 also inhibit other tyrosine kinases such as platelet-derived growth factor receptor (PDGFR), epidermal growth factor receptor (EGFR), FGFR, c-KIT, Raf-1, FMS-like tyrosine kinase 3 (FLT3) and rearranged during transfection (RET) (as specified in Tugues *et al.* (2011) and Figure 7.7). The long list of TKIs includes: sorafenib/Bay43-9006 (Nexavar; from Bayer/Schering), sunitinib/SU11248 (Sutent; from Pfizer), pazopanib (Votrient; from Glaxo-SmithKline), axitinib/AG013736 (from Pfizer), vandetanib/ZD6474 (Zactima; from AstraZeneca), cediranib/AZD2171 (Resentin; from AstraZeneca), brivanib alanitate (from Bristol-Myers Squibb), motesanib/AMG706 (from Amgen), linifanib/ABT869 (from Abbott), tivozanib/AV-951 (from Abbott), vatalanib/PTK787 (from Novartis Pharmaceutical) (all referenced in Tugues *et al.*, 2011). Sorafenib, sunitinib and pazopanib have been approved by the FDA for treatment of some cancers, for example, advanced renal cell carcinomas (Tugues *et al.*, 2011). Sorafenib showed promising results in a trial for inoperable hepatocellular carcinomas, where it extended the patient median survival and the time to radiologic progression for 3 months in comparison with patients receiving placebo (Llovet *et al.*, 2008). In patients with clear renal cell carcinoma, which failed to respond to previous treatments, sorafenib extended progression free survival but had adverse effects and was highly toxic (Escudier *et al.*, 2007). In addition to targeting vasculature, sorafenib exhibits antiviral and inhibitory effects towards T cells and dendritic cells (Himmelsbach *et al.*, 2009; Seliger *et al.*, 2010). Pazopanib, another TKI used in the clinic to treat advanced renal cell carcinoma, is showing promising results in term of progression free survival and is well tolerated with the smaller toxicity when compared with other TKIs (Zivi *et al.*, 2012).

Various anti-VEGFR TKIs are being tested in combination with other drugs and also they have a high likelihood of working as monotherapies, since they hit more than one signalling pathway. This is supported by the results obtained with sorafenib and sunitinib, which when used alone show tumour-inhibiting results in metastatic renal cell carcinomas (Ruegg and Mutter, 2007). However, many more studies need to be undertaken to maximise the outcome of treatments with anti-angiogenic drugs. For example, continuous daily administration of sunitinib had a beneficiary effect on progression free and overall survival of patients with advanced pancreatic neuroendocrine tumours (Raymond *et al.*, 2011). On the other hand, when given to mice for short periods of time, sunitinib significantly accelerated metastasis of various tumours tested and decreased overall survival (Ebos *et al.*, 2009).

7.6.2   Future strategies

Although targeting VEGF/VEGFR signalling as an anti-angiogenic strategy in cancer treatment gives very promising results in the pre-clinical studies (Tugues *et al.*, 2011), it still faces significant challenges as seen by the mild effects in the final patient outcomes. It needs improvement of the efficacy of these therapies and an increase in the overall patient survival rates. Many of the anti-VEGF/VEGFR drugs developed so far require further optimisation studies for dosing and timing in order to minimise the adverse effects and maximise the clinical efficacy.

A possible way to improve the efficacy of current anti-VEGF/VEGFR drugs is to use them in combination with other anticancer treatments. The use of bevacizumab in combination with chemotherapy has already been more promising in treating colorectal cancer, when compared with single therapies (Hurwitz *et al.*, 2004; Ainsworth *et al.*, 2009). Moreover, additive anticancer effects might be seen when drugs that hit various signalling pathways or different cell types within the tumour microenvironment are combined. A very recent study demonstrated that using paclitaxel, which inhibits mitosis by stabilising microtubules, followed by administration of sorafenib had a synergistic effect in treating NSCLC, as shown by decreased proliferation, increased apoptosis, reduced vascular area and delayed tumour growth (Zhang *et al.*, 2012). This study, as with many other pre-clinical studies, was carried out in animals, where tumours are injected subcutaneously. In such cases more promising results are often obtained, as injected tumour cells have a challenge in the first place to grow and drive the formation of the vasculature 'from scratch'. Therefore they are likely to be affected by the anti-angiogenic treatment. Clearly, pre-clinical studies are crucial as they give insights into whether the new drug is likely to inhibit tumour growth. However, in the real patient scenarios this situation is more complicated. Very often at the time of diagnosis cancer is an established heterogeneous mass of cells with the on-going angiogenesis. On top of that, when we consider that the cancer may have already metastasised, the likelihood of observing the beneficial effects of anti-angiogenic therapy on overall patient survival becomes significantly reduced. Thus it is important to extract as much information about the cancer stage as possible, in order to decide on the best cure, including suitable anti-angiogenic therapy, most likely combined with chemotherapy or other treatments. The development of biomarkers, which would allow assessing the stage of diseases and how well the patient is likely to respond to anti-angiogenic inhibitors, is therefore a priority for future research.

References

Aase, K., von Euler, G., Li, X. *et al.* (2001) Vascular endothelial growth factor-B-deficient mice display an atrial conduction defect. *Circulation*, **104** (3), 358–364.

Abu-Ghazaleh, R., Kabir, J., Jia, H. *et al.* (2001) Src mediates stimulation by vascular endothelial growth factor of the phosphorylation of focal adhesion kinase at tyrosine 861, and migration and anti-apoptosis in endothelial cells. *Biochemical Journal*, **360** (Pt 1), 255–264.

Ahmad, S., Hewett, P.W., Wang, P. *et al.* (2006) Direct evidence for endothelial vascular endothelial growth factor receptor-1 function in nitric oxide-mediated angiogenesis. *Circulation Research*, **99** (7), 715–722.

Ainsworth, N.L., Lee, J.S. and Eisen, T. (2009) Impact of anti-angiogenic treatments on metastatic renal cell carcinoma. *Expert Review of Anticancer Therapy*, **9** (12), 1793–1805.

Albuquerque, R.J., Hayashi, T., Cho, W.G. *et al.* (2009) Alternatively spliced vascular endothelial growth factor receptor-2 is an essential endogenous inhibitor of lymphatic vessel growth. *Nature Medicine*, **15** (9), 1023–1030.

Autiero, M., Waltenberger, J., Communi, D. *et al.* (2003) Role of PlGF in the intra- and intermolecular cross talk between the VEGF receptors Flt1 and Flk1. *Nature Medicine*, **9** (7), 936–943.

Barleon, B., Sozzani, S., Zhou, D. *et al.* (1996) Migration of human monocytes in response to vascular endothelial growth factor (VEGF) is mediated via the VEGF receptor flt-1. *Blood*, **87** (8), 3336–3343.

Bates, D.O., Cui, T.G., Doughty, J.M. *et al.* (2002) VEGF165b, an inhibitory splice variant of vascular endothelial growth factor, is down-regulated in renal cell carcinoma. *Cancer Research*, **62** (14), 4123–4131.

Becker, P.M., Waltenberger, J., Yachechko, R. *et al.* (2005) Neuropilin-1 regulates vascular endothelial growth factor-mediated endothelial permeability. *Circulation Research*, **96** (12), 1257–1265.

Bellik, L., Vinci, M.C., Filippi, S. *et al.* (2005) Intracellular pathways triggered by the selective FLT-1-agonist placental growth factor in vascular smooth muscle cells exposed to hypoxia. *British Journal of Pharmacology*, **146** (4), 568–575.

Bellomo, D., Headrick, J.P., Silins, G.U. *et al.* (2000) Mice lacking the vascular endothelial growth factor-B gene (Vegfb) have smaller hearts, dysfunctional coronary vasculature, and impaired recovery from cardiac ischemia. *Circulation Research*, **86** (2), E29–E35.

Bhattacharya, R., Kang-Decker, N., Hughes, D.A. *et al.* (2005) Regulatory role of dynamin-2 in VEGFR-2/KDR-mediated endothelial signaling. *FASEB Journal*, **19** (12), 1692–1694.

Borges, E., Jan, Y. and Ruoslahti, E. (2000) Platelet-derived growth factor receptor beta and vascular endothelial growth factor receptor 2 bind to the beta 3 integrin through its extracellular domain. *Journal of Biological Chemistry*, **275** (51), 39867–39873.

Cai, J., Ahmad, S., Jiang, W.G., *et al.* (2003) Activation of vascular endothelial growth factor receptor-1 sustains angiogenesis and Bcl-2 expression via the phosphatidylinositol 3-kinase pathway in endothelial cells. *Diabetes*, **52** (12), 2959–2968.

Carmeliet, P. (2003) Angiogenesis in health and disease. *Nature Medicine*, **9** (6), 653–660.

Carmeliet, P. and Jain, R.K. (2011) Molecular mechanisms and clinical applications of angiogenesis. *Nature*, **473** (7347), 298–307.

Carmeliet, P., Ferreira, V., Breier, G. *et al.* (1996) Abnormal blood vessel development and lethality in embryos lacking a single VEGF allele. *Nature*, **380** (6573), 435–439.

Carmeliet, P., Moons, L., Luttun, A. *et al.* (2001a) Synergism between vascular endothelial growth factor and placental growth factor contributes to angiogenesis and plasma extravasation in pathological conditions. *Nature Medicine*, **7** (5), 575–583.

Carmeliet, P., Moons, L., Luttun, A. *et al.* (2001b) Synergism between vascular endothelial growth factor and placental growth factor contributes to angiogenesis and plasma extravasation in pathological conditions. *Nature Medicine*, **7** (5), 575–583.

Caron, C., Spring, K., Laramee, M. *et al.* (2009) Non-redundant roles of the Gab1 and Gab2 scaffolding adapters in VEGF-mediated signalling, migration, and survival of endothelial cells. *Cell Signal*, **21** (6), 943–953.

Cassidy, J., Saltz, L.B., Giantonio, B.J. *et al.* (2010) Effect of bevacizumab in older patients with metastatic colorectal cancer: pooled analysis of four randomized studies. *Journal of Cancer Research and Clinical Oncology*, **136** (5), 737–743.

Chabot, C., Spring, K., Gratton, J.P. *et al.* (2009) New role for the protein tyrosine phosphatase DEP-1 in Akt activation and endothelial cell survival. *Molecular and Cellular Biology*, **29** (1), 241–253.

Chau, C.H. and Figg, W.D. (2012) Aflibercept in pediatric solid tumors: moving beyond the trap. *Clinical Cancer Research*, **18** (18), 4868–4871.

Chen, X.L., Nam, J.O., Jean, C. *et al.* (2012) VEGF-induced vascular permeability is mediated by FAK. *Developmental Cell*, **22** (1), 146–157.

Ciurea, R., Margaritescu, C., Simionescu, C. *et al.* (2011) VEGF and his R1 and R2 receptors expression in mast cells of oral squamous cells carcinomas and their involvement in tumoral angiogenesis. *Romanian Journal of Morphology and Embryology*, **52** (4), 1227–1232.

Claesson-Welsh, L. (2012) Blood vessels as targets in tumor therapy. *Upsala Journal of Medical Science*, **117** (2), 178–186.

Coso, S., Zeng, Y., Opeskin, K. and Williams, E.D. (2012) Vascular endothelial growth factor receptor-3 directly interacts with phosphatidylinositol 3-kinase to regulate lymphangiogenesis. *PLoS One*, **7** (6), e39558.

Cunningham, S.A., Waxham, M.N., Arrate, P.M. and Brock, T.A. (1995) Interaction of the Flt-1 tyrosine kinase receptor with the p85 subunit of phosphatidylinositol 3-kinase. Mapping of a novel site involved in binding. *Journal of Biological Chemistry*, **270** (35), 20254–20257.

Cunningham, S.A., Arrate, M.P., Brock, T.A. *et al.* (1997) Interactions of FLT-1 and KDR with phospholipase C gamma: identification of the phosphotyrosine binding sites. *Biochemical and Biophysical Research Communications*, **240** (3), 635–639.

David Dong, Z.M., Aplin, A.C. and Nicosia, R.F. (2009) Regulation of angiogenesis by macrophages, dendritic cells, and circulating myelomonocytic cells. *Current Pharmaceutical Design*, **15** (4), 365–379.

Dayanir, V., Meyer, R.D., Lashkari, K. and Rahimi, N. (2001) Identification of tyrosine residues in vascular endothelial growth factor receptor-2/FLK-1 involved in activation of phosphatidylinositol 3-kinase and cell proliferation. *Journal of Biological Chemistry*, **276** (21), 17686–17692.

De Falco, S. (2012) The discovery of placenta growth factor and its biological activity. *Experimental and Molecular Medicine*, **44** (1), 1–9.

Del Valle-Perez, B., Martinez, V.G., Lacasa-Salavert, C. *et al.* (2010) Filamin B plays a key role in vascular endothelial growth factor-induced endothelial cell motility through its interaction with Rac-1 and Vav-2. *Journal of Biological Chemistry*, **285** (14), 10748–10760.

Denekamp, J. (1990) Vascular attack as a therapeutic strategy for cancer. *Cancer and Metastasis Reviews*, **9** (3), 267–282.

Dhakal, H.P., Naume, B., Synnestvedt, M. *et al.* (2012) Expression of vascular endothelial growth factor and vascular endothelial growth factor receptors 1 and 2 in invasive breast carcinoma: prognostic significance and relationship with markers for aggressiveness. *Histopathology*, **61** (3), 350–364.

Dimmeler, S., Fleming, I., Fisslthaler, B. *et al.* (1999) Activation of nitric oxide synthase in endothelial cells by Akt-dependent phosphorylation. *Nature*, **399** (6736), 601–605.

Ding, Y., Huang, Y., Song, N. *et al.* (2010) NFAT1 mediates placental growth factor-induced myelomonocytic cell recruitment via the induction of TNF-alpha. *Journal of Immunology*, **184** (5) 2593–2601.

DiSalvo, J., Bayne, M.L., Conn, G. *et al.* (1995) Purification and characterization of a naturally occurring vascular endothelial growth factor.placenta growth factor heterodimer. *Journal of Biological Chemistry*, **270** (13), 7717–7123.

Dubash, A.D., Menold, M.M., Samson, T. *et al.* (2009) Focal adhesions: new angles on an old structure. Chapter 1. *International Review of Cell and Molecular Biology*, **277**, 1–65.

Dumont, D.J., Jussila, L., Taipale, J. *et al.* (1998) Cardiovascular failure in mouse embryos deficient in VEGF receptor-3. *Science*, **282** (5390), 946–949.

Dvorak, H.F., Orenstein, N.S., Carvalho, A.C. *et al.* (1979) Induction of a fibrin-gel investment: an early event in line 10 hepatocarcinoma growth mediated by tumor-secreted products. *Journal of Immunology*, **122** (1), 166–174.

Ebos, J.M., Lee, C.R., Cruz-Munoz, W. *et al.* (2009) Accelerated metastasis after short-term treatment with a potent inhibitor of tumor angiogenesis. *Cancer Cell*, **15** (3), 232–239.

Escudier, B., Eisen, T., Stadler, W.M. *et al.* (2007) Sorafenib in advanced clear-cell renal-cell carcinoma. *New England Journal of Medicine*, **356** (2), 125–134.

Evans, I.M., Britton, G. and Zachary, I.C. (2008) Vascular endothelial growth factor induces heat shock protein (HSP) 27 serine 82 phosphorylation and endothelial tubulogenesis via protein kinase D and independent of p38 kinase. *Cell Signal*, **20** (7), 1375–1384.

Ewan, L.C., Jopling, H.M., Jia, H.Y. *et al.* (2006) Intrinsic tyrosine kinase activity is required for vascular endothelial growth factor receptor 2 ubiquitination, sorting and degradation in endothelial cells. *Traffic*, **7** (9), 1270–1282.

Favier, B., Alam, A., Barron, P. *et al.* (2006) Neuropilin-2 interacts with VEGFR-2 and VEGFR-3 and promotes human endothelial cell survival and migration. *Blood*, **108** (4), 1243–1250.

Ferrara, N. and Kerbel, R.S. (2005) Angiogenesis as a therapeutic target. *Nature*, **438** (7070), 967–974.

Ferrara, N., Carver-Moore, K., Chen, H. *et al.* (1996) Heterozygous embryonic lethality induced by targeted inactivation of the VEGF gene. *Nature*, **380** (6573), 439–442.

Folkman, J. (1971) Tumor angiogenesis: therapeutic implications. *New England Journal of Medicine*, **285** (21), 1182–1186.

Folkman, J., Watson, K., Ingber, D. and Hanahan, D. (1989) Induction of angiogenesis during the transition from hyperplasia to neoplasia. *Nature*, **339** (6219), 58–61.

Fong, G.H., Rossant, J., Gertsenstein, M. and Breitman, M. L. (1995) Role of the Flt-1 receptor tyrosine kinase in regulating the assembly of vascular endothelium. *Nature*, **376** (6535), 66–70.

Fujio, Y. and Walsh, K. (1999) Akt mediates cytoprotection of endothelial cells by vascular endothelial growth factor in an anchorage-dependent manner. *Journal of Biological Chemistry*, **274** (23), 16349–16354.

Fukumura, D., Gohongi, T., Kadambi, A. *et al.* (2001) Predominant role of endothelial nitric oxide synthase in vascular endothelial growth factor-induced angiogenesis and vascular permeability. *Proceedings of the National Academy of Sciences, USA*, **98** (5), 2604–2609.

Fulton, D., Gratton, J.P., McCabe, T.J. *et al.* (1999) Regulation of endothelium-derived nitric oxide production by the protein kinase Akt. *Nature*, **399** (6736), 597–601.

Galland, F. *et al.* (1993) The FLT4 gene encodes a transmembrane tyrosine kinase related to the vascular endothelial growth factor receptor. *Oncogene*, **8**(5), 1233–1240.

Galvagni, F., Pennacchini, S., Salameh, A. *et al.* (2010) Endothelial cell adhesion to the extracellular matrix induces c-Src-dependent VEGFR-3 phosphorylation without the activation of the receptor intrinsic kinase activity. *Circulation Research*, **106** (12), 1839–1848.

Gampel, A., Moss, L., Jones, M.C. *et al.* (2006) VEGF regulates the mobilization of VEGFR2/KDR from an intracellular endothelial storage compartment. *Blood*, **108** (8), 2624–2631.

Gavard, J. and Gutkind, J.S. (2006) VEGF controls endothelial-cell permeability by promoting the beta-arrestin-dependent endocytosis of VE-cadherin. *Nature Cell Biology*, **8** (11), 1223–1234.

Gaya, A. and Tse, V. (2012) A preclinical and clinical review of aflibercept for the management of cancer. *Cancer Treatment Reviews*, **38** (5), 484–493.

Giatromanolaki, A., Bai, M., Margaritis, D. *et al.* (2007) Activated VEGFR2/KDR pathway in tumour cells and tumour associated vessels of colorectal cancer. *European Journal of Clinical Investigation*, **37** (11), 878–886.

Giatromanolaki, A., Koukourakis, M.I., Sivridis, E. *et al.* (2010) Hypoxia and activated VEGF/receptor pathway in multiple myeloma. *Anticancer Research*, **30** (7), 2831–2836.

Gille, H., Kowalski, J., Yu, L. *et al.* (2000) A repressor sequence in the juxtamembrane domain of Flt-1 (VEGFR-1) constitutively inhibits vascular endothelial growth factor-dependent phosphatidylinositol 3′-kinase activation and endothelial cell migration. *EMBO Journal*, **19** (15), 4064–4073.

Graells, J., Vinyals, A., Figueras, A. *et al.* (2004) Overproduction of VEGF concomitantly expressed with its receptors promotes growth and survival of melanoma cells through MAPK and PI3K signaling. *Journal of Investigative Dermatology*, **123** (6), 1151–1161.

Gratzinger, D., Advani, R., Zhao, S. *et al.* (2010) Lymphoma cell VEGFR2 expression detected by immunohistochemistry predicts poor overall survival in diffuse large B cell lymphoma treated with immunochemotherapy (R-CHOP). *British Journal of Haematology*, **148** (2), 235–244.

Grazia Lampugnani, M., Zanetti, A., Corada, M. *et al.* (2003) Contact inhibition of VEGF-induced proliferation requires vascular endothelial cadherin, beta-catenin, and the phosphatase DEP-1/CD148. *Journal of Cell Biology*, **161** (4), 793–804.

Grunewald, F.S., Prota, A.E., Giese, A. and Ballmer-Hofer, K. (2010) Structure-function analysis of VEGF receptor activation and the role of coreceptors in angiogenic signaling. *Biochimica et Biophysica Acta*, **1804** (3), 567–580.

Guo, S., Colbert, L.S., Fuller, M. *et al.* (2010) Vascular endothelial growth factor receptor-2 in breast cancer. *Biochimica et Biophysica Acta*, **1806** (1), 108–121.

Ha, C.H., Wang, W., Jhun, B.S. *et al.* (2008) Protein kinase D-dependent phosphorylation and nuclear export of histone deacetylase 5 mediates vascular endothelial growth factor-induced gene expression and angiogenesis. *Journal of Biological Chemistry*, **283** (21), 14590–14599.

Hagberg, C.E., Falkevall, A., Wang, X. *et al.* (2010) Vascular endothelial growth factor B controls endothelial fatty acid uptake. *Nature*, **464** (7290), 917–921.

Haiko, P., Makinen, T., Keskitalo, S. *et al.* (2008) Deletion of Vascular endothelial growth factor C (VEGF-C) and VEGF-D is not equivalent to VEGF receptor 3 deletion in mouse embryos. *Molecular and Cellular Biology*, **28** (15), 4843–4850.

Heath, V.L. and Bicknell, R. (2009) Anticancer strategies involving the vasculature. *Nature Reviews Clinical Oncology*, **6** (7), 395–404.

Himmelsbach, K., Sauter, D., Baumert, T.F. *et al.* (2009) New aspects of an anti-tumour drug: sorafenib efficiently inhibits HCV replication. *Gut*, **58** (12), 1644–1653.

Hiratsuka, S., Minowa, O., Kuno, J. *et al.* (1998) Flt-1 lacking the tyrosine kinase domain is sufficient for normal development and angiogenesis in mice. *Proceedings of the National Academy of Sciences, USA*, **95** (16), 9349–9354.

Holmqvist, K., Cross, M., Riley, D. and Welsh, M. (2003) The Shb adaptor protein causes Src-dependent cell spreading and activation of focal adhesion kinase in murine brain endothelial cells. *Cell Signal*, **15** (2), 171–179.

Huang, K., Andersson, C., Roomans, G.M., *et al.* (2001) Signaling properties of VEGF receptor-1 and-2 homo- and heterodimers. *International Journal of Biochemistry and Cell Biology*, **33** (4), 315–324.

Huang, J., Zhang, X., Tang, Q. *et al.* (2011) Prognostic significance and potential therapeutic target of VEGFR2 in hepatocellular carcinoma. *Journal of Clinical Pathology*, **64** (4), 343–348.

Hurwitz, H., Fehrenbacher, L., Novotny, W. *et al.* (2004) Bevacizumab plus irinotecan, fluorouracil, and leucovorin for metastatic colorectal cancer. *New England Journal of Medicine*, **350** (23), 2335–2342.

Ichise, T., Yoshida, N. and Ichise, H. (2010) H-, N- and Kras cooperatively regulate lymphatic vessel growth by modulating VEGFR3 expression in lymphatic endothelial cells in mice. *Development*, **137** (6), 1003–1013.

Igarashi, K., Isohara, T., Kato, T. *et al.* (1998) Tyrosine 1213 of Flt-1 is a major binding site of Nck and SHP-2. *Biochemical and Biophysical Research Communications*, **246** (1), 95–99.

Ikeda, S., Ushio-Fukai, M., Zuo, L. *et al.* (2005) Novel role of ARF6 in vascular endothelial growth factor-induced signaling and angiogenesis. *Circulation Research*, **96** (4), 467–475.

Ilic, D., Furuta, Y., Kanazawa, S. *et al.* (1995) Reduced cell motility and enhanced focal adhesion contact formation in cells from FAK-deficient mice. *Nature*, **377** (6549), 539–544.

Ito, N., Wernstedt, C., Engstrom, U. and Claesson-Welsh, L. (1998) Identification of vascular endothelial growth factor receptor-1 tyrosine phosphorylation sites and binding of SH2 domain-containing molecules. *Journal of Biological Chemistry*, **273** (36), 23410–23418.

Jain, R.K. (2001) Normalizing tumor vasculature with anti-angiogenic therapy: a new paradigm for combination therapy. *Nature Medicine*, **7** (9), 987–989.

Jain, R.K. (2005) Normalization of tumor vasculature: an emerging concept in antiangiogenic therapy. *Science*, **307** (5706), 58–62.

Jakobsson, L., Kreuger, J., Holmborn, K. *et al.* (2006) Heparan sulfate in trans potentiates VEGFR-mediated angiogenesis. *Developmental Cell*, **10** (5), 625–634.

Jorgensen, J.M., Sorensen, F.B., Bendix, K. *et al.* (2009) Expression level, tissue distribution pattern, and prognostic impact of vascular endothelial growth factors VEGF and VEGF-C and their receptors Flt-1, KDR, and Flt-4 in different subtypes of non-Hodgkin lymphomas. *Leukemia and Lymphoma*, **50** (10), 1647–1660.

Kampen, K.R. (2012) The mechanisms that regulate the localization and overexpression of VEGF receptor-2 are promising therapeutic targets in cancer biology. *Anticancer Drugs*, **23** (4), 347–354.

Kappas, N.C., Zeng, G.F., Chappell, J.C. *et al.* (2008) The VEGF receptor Flt-1 spatially modulates Flk-1 signaling and blood vessel branching. *Journal of Cell Biology*, **181** (5), 847–858.

Kappert, K., Peters, K.G., Bohmer, F.D. and Ostman, A. (2005) Tyrosine phosphatases in vessel wall signaling. *Cardiovascular Research*, **65** (3), 587–598.

Kawamura, H., Li, X., Goishi, K. *et al.* (2008) Neuropilin-1 in regulation of VEGF-induced activation of p38MAPK and endothelial cell organization. *Blood*, **112** (9), 3638–3649.

Kearney, J.B., Kappas, N.C., Ellerstrom, C. *et al.* (2004) The VEGF receptor flt-1 (VEGFR-1) is a positive modulator of vascular sprout formation and branching morphogenesis. *Blood*, **103** (12), 4527–4535.

Kendall, R.L. and Thomas, K.A. (1993) Inhibition of vascular endothelial cell growth factor activity by an endogenously encoded soluble receptor. *Proceedings of the National Academy of Sciences, USA*, **90** (22), 10705–10709.

Kendall, R.L., Wang, G., DiSalvo, J. and Thomas, K.A. (1994) Specificity of vascular endothelial cell growth factor receptor ligand binding domains. *Biochemical and Biophysical Research Communications*, **201** (1), 326–330.

Kerbel, R. and Folkman, J. (2002) Clinical translation of angiogenesis inhibitors. *Nature Review Cancer*, **2** (10), 727–739.

Kerber, M., Reiss, Y., Wickersheim, A. *et al.* (2008) Flt-1 signaling in macrophages promotes glioma growth *in vivo*. *Cancer Research*, **68** (18), 7342–7351.

Kobayashi, S., Sawano, A., Nojima, Y. *et al.* (2004) The c-Cbl/CD2AP complex regulates VEGF-induced endocytosis and degradation of Flt-1 (VEGFR-1). *FASEB Journal*, **18** (7), 929–931.

Koch, S. (2012) Neuropilin signalling in angiogenesis. *Biochemical Society Transactions*, **40** (1), 20–25.

Koch, S., Tugues, S., Li, X. *et al.* (2011) Signal transduction by vascular endothelial growth factor receptors. *Biochemical Journal*, **437** (2), 169–183.

Kou, R., SenBanerjee, S., Jain, M.K., and Michel, T. (2005) Differential regulation of vascular endothelial growth factor receptors (VEGFR) revealed by RNA interference: interactions of VEGFR-1 and VEGFR-2 in endothelial cell signaling. *Biochemistry*, **44** (45), 15064–15073.

Kranenburg, O., Gebbink, M.F. and Voest, E.E. (2004) Stimulation of angiogenesis by Ras proteins. *Biochimica et Biophysica Acta*, **1654** (1), 23–37.

Krysiak, O., Bretschneider, A., Zhong, E. *et al.* (2005) Soluble vascular endothelial growth factor receptor-1 (sFLT-1) mediates downregulation of FLT-1 and prevents activated neutrophils from women with preeclampsia from additional migration by VEGF. *Circulation Research*, **97** (12), 1253–1261.

Labrecque, L., Royal, I., Surprenant, D.S. *et al.* (2003) Regulation of vascular endothelial growth factor receptor-2 activity by caveolin-1 and plasma membrane cholesterol. *Molecular and Cellular Biology*, **14** (1), 334–347.

Ladomery, M.R., Harper, S.J and Bates, D.O. (2007) Alternative splicing in angiogenesis: the vascular endothelial growth factor paradigm. *Cancer Letters*, **249** (2), 133–142.

Lamalice, L., Houle, F. and Huot, J. (2006) Phosphorylation of Tyr1214 within VEGFR-2 triggers the recruitment of Nck and activation of Fyn leading to SAPK2/p38 activation and endothelial cell migration in response to VEGF. *Journal of Biological Chemistry*, **281** (45), 34009–34020.

Lampugnani, M.G., Orsenigo, F., Gagliani, M.C. *et al.* (2006) Vascular endothelial cadherin controls VEGFR-2 internalization and signaling from intracellular compartments. *Journal of Cell Biology*, **174** (4), 593–604.

Lanahan, A.A., Hermans, K., Claes, F. *et al.* (2010) VEGF receptor 2 endocytic trafficking regulates arterial morphogenesis. *Developmental Cell*, **18** (5), 713–724.

Laramee, M., Chabot, C., Cloutier, M. *et al.* (2007) The scaffolding adapter Gab1 mediates vascular endothelial growth factor signaling and is required for endothelial cell migration and capillary formation. *Journal of Biological Chemistry*, **282** (11), 7758–7769.

Le Boeuf, F., Houle, F., Sussman, M. and Huot, J. (2006) Phosphorylation of focal adhesion kinase (FAK) on Ser732 is induced by rho-dependent kinase and is essential for proline-rich tyrosine kinase-2-mediated phosphorylation of FAK on Tyr407 in response to vascular endothelial growth factor. *Molecular and Cellular Biology*, **17** (8), 3508–3520.

Lesslie, D.P., Summy, J.M., Parikh, N.U. *et al.* (2006) Vascular endothelial growth factor receptor-1 mediates migration of human colorectal carcinoma cells by activation of Src family kinases. *British Journal of Cancer*, **94** (11), 1710–1707.

Levine, A.M., Tulpule, A., Quinn, D.I. *et al.* (2006) Phase I study of antisense oligonucleotide against vascular endothelial growth factor: decrease in plasma vascular endothelial growth factor with potential clinical efficacy. *Journal of Clinical Oncology*, **24** (11), 1712–1719.

Li, X., Tjwa, M., Van Hove, I. *et al.* (2008) Reevaluation of the role of VEGF-B suggests a restricted role in the revascularization of the ischemic myocardium. *Arteriosclerosis, Thrombosis, and Vascular Biology*, **28** (9), 1614–1620.

Li, B., Wang, C., Zhang, Y., *et al.* (2012) Elevated PLGF contributes to small-cell lung cancer brain metastasis. *Oncogene*, doi: 10.1038/onc.2012.

Li, T., Zhang, X., Tang, Q. *et al.* (2012) Expression and prognostic significance of vascular endothelial growth factor receptor 1 in hepatocellular carcinoma. *Journal of Clinical Pathology*, **65** (9), 808–814.

Liu, L., Ratner, B.D., Sage, E.H. and Jiang, S. (2007) Endothelial cell migration on surface-density gradients of fibronectin, VEGF, or both proteins. *Langmuir*, **23** (22), 11168–11173.

Llovet, J.M., Ricci, S., Mazzaferro, V. *et al.* (2008) Sorafenib in advanced hepatocellular carcinoma. *New England Journal of Medicine*, **359**(4), 378–390.

Loganathan, S., Kanteti, R., Siddiqui, S.S. *et al.* (2011) Role of protein kinase C beta and vascular endothelial growth factor receptor in malignant pleural mesothelioma: Therapeutic implications and the usefulness of *Caenorhabditis elegans* model organism. *Journal of Carcinogenesis*, **10**, 4.

Mac Gabhann, F. and. Popel, A.S (2007) Dimerization of VEGF receptors and implications for signal transduction: A computational study. *Biophysical Chemistry*, **128** (2–3), 125–139.

Mahabeleshwar, G.H., Feng, W., Phillips, D.R. and Byzova, T.V. (2006) Integrin signaling is critical for pathological angiogenesis. *Journal of Experimental Medicine*, **203** (11), 2495–2507.

Mahabeleshwar, G.H., Chen, J., Feng, W. *et al.* (2008) Integrin affinity modulation in angiogenesis. *Cell Cycle*, **7** (3), 335–347.

Makinen, T., Veikkola, T., Mustjoki, S. *et al.* (2001) Isolated lymphatic endothelial cells transduce growth, survival and migratory signals via the VEGF-C/D receptor VEGFR-3. *Embo Journal*, **20** (17), 4762–4773.

Matsumoto, T., Bohman, S., Dixelius, J. *et al.* (2005) VEGF receptor-2 Y951 signaling and a role for the adapter molecule TSAd in tumor angiogenesis. *EMBO Journal*, **24** (13), 2342–2353.

Meadows, K.N., Bryant, P. and Pumiglia, K. (2001) Vascular endothelial growth factor induction of the angiogenic phenotype requires Ras activation. *Journal of Biological Chemistry*, **276** (52), 49289–49298.

Meadows, K.N., Bryant, P., Vincent, P.A., and Pumiglia, K.M. (2004) Activated Ras induces a proangiogenic phenotype in primary endothelial cells. *Oncogene*, **23** (1), 192–200.

Meyer, R.D., Mohammadi, M. and Rahimi, N. (2006) A single amino acid substitution in the activation loop defines the decoy characteristic of VEGFR-1/FLT-1. *Journal of Biological Chemistry*, **281** (2), 867–875.

Meyer, R.D., Sacks, D.B. and Rahimi, N. (2008) IQGAP1-dependent signaling pathway regulates endothelial cell proliferation and angiogenesis. *PLoS One*, **3** (12), e3848.

Miao, H.Q., Soker, S., Feiner, L. *et al.* (1999) Neuropilin-1 mediates collapsin-1/semaphorin III inhibition of endothelial cell motility: functional competition of collapsin-1 and vascular endothelial growth factor-165. *Journal of Cell Biology*, **146** (1), 233–242.

Muramatsu, M., Yamamoto, S., Osawa, T. and Shibuya, M. (2010) Vascular endothelial growth factor receptor-1 signaling promotes mobilization of macrophage lineage cells from bone marrow and stimulates solid tumor growth. *Cancer Research*, **70** (20), 8211–8221.

Murohara, T., Horowitz, J.R., Silver, M. *et al.* (1998) Vascular endothelial growth factor/vascular permeability factor enhances vascular permeability via nitric oxide and prostacyclin. *Circulation*, **97** (1), 99–107.

Nilsson, I., Bahram, F., Li, X.J. *et al.* (2010) VEGF receptor 2/-3 heterodimers detected in situ by proximity ligation on angiogenic sprouts. *Embo Journal*, **29** (8), 1377–1388.

Nowak, D.G., Woolard, J., Amin, E.M. *et al.* (2008) Expression of pro- and anti-angiogenic isoforms of VEGF is differentially regulated by splicing and growth factors. *Journal of Cell Science*, **121** (Pt 20), 3487–3495.

Ogawa, S., Oku, A., Sawano, A. *et al.* (1998) A novel type of vascular endothelial growth factor, VEGF-E (NZ-7 VEGF), preferentially utilizes KDR/Flk-1 receptor and carries a potent mitotic activity without heparin-binding domain. *Journal of Biological Chemistry*, **273** (47), 31273–31282.

Olsson, A.K. Dimberg, A., Kreuger, J. and Claesson-Welsh, L. (2006) VEGF receptor signalling - in control of vascular function. *Nature Reviews Molecula and Celllar Biology*, **7** (5), 359–371.

Osada-Oka, M., Ikeda, T., Imaoka, S. *et al.* (2008) VEGF-enhanced proliferation under hypoxia by an autocrine mechanism in human vascular smooth muscle cells. *Journal of Atherosclerosis and Thrombosis*, **15** (1), 26–33.

Osaki, T., Nagashima, A., Yoshimatsu, T. *et al.* (2004) Survival and characteristics of lymph node involvement in patients with N1 non-small cell lung cancer. *Lung Cancer*, **43** (2), 151–157.

Padro, T., Bieker, R., Ruiz, S. *et al.* (2002) Overexpression of vascular endothelial growth factor (VEGF) and its cellular receptor KDR (VEGFR-2) in the bone marrow of patients with acute myeloid leukemia. *Leukemia*, **16** (7), 1302–1310.

Pajares, M.J., Agorreta, J., Larrayoz, M. *et al.* (2012) Expression of tumor-derived vascular endothelial growth factor and its receptors is associated with outcome in early squamous cell carcinoma of the lung. *Journal of Clinical Oncology*, **30** (10), 1129–1136.

Pavlakovic, H., Becker, J., Albuquerque, R. *et al.* (2010) Soluble VEGFR-2: an anti-lymphangiogenic variant of VEGF receptors. *Annals of the New York Academy of Sciences*, **1207** (Suppl 1), E7–E15.

Petrova, T.V., Bono, P., Holnthoner, W. *et al.* (2008) VEGFR-3 expression is restricted to blood and lymphatic vessels in solid tumors. *Cancer Cell*, **13** (6), 554–556.

Ping, S.Y., Shen, K.H. and Yu, D.S. (2012) Epigenetic regulation of vascular endothelial growth factor a dynamic expression in transitional cell carcinoma. *Molecular Carcinogenesis*, doi: 10.1002/mc.21892.

Pritchard-Jones, R.O., Harper, S. J. and Bates, D.O. (2007) Expression of VEGF(xxx)b, the inhibitory isoforms of VEGF, in malignant melanoma. *British Journal of Cancer*, **97** (2), 223–230.

Qin, L., Zeng, H. and Zhao, D. (2006) Requirement of protein kinase D tyrosine phosphorylation for VEGF-A165-induced angiogenesis through its interaction and regulation of phospholipase Cgamma phosphorylation. *Journal of Biological Chemistry*, **281** (43), 32550–32558.

Quentmeier, H., Eberth, S., Romani, J. *et al.* (201) DNA methylation regulates expression of VEGF-R2 (KDR) and VEGF-R3 (FLT4). *BMC Cancer*, **12** (2), 19.

Rahimi, N., Dayanir, V. and Lashkari, K. (2000) Receptor chimeras indicate that the vascular endothelial growth factor receptor-1 (VEGFR-1) modulates mitogenic activity of VEGFR-2 in endothelial cells. *Journal of Biological Chemistry*, **275** (22), 16986–16992.

Rak, J. and Kerbel, R.S. (2001) Ras regulation of vascular endothelial growth factor and angiogenesis. *Methods in Enzymology*, **333**, 267–283.

Randi, A.M., Sperone, A., Dryden, N.H. and Birdsey, G.M. (2009) Regulation of angiogenesis by ETS transcription factors. *Biochemical Society Transactions*, **37** (Pt 6), 1248–1253.

Rankin, E.B. and Giaccia, A.J. (2008) The role of hypoxia-inducible factors in tumorigenesis. *Cell Death and Differentiation*, **15** (4), 678–685.

Raymond, E., Dahan, L., Raoul, J.L. *et al.* (2011) Sunitinib malate for the treatment of pancreatic neuroendocrine tumors. *New England Journal of Medicine*, **364** (6), 501–513.

Rodriguez-Antona, C., Pallares, J., Montero-Conde, C. *et al.* (2010) Overexpression and activation of EGFR and VEGFR2 in medullary thyroid carcinomas is related to metastasis. *Endocrine-Related Cancer*, **17** (1), 7–16.

Roma, A.A., Magi-Galluzzi, C., Kral, M.A. *et al.* (2006) Peritumoral lymphatic invasion is associated with regional lymph node metastases in prostate adenocarcinoma. *Modern Pathology*, **19** (3), 392–398.

Ruegg, C. and Mutter, N. (2007) Anti-angiogenic therapies in cancer: achievements and open questions. *Bulletin du Cancer*, **94** (9), 753–762.

Ruhrberg, C., Gerhardt, H., Golding, M. *et al.* (2002) Spatially restricted patterning cues provided by heparin-binding VEGF-A control blood vessel branching morphogenesis. *Genes and Development*, **16** (20), 2684–2698.

Salameh, A., Galvagni, F., Bardelli, M. *et al.* (2005) Direct recruitment of CRK and GRB2 to VEGFR-3 induces proliferation, migration, and survival of endothelial cells through the activation of ERK, AKT, and JNK pathways. *Blood*, **106** (10), 3423–3431.

Sawano, A., Takahashi, T., Yamaguchi, S. and Shibuya, M. (1997) The phosphorylated 1169-tyrosine containing region of flt-1 kinase (VEGFR-1) is a major binding site for PLCgamma. *Biochemical and Biophysical Research Communications*, **238** (2), 487–491.

Scott, A. and Mellor, H. (2009) VEGF receptor trafficking in angiogenesis. *Biochemical Society Transactions*, **37** (Pt 6), 1184–1188.

Seliger, B., Massa, C., Rini, B., Ko, J. and Finke, J. (2010) Antitumour and immune-adjuvant activities of protein-tyrosine kinase inhibitors. *Trends in Molecular Medicine*, **16** (4), 184–192.

Senger, D.R., Galli, S.J., Dvorak, A.M. *et al.* (1983) Tumor cells secrete a vascular permeability factor that promotes accumulation of ascites fluid. *Science*, **219** (4587), 983–985.

Shalaby, F., Rossant, J., Yamaguchi, T.P. *et al.* (1995) Failure of blood-island formation and vasculogenesis in Flk-1-deficient mice. *Nature*, **376** (6535), 62–66.

Shattil, S.J., Kim, C. and Ginsberg, M.H. (2010) The final steps of integrin activation: the end game. *Nature Review Molecular and Cellular Biology*, **11** (4), 288–300.

Shinkai, A., Ito, M., Anazawa, H. *et al.* (1998) Mapping of the sites involved in ligand association and dissociation at the extracellular domain of the kinase insert domain-containing receptor for vascular endothelial growth factor. *Journal of Biological Chemistry*, **273** (47), 31283–31288.

Small, A.R., Neagu, A., Amyot, F. *et al.* (2008) Spatial distribution of VEGF isoforms and chemotactic signals in the vicinity of a tumor. *Journal of Theoretical Biology*, **252** (4), 593–607.

Spannuth, W.A., Nick, A.M., Jennings, N.B. *et al.* (2009) Functional significance of VEGFR-2 on ovarian cancer cells. *International Journal of Cancer*, **124** (5), 1045–1053.

Spratlin, J. (2011) Ramucirumab (IMC-1121B): Monoclonal antibody inhibition of vascular endothelial growth factor receptor-2. *Current Oncology Reports*, **13** (2), 97–102.

Stinga, A.C., Margaritescu, O., Stinga, A.S. *et al.* (2011) VEGFR1 and VEGFR2 immunohistochemical expression in oral squamous cell carcinoma: a morphometric study. *Romanian Journal of Morphology and Embryology*, **52** (4), 1269–1275.

Stringer, S.E. (2006) The role of heparan sulphate proteoglycans in angiogenesis. *Biochemical Society Transactions*, **34** (Pt 3), 451–453.

Stuttfeld, E. and Ballmer-Hofer, K. (2009) Structure and function of VEGF receptors. *IUBMB Life*, **61** (9), 915–922.

Sun, Z., Li, X., Massena, S. *et al.* (2012) VEGFR2 induces c-Src signaling and vascular permeability *in vivo* via the adaptor protein TSAd. *Journal of Experimental Medicine*, **209** (7), 1363–1377.

Takahashi, T., Ueno, H.and Shibuya, M. (1999) VEGF activates protein kinase C-dependent, but Ras-independent Raf-MEK-MAP kinase pathway for DNA synthesis in primary endothelial cells. *Oncogene*, **18** (13), 2221–2230.

Taylor, A.P., Leon, E. and Goldenberg, D.M. (2010) Placental growth factor (PlGF) enhances breast cancer cell motility by mobilising ERK1/2 phosphorylation and cytoskeletal rearrangement. *British Journal of Cancer*, **103** (1), 82–89.

Tchaikovski, V., Fellbrich, G. and Waltenberger, J. (2008) The molecular basis of VEGFR-1 signal transduction pathways in primary human monocytes. *Arteriosclerosis, Thrombosis, and Vascular Biology*, **28** (2), 322–328.

Teng, L.S., Jin, K.T., He, K.F. *et al.* (2010) Clinical applications of VEGF-trap (aflibercept) in cancer treatment. *Journal of the Chinese Medical Association*, **73** (9), 449–456.

Thibeault, S., Rautureau, Y., Oubaha, M. *et al.* (2010) *S*-Nitrosylation of beta-catenin by eNOS-derived NO promotes VEGF-induced endothelial cell permeability. *Molecular Cell*, **39** (3), 468–476.

Trinh, X.B., Tjalma, W.A., Vermeulen, P.B. *et al.* (2009) The VEGF pathway and the AKT/mTOR/p70S6K1 signalling pathway in human epithelial ovarian cancer. *British Journal of Cancer*, **100** (6), 971–978.

Tugues, S., Koch, S., Gualandi, L. *et al.* (2011) Vascular endothelial growth factors and receptors: anti-angiogenic therapy in the treatment of cancer. *Molecular Aspects of Medicine*, **32** (2), 88–111.

Turunen, M.P., Lehtola, T., Heinonen, S.E. *et al.* (2009) Efficient regulation of VEGF expression by promoter-targeted lentiviral shRNAs based on epigenetic mechanism: a novel example of epigenetherapy. *Circulation Research*, **105** (6), 604–609.

Turunen, M.P. and Yla-Herttuala, S. (2011) Epigenetic regulation of key vascular genes and growth factors. *Cardiovascular Research*, **90** (3), 441–446.

Uniewicz, K.A. and Fernig, D.G. (2008) Neuropilins: a versatile partner of extracellular molecules that regulate development and disease. *Frontiers in Bioscience*, **13**, 4339–4360.

Ushio-Fukai, M. and Nakamura, Y. (2008) Reactive oxygen species and angiogenesis: NADPH oxidase as target for cancer therapy. *Cancer Letters*, **266** (1), 37–52.

Van Meter, M.E. and Kim, E.S. (2010) Bevacizumab: current updates in treatment. *Current Opinion in Oncology*, **22** (6), 586–591.

Vander Kooi, C.W., Jusino, M.A., Perman, B. *et al.* (2007) Structural basis for ligand and heparin binding to neuropilin B domains. *Proceedings of the National Academy of Sciences, USA*, **104** (15), 6152–6157.

Varey, A.H., Rennel, E.S., Qiu, Y. *et al.* (2008) VEGF 165 b, an antiangiogenic VEGF-A isoform, binds and inhibits bevacizumab treatment in experimental colorectal carcinoma: balance of pro- and antiangiogenic VEGF-A isoforms has implications for therapy. *British Journal of Cancer*, **98** (8), 1366–1379.

Wang, G.L., Jiang, B.H., Rue, E.A. and Semenza, G.L. (1995) Hypoxia-inducible factor 1 is a basic-helix-loop-helix-PAS heterodimer regulated by cellular O_2 tension. *Proceedings of the National Academy of Sciences, USA*, **92** (12), 5510–5514.

Wang, L., Zeng, H., Wang, P. *et al.* (2003) Neuropilin-1-mediated vascular permeability factor/vascular endothelial growth factor-dependent endothelial cell migration. *Journal of Biological Chemistry*, **278** (49), 48848–48860.

Wang, S., Li, X., Parra, M. *et al.* (2008) Control of endothelial cell proliferation and migration by VEGF signaling to histone deacetylase 7. *Proceedings of the National Academy of Sciences, USA*, **105** (22), 7738–7743.

Wang, Y.D., Nakayama, M., Pitulescu, M.E. *et al.* (2010) Ephrin-B2 controls VEGF-induced angiogenesis and lymphangiogenesis. *Nature*, **465** (7297), 483–486.

Wang, F., Yamauchi, M., Muramatsu, M. *et al.* (2011) RACK1 regulates VEGF/Flt1-mediated cell migration via activation of a PI3K/Akt pathway. *Journal of Biological Chemistry*, **286** (11), 9097–9106.

Wang, Z., Chen, Y., Li, X. *et al.* (2012) Expression of VEGF-C/VEGFR-3 in human laryngeal squamous cell carcinomas and its significance for lymphatic metastasis. *Asian Pacific Journal of Cancer Prevention*, **13** (1), 27–31.

Webb, D.J., Donais, K., Whitmore, L.A. *et al.* (2004) FAK-Src signalling through paxillin, ERK and MLCK regulates adhesion disassembly. *Nature Cell Biology*, **6** (2) 154–161.

Weigand, M., Hantel, P., Kreienberg, R. and Waltenberger, J. (2005) Autocrine vascular endothelial growth factor signalling in breast cancer. Evidence from cell lines and primary breast cancer cultures *in vitro*. *Angiogenesis*, **8** (3), 197–204.

Wellner, M., Maasch, C., Kupprion, C. *et al.* (1999) The proliferative effect of vascular endothelial growth factor requires protein kinase C-alpha and protein kinase C-zeta. *Arteriosclerosis, Thrombosis, and Vascular Biology*, **19** (1), 178–185.

Wong, C. and Jin, Z.G. (2005) Protein kinase C-dependent protein kinase D activation modulates ERK signal pathway and endothelial cell proliferation by vascular endothelial growth factor. *Journal of Biological Chemistry*, **280** (39), 33262–33269.

Woolard, J., Wang, W.Y., Bevan, H.S., *et al.* (2004) VEGF165b, an inhibitory vascular endothelial growth factor splice variant: mechanism of action, *in vivo* effect on angiogenesis and endogenous protein expression. *Cancer Research*, **64** (21), 7822–7835.

Wu, H.M., Huang, Q., Yuan, Y. and Granger, H.J. (1996) VEGF induces NO-dependent hyperpermeability in coronary venules. *American Journal of Physiology*, **271** (6 Pt 2), H2735–H2739.

Wu, Y., Zhong, Z., Huber, J. *et al.* (2006) Anti-vascular endothelial growth factor receptor-1 antagonist antibody as a therapeutic agent for cancer. *Clinical Cancer Research*, **12** (21), 6573–6584.

Xia, P., Aiello, L.P., Ishii, H. *et al.* (1996) Characterization of vascular endothelial growth factor's effect on the activation of protein kinase C, its isoforms, and endothelial cell growth. *Journal of Clinical Investigation*, **98** (9), 2018–2026.

Xia, G., Kumar, S.R., Hawes, D. *et al.* (2006) Expression and significance of vascular endothelial growth factor receptor 2 in bladder cancer. *Journal of Urology*, **175** (4), 1245–1252.

Xu, D., Fuster, M.M., Lawrence, R. and Esko, J. D. (2011) Heparan sulfate regulates VEGF165- and VEGF121-mediated vascular hyperpermeability. *Journal of Biological Chemistry*, **286** (1), 737–745.

Yamaoka-Tojo, M., Tojo, T., Kim, H.W. *et al.* (2006) IQGAP1 mediates VE-cadherin-based cell-cell contacts and VEGF signaling at adherence junctions linked to angiogenesis. *Arteriosclerosis, Thrombosis, and Vascular Biology*, **26** (9) 1991–1997.

Yamazaki, Y. Tokunaga, Y., Takani, K. and Morita, T. (2005) C-terminal heparin-binding peptide of snake venom VEGF specifically blocks VEGF-stimulated endothelial cell proliferation. *Pathophysiology of Haemostasis and Thrombosis*, **34** (4–5), 197–199.

Yang, F., Tang, X., Riquelme, E. *et al.* (2011) Increased VEGFR-2 gene copy is associated with chemoresistance and shorter survival in patients with non-small-cell lung carcinoma who receive adjuvant chemotherapy. *Cancer Research*, **71** (16), 5512–5521.

Yu, Y., Hulmes, J.D., Herley, M.T. *et al.* (2001) Direct identification of a major autophosphorylation site on vascular endothelial growth factor receptor Flt-1 that mediates phosphatidylinositol 3'-kinase binding. *Biochemical Journal*, **358** (Pt 2), 465–472.

Zhang, L.Q., Zhou, F., Han, W.C. *et al.* (2010) VEGFR-3 ligand-binding and kinase activity are required for lymphangiogenesis but not for angiogenesis. *Cell Research*, **20** (12), 1319–1331.

Zhang, X.H., Shin, J.Y., Kim, J.O. *et al.* (2012) Synergistic antitumor efficacy of sequentially combined paclitaxel with sorafenib *in vitro* and *in vivo* NSCLC models harboring KRAS or BRAF mutations. *Cancer Letters*, **322** (2), 213–222.

Zivi, A., Cerbone, L., Recine, F. and Sternberg, C.N. (2012) Safety and tolerability of pazopanib in the treatment of renal cell carcinoma. *Expert Opinion on Drug Safety*, **11** (5), 851–859.

8

Progesterone receptor signalling in breast cancer models

Andrea R. Daniel, Todd P. Knutson, Christy R. Hagan
and Carol A. Lange

*Departments of Medicine (Division of Hematology, Oncology, and
Transplantation) and Pharmacology, Masonic Cancer Center,
University of Minnesota*

In the clinical setting, progesterone receptors (PR) are primarily used as
biomarkers of luminal-A type or endocrine-sensitive breast cancers. PR expression in oestrogen receptor (ER) positive breast cancers is associated with good
prognosis, as it is indicative of the presence of functional ER; ER+/PR+ breast
cancers are more likely to respond to anti-oestrogen therapies relative to those
(luminal-B) that have become PR-null (Osborne *et al.*, 2005). However, historical
dogma that PR serve largely as useful biomarkers of ER action is steadily
being replaced with the concept that PR isoforms indeed contribute to breast
cancer progression as key mediators of mammary epithelial cell proliferation and
pro-survival as well as regulators of the mammary stem cell niche. As a result,
considerable effort has been directed towards a more complete understanding of
PR biochemistry and the mechanisms of signalling (i.e. promoter selection) as
they relate to mammary gland development and during breast cancer initiation
and early progression. PR/progestin action in breast tumours appears to be fairly
distinct from that in the normal adult breast (Clarke and Graham, 2012; Graham
et al., 2009). However, given the appropriate proliferative bursts directed by
PR-B during mammary gland development, menstruation and in pregnancy,
it is likely that PR retains the potential to inappropriately drive dangerous
growth programmes in a malignant environment (Knutson *et al.*, 2012). As such,
anti-progestins represent a timely opportunity to improve modern endocrine
therapies. Emerging evidence suggests that steroid hormone receptors are
highly context-dependent transcription factors; these molecules are heavily
post-translationally modified and influenced by a variety of cofactors. Given the

Cancer Cell Signalling, First Edition. Edited by Amanda Harvey.
© 2013 John Wiley & Sons, Ltd. Published 2013 by John Wiley & Sons, Ltd.

heterogeneity of human breast cancer, perhaps the next challenge for the PR/ progestin field is to identify which tumours are most likely driven by active PR, and thus well-suited for endocrine therapies that may include a highly selective anti-progestin. Herein, we discuss the context-dependent actions of PR, and provide biochemical hints as to what molecular environments may drive PR signalling toward the emergence of malignant phenotypes.

8.1 Progesterone receptor function

Progesterone, an ovarian steroid hormone, is produced during the luteal phase of the menstrual cycle and throughout pregnancy. Progesterone binds progesterone receptors (PR) to elicit a biological response. PR are expressed in multiple human tissues including the uterus, mammary gland, brain, pancreas, thymus, bone, ovary, testes and in the urinary tract (Scarpin *et al.*, 2009). Two primary PR protein isoforms exist (PR-A and PR-B) that are derived from a single gene with unique promoters (Kastner *et al.*, 1990). PR-B is the full-length receptor that contains an additional 164 amino acids at the *N*-terminus that is absent in PR-A; otherwise these protein isoforms have the same peptide sequence (Hill *et al.*, 2012). Both receptors contain a DBD (DNA binding domain), an LBD (ligand binding domain) separated by a hinge region (also known as the CTE, carboxy terminal extension) and two AF (activation function) domains (Figure 8.1). PR-B contains a third AF domain located in its *N*-terminus that is not present in PR-A (Sartorius *et al.*, 1994). The AF domains function to interact with co-regulatory molecules to enhance PR transcriptional activation of genes.

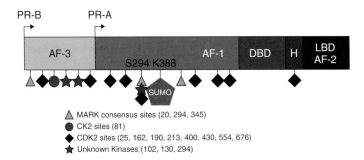

Figure 8.1   The progesterone receptor is post-translationally modified by phosphorylation and sumoylation. Both progesterone receptor (PR) protein isoforms, PR-A and PR-B, are heavily phosphorylated by multiple kinases, including MAPK, CK2 and CDK2. Both receptors contain DNA binding domains (DBD), ligand binding domains (LBD), hinge regions (H) and two activation function (AF) domains. PR-B contains an additional 164 amino acids at its *N*-terminus and a third AF domain. PR phosphorylation at Ser294 antagonises PR sumoylation at Lys388.

Both PR isoforms also contain an *N*-terminal inhibitory function (IF) domain that acts to recruit corepressor molecules; IF activity is only revealed in the context of PR-A (Giangrande and McDonnell, 1999). Following ligand binding, PR undergo a conformational change that initiates unique actions. Isoforms dimerise (A:A, B:B or A:B) and are retained in the nucleus. Nuclear PR activates transcription of target genes, either directly through binding to progesterone response elements (PREs), or indirectly through tethering interactions with other transcription factors (AP1, SP1, STATs) (Owen *et al.*, 1998; Stoecklin *et al.*, 1999; Cicatiello *et al.*, 2004). To initiate transcription (ligand-dependent or -independent) PR recruits co-regulator proteins and basal transcriptional machinery to enhancer and promoter regions of genes (McKemma *et al.*, 1999). These responsive elements are located in chromatin at proximal and distal sites. Recent cistrome (whole genome binding site) analysis demonstrated that these responsive elements may be located up to 50 kb (kilobases) upstream or downstream of the TSS (transcriptional start site) (Tang *et al.*, 2011). PR genomic (transcriptional) activities are integrated with nongenomic actions, where PR is a node within cytoplasmic kinase signalling cascades (for reviews, see Losel and Wehling, 2003; Edwards, 2005; Lange, 2008; Bjornstrom and Sjoberg, 2005); as reported for oestrogen receptor (ER), PR is able to associate with signalling molecules to activate kinase pathways in response to progesterone and to enhance responses to growth factors (Beguelin *et al.*, 2010; Daniel and Hagan, 2011; Labriola *et al.*, 2003).

In the human breast, PR action is critical for maintaining the population of mammary stem cells (via paracrine signalling) (Gonzalez-Suarez *et al.*, 2010; Joshi *et al.*, 2010) and for coordinating the dynamic (proliferative) regulation of glandular structures during menstrual cycling and pregnancy (via both paracrine and autocrine signalling (Beleut *et al.*, 2010; Daniel *et al.*, 2011). Deregulation of the normal proliferative actions of PR in the breast may contribute to the increased risk of breast cancer revealed in clinical trials using progestin containing hormone replacement therapy (Beral, 2003; Chlebowski *et al.*, 2003). In these large trials, oestrogen alone, when given to post-menopausal women protected against breast cancer, while oestrogen plus progestin (E+P) was associated with a higher breast cancer risk and the appearance of larger more aggressive tumours (Chlebowski *et al.*, 2012). These effects were reversed upon cessation of E+P hormone use (Chlebowski *et al.*, 2009), suggesting a tumour-promoting effect of progestin and that E+P may have stimulated increased growth and progression of occult pre-existing breast lesions in these relatively short-term (~4 year) trials. However, lifetime exposure to elevated levels of steroid hormones (including oestrogens, progestins and androgens) also increases the relative risk of breast cancer incidence in post-menopausal women (Key *et al.*, 2002; Clemons and Goss, 2001). Similarly, in mouse studies, inhibiting PR actions with RU486 (PR antagonist/partial agonist) during a 14-day window of time dramatically precluded virgin BRCA1/p53 mutant mice from developing mammary tumours (Poole *et al.*, 2006). In other mouse studies, treatment with the PR agonist MPA (medroxyprogesterone acetate) showed definitively that progestins/PR actions contribute to increased mammary tumour formation (Lanari *et al.*, 2009). Furthermore, PR knockout mice were resistant to mammary tumour development after challenges with chemical carcinogens (Lydon *et al.*, 1999). These and other studies (reviewed in Daniel *et al.*, 2011; Hagan *et al.*, 2012; Lange *et al.*, 2008) have provoked great interest in PR function and its role in breast cancer. Herein, we review basic studies on PR biochemistry as a means to provide further insight into its context-dependent actions and emerging relevance to mechanisms of (luminal) breast cancer initiation and progression.

8.2 Model systems: context for studying PR biochemistry

Studies of PR biochemistry have primarily used a limited number of ER+/PR+ (luminal) human breast cancer cell lines (MCF-7, T47D and ZR75). Notably, PR is a classic ER target gene. Thus, PR mRNA expression in mammary epithelial cells is primarily driven by oestrogen-bound ER, making the study of PR action (in isolation) difficult without the confounding (mitogenic) effects of added oestrogen. The Horwitz lab derived a breast cancer cell model system for studying PR/progestins by first identifying a variant of T47D cells in which PR is constitutively expressed and independent of oestrogen stimulation, termed T47Dco cells (Horwitz *et al.*, 1982). A naturally occurring PR-null variant of these cells, T47D-Y, provided a useful tool for making stable cell lines containing PR-A only, PR-B only, or various mutant version of PR isoforms (Richer *et al.*, 1998). An advantage of this model system is that PR expression levels in stable clones can be selected to closely resemble the levels found in unmodified parental cells (T47Dco). Indeed, PR expression in stable cell lines at levels similar to endogenous expression has been shown to be critical for appropriate PR transcriptional activation, particularly with regard to the actions of PR phospho-mutants. Namely, S294A (Ser294 to Ala) mutant PR-B is heavily sumoylated and transcriptionally repressed relative to wt PR-B when either receptor is expressed stably in T47D-Y cells and at levels similar to that seen in T47Dco cells. However, when overexpressed in transient systems such as COS or HeLa cells this mutant can activate transcription in PRE-luciferase reporter assays, much like wt PR-B (Qui and Lange, 2003). Notably, endogenous factors that may influence PR transcriptional activity are limiting (kinases, co-factors, SUMO molecules and/or PIAS proteins that act as SUMO conjugating enzymes, etc.) (Daniel *et al.*, 2007). Others have reported major functional differences between stably and transiently expressed PRs. For example, transiently expressed PR is unable to induce chromatin remodelling changes necessary to activate an integrated MMTV promoter, while stably expressed PR is fully capable of transactivation (Smith *et al.*, 1993, 1997, 2000). These data highlight the need for model systems that provide appropriate levels of myriad regulatory molecules which interact with and alter steroid receptors. Additionally, they caution against over-interpretation of exogenous expression models only, particularly in the case of receptor regulation by phosphorylation events and other dynamic post-translational modifications, such as sumoylation (Abdel-Hafiz and Horwitz, 2012; Abdel-Hafiz *et al.*, 2009).

Recently, PR mRNA expression in a selected sub-population of stem-like progenitor cells in the human breast was shown to be fully independent of ER (Hilton *et al.*, 2012), suggesting that PR expression in this specialised compartment is sensitive to factors other than oestrogen perhaps cAMP (Jacobsen and Horwitz, 2012). PR protein expression as measured by IHC (immunohistochemistry) was detectable in basal cells of the mammary gland, while PR and ER expression was only detected in adult luminal cells (Hilton *et al.*, 2012). It will be important to further establish additional *ex vivo* models to further understand the mechanisms of ER-independent PR expression.

8.3   Progesterone receptor signalling

PR participation in signalling complexes serves as a 'fine-tuning' mechanism to precisely adjust hormone responses according to specific cellular conditions. Notably, PR-B, but not PR-A, functions outside of the nucleus to rapidly activate protein kinases (MAPK, Akt, c-Src) in part by a ligand-induced interaction between PR and c-Src kinase (Migliaccio *et al.*, 1998; Boonyaratanakornkit *et al.*, 2001; Saitoh *et al.*, 2005; Boonyaratanakornkit *et al.*, 2007). Rapid progesterone-induced c-Src/MAPK activation serves to phosphorylate PR Ser345, and thereby potentiates nuclear PR tethering to SP1 transcription factors to regulate genes required for cell cycle progression and anchorage-independent growth (Faivre and Lange, 2007; Skildum *et al.*, 2005). This 'feed-forward' loop underscores the profound effect that activated kinases have on the nuclear functions of PR; particularly with regard to promoter selectivity (i.e. phospho-PRs target or select specific gene subsets, perhaps in cooperation with co-factors that preferentially recognise receptor phospho-species). Progestin bound PR-B induces sustained activation of MAPK signalling (18–24 h) mediated by EGFR transactivation through matrix metalloproteinase mediated release of EGFR ligands, resulting in Wnt1 up-regulation (genomic PR action) and proliferation (Faivre and Lange, 2007). PR rapid activation of MAPK signalling (Msk1) is also mediated via an interaction with ER/c-Src complexes in response to progestins (Migliaccio *et al.*, 1998; Vicent *et al.*, 2006a; Ballare *et al.*, 2003). These PR/ER/Msk1 complexes are recruited to the MMTV promoter in response to progestin (Vicent *et al.*, 2006b). In recent studies, progestin induced PR/ER complexes were shown to bind the c-myc and cyclin D1 endogenous gene promoters and enhance their transcriptional activity (Giulianelli *et al.*, 2012).

Additionally, progestin/PR activation of c-Src induces Jak1/2 phosphorylation leading to downstream STAT3 transcriptional activation (Proietti *et al.*, 2005). PR interacts with FGFR2 and STAT5 to induce transcriptional changes in the cell (Cerliani *et al.*, 2011), and also participates in signalling complexes with a variety of signalling molecules including cyclins, caveolin-1 and ErbB receptors (Beguelin *et al.*, 2010; Labriola *et al.*, 2003; Balana *et al.*, 2001; Proietti *et al.*, 2011; Salatini *et al.*, 2006; Narayanan *et al.*, 2005a, 2005b; Pierson-Mullany *et al.*, 2004; Pierson-Mullany *et al.*, 2003). These signalling events are influenced by cellular context (i.e. abundance/location of signalling molecules, cell cycle phase, growth factor availability) in addition to the availability of progesterone and incur specific biological outcomes for the cell.

8.4   Regulation of signalling

8.4.1   Post-translational modifications: mediators of context dependent PR action

Post-translational modifications (PTMs) are a class of covalently attached moieties that induce conformational changes in substrate proteins that can dramatically impact enzyme activity, location and/or protein–protein interactions: PTMs have been defined in basic processes including DNA repair, replication, transcription, chromosome segregation, genomic stability and intracellular trafficking (for reviews, see Gill, 2003; Hay, 2005; Johnson, 2004; Gareau and Lima, 2010). PR isoforms are post-translationally modified by phosphorylation, ubiquitination, sumoylation and acetylation (Hagan *et al.*, 2012; Abdel-Hafiz *et al.*, 2002; Lange *et al.*, 2000; Daniel *et al.*, 2010). These regulated modifications are highly dynamic, depend on cellular context and refine PR transcriptional activity by altering PR subcellular localisation, protein stability/turnover and interactions with other proteins and with DNA (Dressing *et al.*, 2009).

Acetylation and nuclear localisation

The hinge region of PR contains a conserved motif of lysine residues (RKXKK) that are rapidly acetylated in response to ligand binding (Daniel *et al.*, 2010). These residues also make up part of the bipartite nuclear localisation signal (NLS) that is required for efficient PR localisation in the nucleus and thus required for PR transcriptional activity (Tyagi *et al.*, 1998; Guiochon-Mantel, *et al.*, 1991, 1992. Mutations within the NLS that mimic acetylation (Q and T) also disrupt the ability of PR to accumulate in the nucleus, indicating that the regulation of PR acetylation and nuclear localisation are intimately linked (Daniel *et al.*, 2010). Rapid ligand induced PR nuclear accumulation is critical for certain PR phosphorylation events and for regulating PR early response genes (1 h) such as c-myc. Additionally, acetylation of PR reduced progestin responsiveness on select latent (18 h) target promoters (Daniel *et al.*, 2010). Notably, other disruptions within this conserved sequence alter PR DNA binding and cofactor recruitment (Hill *et al.*, 2009; Roemer *et al.*, 2006, 2008), indicating the PR hinge region is a critical regulator of PR genomic functions.

Upon ligand binding and nuclear accumulation, PR molecules aggregate with DNA and form transcription factor complexes in discrete foci to activate transcription (Arnett-Mansfield *et al.*, 2004, 2007). These complexes are tethered to the nuclear matrix and contain nascent RNA, activated RNAPolII, p300, and specific chromatin associated with transcriptional activation (Graham *et al.*, 2009; Arnett-Mansfield *et al.*, 2007). Treatment of cells with the CDK2 inhibitor Roscovitine prevents formation of these foci, indicating a kinase signalling dependence (in addition to the presence of progestins) of PR transcriptional activity occurring in these complexes (Scarpin *et al.*, 2009).

8.4.2 Constitutive kinases

PR contains at least 14 serine residues that are phosphorylated by multiple kinases (e.g. MAPK, CK2 and CDK2) either basally or in response to ligand binding (Figure 8.1) (Moore *et al.*, 2007). In conditions where kinases are up-regulated, such as breast cancer, amplified signalling mediates PR-B hypersensitivity to hormone and ligand-independence, thus leading to inappropriate activation of PR-B dependent transcription and expression of growth and pro-survival genes (Qui and Lange, 2003; Pieson-Mullany and Lange, 2004; Santen *et al.*, 2005). Importantly, PR hypersensitivity to ligand may be increasingly relevant to cancer as evidence suggests local production of progestins may occur in the tumour microenvironment (Inoue *et al.*, 2002; Lewis *et al.*, 2004). Mechanisms of kinase induced PR hyperactivation are discussed in the following sections.

CK2

PR Ser81 is a known CK2 site in the PR-B *N*-terminus (not in PR-A) (Zhang *et al.*, 1994; Hagan *et al.*, 2011). CK2 is a ubiquitously expressed, constitutively active kinase that is over-expressed in every cancer examined thus far, including breast cancer. Our recent work (using Ser81-specific phospho-antibodies) demonstrated that PR-B was basally phosphorylated at Ser81 in breast cancer cells. Progestin exposure, in addition to synchronisation of cells at the G1/S phase border, induced robust phosphorylation at this site; both effects were CK2-dependent (Hagan *et al.*, 2011). Cells expressing a PR mutant (S79/81A PR) that cannot be phosphorylated at Ser81 had decreased ligand-independent cell survival in soft agar assays. Phospho-mutant-PR-B also exhibited defects in recruitment to select PR-B-target genes (i.e. *BIRC3*) important for proliferation and survival, both in the presence and absence of ligand. ChIP assays revealed that in contrast to wt PR-B, a phospho-Ser81 mutant receptor (S79/81A PR-B) was also impaired in its ability to recruit CK2 to PR-associated enhancer sites of the *BIRC3* gene. CK2 is not thought to be oncogenic on its own, but appears to increase the oncogenic potential of cancer-promoting substrates and pro-growth signals (such as progestin/PR in the breast) (Tawfic *et al.*, 2001; Trembley *et al.*, 2009). In the context of breast cancer, where progestins have been implicated as a risk factor for tumour development and early progression (Beral, 2003; Chlebowski *et al.*, 2003; Anderson *et al.*, 2004), over-expressed CK2 could further enhance the oncogenic potential of PR through inappropriate phosphorylation (on Ser81), thereby directing phospho-Ser81 PR-B to growth-promoting genes. These data suggest that the interaction of PR-B with kinases, and ultimately Ser81 phosphorylation, may be a key determinant in dictating PR-A versus PR-B target-gene specificity.

CDK2

There is a complex interplay between PR activity and cell cycle regulation. In response to progestin or mitogen treatment, CDK2 signalling is activated and the G1/S-phase transition is initiated. CDK2 has been shown to phosphorylate PR at multiple sites that regulate PR transcriptional activity (Pierson-Mullany and Lange, 2004; Zhang *et al.*, 1997; Daniel and Lange, 2009). PR is basally phosphorylated on Ser400 in resting cells and highly phosphorylated by CDK2 in response to progestins (Zhang *et al.*, 1997). In addition, treatment with mitogenic growth factors known to activate CDK2 activity, or expression of constitutively active CDK2 *in vitro*, induces ligand-independent PR transcriptional activity. In T47D breast cancer cells, high expression of the cell cycle inhibitor p27 also blocked CDK2-induced PR Ser400 phosphorylation and ligand-independent PR transcriptional action (Pierson-Mullany and Lange, 2004). These data suggest phosphorylation at PR Ser400 by activated CDK2 regulates the transcriptional activity of PR during the cell cycle and this may be deregulated in tumour cells, especially when cell cycle check point control is compromised by high CDK2, over-expression of cyclins D, A or E, or loss of cell cycle inhibitor proteins (p15, p16, p21, p27).

PR also interacts with cyclin E/CDK2 (Pierson-Mullany and Lange, 2004; Pierson-Mullany *et al.*, 2003) and cyclinA/CDK2 complexes; PR bound to cyclinA/CDK2 increases SRC-1 phosphorylation and PR binding to the MMTV promoter (Narayanan *et al.*, 2005a, 2005b). PR displays increased transcriptional activation during S phase, an effect dependent on CDK2 activity (Narayanan *et al.*, 2005a). Cancer cells often down-regulate cell cycle inhibitors (p27 and p21) thereby increasing CDK activity and traverse of the cell cycle, thus inducing rapid proliferation (Abukhdeir and Park, 2008; Musgrove *et al.*, 2004). A cancer cell environment with low cell cycle inhibitor activity predicts PR ligand-independent activity and hypersensitivity to low concentrations of progestins. In these circumstances, low levels of locally produced progesterone (Inoue *et al.*, 2002; Lewis *et al.*, 2004) may be sufficient to drive tumour proliferation, leading to increased tumour progression.

MAPK

PR phosphorylation at PR Ser294 has been intensely studied. In the presence of progestins or growth factors (EGF or HRG) (Labriola *et al.*, 2003; Qui and Lange, 2003), PR-B but not PR-A is rapidly phosphorylated at Ser294, accumulates in the nucleus and becomes highly transcriptionally active at multiple genes important for cell cycle progression, proliferation and survival (Daniel and Faivre, 2007; Daniel and Lange, 2009; Shen and Horwitz, 2001; Moore *et al.*, 2000). Ser294 phosphorylation augments PR-B degradation via the ubiquitin-proteasome pathway (Lange *et al.*, 2000). Thus, when PR-B is phosphorylated and is highly sensitive to low concentrations of ligand it undergoes rapid turnover and often becomes more difficult to detect at steady state (by western blotting wt protein) (Lange *et al.*, 2000; Daniel and Lange, 2009; Shen *et al.*, 2001). In the absence of Ser294 phosphorylation, PR is transcriptionally repressed and stabilised (Daniel and Faivre, 2007).

PR phosphorylation on Ser294 in response to progestins or growth factors antagonises sumoylation on Lys388 (Daniel and Faivre, 2007). Sumoylation of PR at this site results in a more stable and transcriptionally repressed PR relative to phospho-Ser294 PR that is desumoylated. The SUMO-deficient PR mutant (K388R) is hypersensitive to low (sub-activating for wt PR) concentrations of progestin (Daniel and Faivre, 2007). A subset of PR target gene promoters is sensitive to PR phosphorylation status (*HBEGF*), while others are insensitive (*Muc1*) (Daniel and Faivre, 2007). PR phosphorylation in the absence of ligand occurs in response to activated kinase pathways (MAPK or CDK2) and increases (desumoylated) PR activity on select ligand-independent gene targets (*SRC1, IRS1*) (Daniel and Lange, 2009). This dynamic regulation of PR Ser294 phosphorylation coupled to Lys388 desumoylation alters PR promoter selectivity, allowing the cell to direct distinct genetic programmes according to changes in the availability of extracellular signals (progesterone and growth factors) (Figure 8.2) (Daniel *et al.*, 2007; Daniel and Lange, 2009).

Recently, an in depth analysis of the target gene profiles of wt PR versus a SUMO-deficient mutant (phospho-Ser294 mimic) PR was performed in breast cancer cells (Knutson *et al.*, 2012). SUMO-sensitive PR target genes largely included molecules that function in pathways responsible for cellular proliferation and survival (Figure 8.3).

Knutson *et al.* demonstrated that desumoylated or phospho-Ser294 PR is recruited to select genes (including *MSX2*) along with coactivator and chromatin remodelling components to induce a permissive chromatin environment and thereby derepress selected target genes (Figure 8.4).

Namely, SUMO-deficient PR was associated with more CBP than PR that could be sumoylated and was able to recruit the methyltransferase MLL2 to promoter regions. PR target gene promoters that were sensitive to the sumoylation/phosphorylation status of PR also displayed increased H3K4 dimethylation and nucleosome remodeling in regions containing PR (desumoylated) bound PREs (Knutson *et al.*, 2012); this methylation mark is associated with the relocation of nucleosomes in transcriptionally active regions of chromatin (He *et al.*, 2010).

Notably, the gene signature specific to desumoylated (Ser294 phosphorylated) PR is associated with HER2 activation in human breast cancers

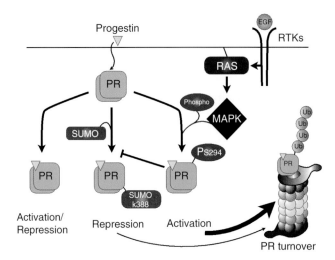

Figure 8.2   Kinase dependent PR Ser294 phosphorylation antagonises PR Lys388 sumoylation and mediates rapid protein turnover. Progestins diffuse through the plasma membrane and bind PR causing rapid sumoylation on Lys388 on a subset of receptors, resulting in transcriptional repression at many cancer relevant genes. Persistent MAPK (or CDK2) pathway activation (e.g. EGF treatment) results in efficient PR Ser294 phosphorylation, inhibition of PR sumoylation and transcriptional activation. Phosphorylated PR is highly ubiquitinated and rapidly degraded by the 26S proteasome; whereas, sumoylated PR is highly stable with a longer half-life.

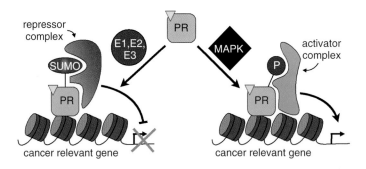

Figure 8.3   PR Ser294 phosphorylation dependent desumoylation drives transcriptional activity at cancer relevant genes. PR undergoes rapid sumoylation upon progestin binding via an enzymatic cascade (left). However, in conditions of high MAPK pathway activation (e.g. EGF treatment or within breast tumours), PR is phosphorylated at Ser294, which antagonises PR sumoylation. Phosphorylated PR Ser294 (desumoylated) regulates unique gene signatures that contribute to cell proliferation and survival.

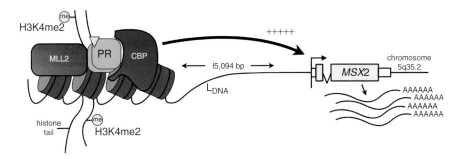

Figure 8.4 **PR regulates *MSX2* gene expression through coactivator recruitment and chromatin modification.** Schematic showing the *MSX2* gene and PRE-containing enhancer region located 15094 bp upstream from the transcriptional start site. High levels of ligand-dependent *MSX2* expression occur in cells expressing SUMO-deficient PR recruitment. In addition, these cells have higher levels of histone acetyltransferase (CBP) and histone methyltransferase (MLL2) recruitment to the *MSX2* enhancer region. This results in higher levels of histone H3 Lys4 dimethylation, a marker of transcriptionally important enhancer regions.

(Knutson *et al.*, 2012). In cell models with HER2 gene amplification, treatment with MEK inhibitors blocked PR SUMO-sensitive gene regulation and decreased cell proliferation in response to progestins (Knutson *et al.*, 2012). In a cohort of ER+ breast tumours, patients whose tumours expressed the SUMO-deficient PR gene signature had reduced distant metastasis free survival (Knutson *et al.*, 2012). These data indicate that PR phosphorylation and sumoylation are able to profoundly alter PR activity and target gene selection in breast cancer cells. Importantly, activated PR gene signatures may be used to identify patients whose tumours are driven by hyperactive PR species and thus likely to benefit from therapies that target PR and upstream kinase pathways in addition to ER.

8.5 Tissue specific PR actions (breast versus reproductive tract)

Progesterone actions vary depending upon the target tissue. Progestins, primarily acting through PR-B, are largely proliferative in the breast. However in the reproductive track, progestins may act primarily through PR-A as potent antagonists of oestrogen-induced hyperplasia (Mulac-Jericevic *et al.*, 2003) and inducers of differentiation (Graham and Clarke, 1997). Recent cistrome analysis comparing PR chromatin binding in T47D breast cancer cells and primary uterine leiomyoma cells in response to RU486 revealed little overlap (Yin *et al.*, 2012). PR-A and PR-B are most often co-expressed in the same tissues, and cells that express only a single PR isoform are rare (Mote *et al.*, 1999, 2002, 2007); the normal 1:1 ratio of PR-A to PR-B is often altered in malignant versus normal breast tissue (Mote *et al.*, 2002; Graham *et al.*, 1995), suggesting that balanced isoform action is crucial to normal (adult) mammary gland biology. Given the equimolar ratios of human PR isoforms in most cells, little is known about the tissue-specific predominance of either isoform and thus the mechanism of tissue selective hormone response. Evidence suggests that PR-A can alter (transrepress) PR-B transcriptional responses to hormone; this may be relevant to altered isoform ratios found in breast cancer and/or to tissue-specific receptor dominance as part of normal physiology (see discussion to follow) (Scarpin *et al.*, 2009). In rat models, PR-A and PR-B are expressed in luminal epithelial cells of the mammary gland and PR-B alone is present in myoepithelial cells, suggesting a unique role for PR-B in regulating myoepithelial processes (Kariagina *et al.*, 2007).

PR-A and PR-B have distinct transcriptional activities (Richer *et al.*, 2002; Jacobsen *et al.*, 2005) and mediate unique developmental processes as determined by PR knockout studies in mice. Mice with both PR-A and PR-B isoforms knocked out develop into adulthood but have drastically impaired female reproductive processes, including: anovulation, uterine hyperplasia, and complete loss of mammary gland ductal and alveolar expansion during pregnancy (Lydon *et al.*, 1995). Selective ablation of PR-A in mice demonstrated that PR-B is the isoform responsible for mammary gland ductal side-branching and lobuloalveolar expansion during pregnancy and regulates a different set of reproductive functions from PR-A (Mulac-Jericevic *et al.*, 2000, 2003). Alternatively, PR-A primarily mediates ovarian and uterine development in response to progestins ((Mulac-Jericevic *et al.*, 2003). Additional work from the PR knockout mouse models showed definitively that PR contributes to mammary gland tumourigenesis (independent of ER action) (Lydon *et al.*, 1995).

While PR-A and PR-B share structural and sequence similarity, they are functionally distinct transcriptional regulators with almost entirely non-overlapping transcriptional profiles, exhibiting recruitment to different subsets of PR-target gene promoters (Richer *et al.*, 2002). Little is understood regarding regulation of PR isoform-specific transcription. The receptors do exhibit unique post-translational modification profiles. PR-B is robustly phosphorylated on Ser294 in response to ligand (and growth factors) while PR-A phosphorylation at this residue is undetectable in intact cells/cell lysates (Clemm *et al.*, 2000). In turn, PR-B is distinctly less sumoylated relative to PR-A (Daniel *et al.*, 2007). PR-A also lacks the *N*-terminal Ser81 phosphorylation site found in PR-B and is therefore blind to CK2 kinase inputs that dramatically alter PR-B gene selectivity (Hagan *et al.*, 2011). Mutation of Ser81 to Ala in PR-B converts its transcriptional response on selected PR-target genes into that of PR-A. Notably, structure-function studies propose that the presence of the BUS (B-upstream segment, including AF3) allows PR-B to adopt distinct conformations which support coactivator binding while PR-A displays an increased affinity for corepressors (Scarpin *et al.*, 2009). Additionally, PR-B, and not PR-A, displays the ability to rapidly signal to c-Src/MAPK (Boonyaratanakornkit *et al.*, 2007). It is thus hypothesised that differential abundance/localisation of coregulator molecules and varying kinase pathway utilisation may account for some of the tissue specificity and context-dependent action of progesterone/PR.

8.6   Progesterone receptor and cancer

Finally, normal versus neoplastic contexts appear to profoundly influence PR action in breast cancer cells, perhaps due, in part, to the biochemical mechanisms described above. Recent comparisons of malignant versus normal primary cell lines of the breast revealed largely distinct gene signatures in response to progestins (Graham *et al.*, 2009). Likewise, cistrome analysis of transformed cell lines expressing exogenous PR versus PR+ neoplastic cell lines confirmed these results. The relatively non-overlapping PR chromatin binding profiles were due, in part, to the differential expression of known steroid receptor pioneer factor FOXA1 (Tang *et al.*, 2011) in the cell lines; the PR cistrome was significantly altered upon expression of FOXA1 in the 'normal' cell line, but this did not predictably approach that found in cancer cells (Clarke and Graham, 2012). Levels of kinase activities increase dramatically in neoplastic settings (Banerji *et al.*, 2012; Dhomen *et al.*, 2012). It is therefore likely that the alterations in PR post-translational modifications and participation in signalling pathways described above cooperate with altered co-factor availability to account for much of the changes seen in PR target genes within the malignant setting.

In the normal breast PR-A and -B are expressed in equimolar ratios, whereas in breast cancers these ratios can be disrupted; altered PR isoform ratios have been shown to be associated with tumour aggressiveness. In early breast lesions PR-A/B ratios are distorted, PR-A expression predominates in DCIS (ductal carcinoma in situ) and invasive lesions (Mote *et al.*, 2002). In breast cancer a high PR-A/B ratio is associated with an undifferentiated phenotype and a poorer prognosis (Bamberger *et al.*, 2000), analysis of these tumours shows this altered ratio is likely due to decreased expression of PR-B rather than increased expression of PR-A (Graham *et al.*, 1995). In the face of phosphorylation events, steady-state levels of activated phospho-PR-B are predicted to be lowered by rapid proteasome-dependent protein turnover (Shen *et al.*, 2004). This context (i.e. cancers with high kinases activities) predicts a higher PR-A/B ratio that favours activation of growth promoting gene programs (Knutson *et al.*, 2012).

8.7   Summary

As highly post-translationally modified transcription factors, PR molecules act as context-dependent 'sensors' for the integration of ever-fluctuating mixtures of steroid hormones and growth factors. Under conditions where growth factors are abundant, phosphorylated PR-B becomes exquisitely sensitive to low concentrations of progesterone; in the normal mammary gland this serves to initiate developmentally appropriate proliferative programmes in order to achieve rapid expansion of ductal structures during pregnancy. In the context of malignant transformation, the up-regulation of kinase signalling coupled to down-regulation of cell cycle inhibitory molecules predicts PR hyperactivation of similar transcriptional programmes. Most notably, phospho-PR target genes include the components of protein kinase pathways such as the growth factors themselves, their cell surface receptors (IGFR, EGFR/erbB2) and required downstream effectors. PR-driven remodelling of proliferative circuitry thus serves to further sensitise cancer cells to local hormones, creating a potent feed forward proliferative response. At peak PR (transcriptional) activity, rapid ligand-dependent down-regulation of phospho-PR predicts low steady-state protein levels (Lange *et al.*, 2000; Shen *et al.*, 2001). Thus, the presence of a PR gene signature (Knutson *et al.*, 2012) rather than PR protein levels, provides a reliable biomarker of PR-driven breast cancer biologies (i.e. proliferation and pro-survival); breast cancer patients with this signature are good candidates for alternative endocrine therapeutics that include an anti-progestin.

References

Abdel-Hafiz, H.A. and Horwitz, K.B. (2012) Control of progesterone receptor transcriptional synergy by SUMOylation and deSUMOylation. *BMC Molecular Biology*, **13**, 10.

Abdel-Hafiz, H., Takimoto, G.S.,Tung, L. and Horwitz, K.B. (2002) The inhibitory function in human progesterone receptor N termini binds SUMO-1 protein to regulate autoinhibition and transrepression. *Journal of Biological Chemistry*, **277**, 33950–33956.

Abdel-Hafiz, H., Dudevoir, M.L. and Horwitz, K.B. (2009) Mechanisms underlying the control of progesterone receptor transcriptional activity by SUMOylation. *Journal of Biological Chemistry*, **284**, 9099–9108.

Abukhdeir, A.M. and Park, B.H. (2008) P21 and p27: roles in carcinogenesis and drug resistance. *Expert Reviews in Molecular Medicine*, **10**, e19.

Anderson, G.L., Limacher, M., Assaf, A.R. *et al.* (2004) Effects of conjugated equine estrogen in postmenopausal women with hysterectomy: the Women's Health Initiative randomized controlled trial. *JAMA*, **291**, 1701–1712.

Arnett-Mansfield, R.L., DeFazio, A., Mote, P.A. and Clarke, C.L. (2004) Subnuclear distribution of progesterone receptors A and B in normal and malignant endometrium. *Journal of Clinical and Endocrinology and Metabolism*, **89**, 1429–1442.

Arnett-Mansfield, R.L., Graham, J.D., Hanson, A.R. *et al.* (2007) Focal subnuclear distribution of progesterone receptor is ligand dependent and associated with transcriptional activity. *Molecular Endocrinology*, **21**, 14–29.

Balana, M.E., Labriola, L., Salatino, M. *et al.* (2001) Activation of ErbB-2 via a hierarchical interaction between ErbB-2 and type I insulin-like growth factor receptor in mammary tumor cells. *Oncogene*, **20**, 34–47.

Ballare, C., Uhrig, M., Bechtold, T. *et al.* (2003) Two domains of the progesterone receptor interact with the estrogen receptor and are required for progesterone activation of the c-Src/Erk pathway in mammalian cells. *Molecular and Cellular Biology*, **23**, 1994–2008.

Bamberger, A.M., Milde-Langosch, K., Schulte, H.M. and Loning, T. (2000) Progesterone receptor isoforms, PR-B and PR-A, in breast cancer: correlations with clini-
copathologic tumor parameters and expression of AP-1 factors. *Hormone Resarch*,
54, 32–37.

Banerji, S., Cibulskis, K., Rangel-Escareno, C. *et al.* (2012) Sequence analysis of
mutations and translocations across breast cancer subtypes. *Nature*, **486**, 405–409.

Beguelin, W., Diaz Flaque, M.C., Proietti, C.J. *et al.* (2010) Progesterone receptor
induces ErbB-2 nuclear translocation to promote breast cancer growth via a novel
transcriptional effect: ErbB-2 function as a coactivator of Stat3. *Molecular and
Cellular Biology*, **30**, 5456–5472.

Beleut, M., Rajaram, R.D., Caikovski, M. *et al.* (2010) Two distinct mechanisms
underlie progesterone-induced proliferation in the mammary gland. *Proceedings of
the National Academy of Sciences, USA*, **107**, 2989–2994.

Beral, V. (2003) Breast cancer and hormone-replacement therapy in the Million
Women Study. *Lancet*, **362**, 419–427.

Bjornstrom, L. Sjoberg, M. (2005) Mechanisms of estrogen receptor signaling: convergence of genomic and nongenomic actions on target genes. *Molecular Endocrinology*, **19**, 833–842.

Boonyaratanakornkit, V., Scott, M.P., Ribon, V. *et al.* (2001) Progesterone receptor
contains a proline-rich motif that directly interacts with SH3 domains and activates
c-Src family tyrosine kinases. *Molecular Cell*, **8**, 269–280.

Boonyaratanakornkit, V., McGowan, E., Sherman, L. *et al.* (2007) The role of extranu-
clear signaling actions of progesterone receptor in mediating progesterone regulation
of gene expression and the cell cycle. *Molecular Endocrinology*, **21**, 359–375.

Cerliani, J.P., Guillardoy, T., Giulianelli, S. *et al.* (2011) Interaction between FGFR-
2, STAT5, and progesterone receptors in breast cancer. *Cancer Research*, **71**,
3720–3731.

Chlebowski, R.T. and Anderson, G.L. (2012) Changing concepts: Menopausal hormone therapy and breast cancer. *Journal of the National Cancer Institute*, **104**,
517–527.

Chlebowski, R.T., Hendrix, S.L., Langer, R.D. *et al.* (2003) Influence of estrogen plus
progestin on breast cancer and mammography in healthy postmenopausal women:
the Women's Health Initiative Randomized Trial. *Jama*, **289**, 3243–3253.

Chlebowski, R.T., Kuller, L.H., Prentice, R.L. *et al.* (2009) Breast cancer after use
of estrogen plus progestin in postmenopausal women. *New England Journal of
Medicine*, **360**, 573–587.

Cicatiello, L., Addeo, R., Sasso, A. *et al.* (2004) Estrogens and progesterone promote
persistent CCND1 gene activation during G1 by inducing transcriptional derepres-
sion via c-Jun/c-Fos/estrogen receptor (progesterone receptor) complex assembly to
a distal regulatory element and recruitment of cyclin D1 to its own gene promoter.
Molecular and Cellular Biology, **24**, 7260–7274.

Clarke, C.L. and Graham, J.D. (2012) Non-overlapping progesterone receptor
cistromes contribute to cell-specific transcriptional outcomes. *PLoS One*, **7**, e35859.

Clemm, D.L., Sherman, L., Boonyaratanakornkit, V. *et al.* (2000) Differential hormone-dependent phosphorylation of progesterone receptor A and B
forms revealed by a phosphoserine site-specific monoclonal antibody. *Molecular
Endocrinology*, **14**, 52–65.

Clemons, M. and Goss, P. (2001) Estrogen and the risk of breast cancer. *New England
Journal of Medicine*, **344**, 276–285.

Daniel, A.R. and Lange, C.A. (2009) Protein kinases mediate ligand-independent dere-pression of sumoylated progesterone receptors in breast cancer cells. *Proceedings of the National Academy of Sciences, USA*, **106**, 14287–14292.

Daniel, A.R., Faivre, E.J. and Lange, C.A. (2007) Phosphorylation-dependent antago-nism of sumoylation derepresses progesterone receptor action in breast cancer cells. *Molecular Endocrinology*, **21**, 2890–2906.

Daniel, A.R., Gaviglio, A.L., Czaplicki, L.M. *et al.* (2010) The progesterone receptor hinge region regulates the kinetics of transcriptional responses through acetyla-tion, phosphorylation, and nuclear retention. *Molecular Endocrinology*, **24** (11), 2126–2138.

Daniel, A.R., Hagan, C.R. and Lange, C.A. (2011) Progesterone receptor action: defin-ing a role in breast cancer. *Expert Reviews of Endocrinology and Metabolism*, **6**, 359–369.

Dhomen, N.S., Mariadason, J., Tebbutt, N., Scott, A.M. Therapeutic targeting of the epidermal growth factor receptor in human cancer. *Crit Rev Oncog* **17** (2012) 31-50.

Dressing, G.E., Hagan, C.R., Knutson, T.P. *et al.* (2009) Progesterone receptors act as sensors for mitogenic protein kinases in breast cancer models. *Endocrine Related Cancer*, **16**, 351–361.

Edwards, D.P. (2005) Regulation of signal transduction pathways by estrogen and progesterone. *Annual Review of Physiology*, **67**, 335–376.

Faivre, E.J. and Lange, C.A. (2007) Progesterone receptors upregulate Wnt-1 to induce epidermal growth factor receptor transactivation and c-Src-dependent sustained acti-vation of Erk1/2 mitogen-activated protein kinase in breast cancer cells. *Molecular and Cellular Biology*, **27**, 466–480.

Gareau, J.R. and Lima, C.D. (2010) The SUMO pathway: emerging mechanisms that shape specificity, conjugation and recognition. *Nature Reviews. Molecular Cell Biology*, **11**, 861–871.

Giangrande, P.H. and McDonnell, D.P. (1999) The A and B isoforms of the hman progesterone receptor: two functionally different transcription factors encoded by a single gene. *Recent Progress in Hormone Research*, **54**, 291–314.

Gill, G. (2003) Post-translational modification by the small ubiquitin-related modifier SUMO has big effects on transcription factor activity. *Current Opinion in Genetics and Development*, **13**, 108–113.

Giulianelli, S., Vaque, J.P., Soldati, R. *et al.* (2012) Estrogen receptor alpha medi-ates progestin-induced mammary tumor growth by interacting with progesterone receptors at the cyclin D1/MYC promoters. *Cancer Research*, **72**, 2416–2427.

Gonzalez-Suarez, E., Jacob, A.P., Jones, J. *et al.* (2010) RANK ligand mediates progestin-induced mammary epithelial proliferation and carcinogenesis. *Nature*, **468**, 103–107.

Graham, J.D. and Clarke, C.L. (1997) Physiological action of progesterone in target tissues. *Endocrine Reviews*, **18**, 502–519.

Graham, J.D., Yeates, C., Balleine, R.L. *et al.* (1995) Characterization of proges-terone receptor A and B expression in human breast cancer. *Cancer Research*, **55**, 5063–5068.

Graham, J.D., Mote, P.A. and Salagame, U. *et al.* (2009) DNA replication licensing and progenitor numbers are increased by progesterone in normal human breast. *Endocrinology*, **150**, 3318–3326.

Guiochon-Mantel, A., Lescop, P., Christin-Maitre, S. *et al.* (1991) Nucleocytoplasmic shuttling of the progesterone receptor. *Embo Journal*, **10**, 3851–3859.

Guiochon-Mantel, A., Loosfelt, H., Lescop, P. *et al.* (1992) Mechanisms of nuclear localization of the progesterone receptor. *Journal of Steroid Biochemistry and Molecular Biology*, **41**, 209–215.

Hagan, C.R., Regan, T.M., Dressing, G.E. and Lange, C.A. (2011) ck2-dependent phosphorylation of progesterone receptors (PR) on Ser81 regulates PR-B isoform-specific target gene expression in breast cancer cells. *Molecular and Cellular Biology*, **31**, 2439–2452.

Hagan, C.R., Daniel, A.R., Dressing, G.E. and Lange, C.A. (2012) Role of phosphorylation in progesterone receptor signaling and specificity. *Molecular and Cellular Endocrinology*, **357**, 43–49.

Hay, R.T. (2005) SUMO: a history of modification. *Molecular Cell*, **18**, 1–12.

He, H.H., Meyer, C.A., Shin, H. *et al.* (2010) Nucleosome dynamics define transcriptional enhancers. *Nature Genetics*, **42**, 343–347.

Hill, K.K., Roemer, S.C., Jones, D.N. *et al.* (2009) A progesterone receptor co-activator (JDP2) mediates activity through interaction with residues in the carboxyl-terminal extension of the DNA binding domain. *Journal of Biological Chemistry*, **284**, 24415–24424.

Hill, K.K., Roemer, S.C., Churchill, M.E. and Edwards, D.P. (2012) Structural and functional analysis of domains of the progesterone receptor. *Molecular and Cellular Endocrinology*, **348**, 418–429.

Hilton, H.N., Graham, J.D., Kantimm, S. *et al.* (2012) Progesterone and estrogen receptors segregate into different cell subpopulations in the normal human breast. *Molecular and Cellular Endocrinology*, **361**(1-2), 191–201.

Horwitz, K.B., Mockus, M.B. and Lessey, B.A. (1982) Variant T47D human breast cancer cells with high progesterone-receptor levels despite estrogen and antiestrogen resistance. *Cell*, **28**, 633–642.

Inoue, T., Akahira, J., Suzuki, T. *et al.* (2002) Progesterone production and actions in the human central nervous system and neurogenic tumors. *Journal of Clinical and Endocrinology and Metabolism*, **87**, 5325–5331.

Jacobsen, B.M. and Horwitz, K.B. (2012) Progesterone receptors, their isoforms and progesterone regulated transcription. *Molecular and Cellular Endocrinology*, **357**, 18–29.

Jacobsen, B.M., Schittone, S.A., Richer, J.K. and Horwitz, K.B. (2005) Progesterone-independent effects of human progesterone receptors (PRs) in estrogen receptor-positive breast cancer: PR isoform-specific gene regulation and tumor biology. *Molecular Endocrinology*, **19**, 574–587.

Johnson, E.S. (2004) Protein modification by SUMO. *Annual Review of Biochemistry*, **73**, 355–382.

Joshi, P.A., Jackson, H.W., Beristain, A.G. *et al.* (2010) Progesterone induces adult mammary stem cell expansion. *Nature*, **465**, 803–807.

Kariagina, A., Aupperlee, M.D. and Haslam, S.Z. (2007) Progesterone receptor isoforms and proliferation in the rat mammary gland during development. *Endocrinology*, **148**, 2723–2736.

Kastner, P., Krust, A., Turcotte, B. *et al.* (1990) Two distinct estrogen-regulated promoters generate transcripts encoding the two functionally different human progesterone receptor forms A and B. *Embo Journal*, **9**, 1603–1614.

Key, T., Appleby, P., Barnes, I. and Reeves, G. (2002) Endogenous sex hormones and breast cancer in postmenopausal women: reanalysis of nine prospective studies. *Journal of the National Cancer Institute*, **94**, 606–616.

Knutson, T.P., Daniel, A.R. and Fan, D. *et al.* (2012) Phosphorylated and sumoylation-deficient progesterone receptors drive proliferative gene signatures during breast cancer progression. *Breast Cancer Research*, **14**, R95.

Labriola, L., Salatino, M., Proietti, C.J. *et al.* (2003) Heregulin induces transcriptional activation of the progesterone receptor by a mechanism that requires functional ErbB-2 and mitogen-activated protein kinase activation in breast cancer cells. *Molecular and Cellular Biology*, **23**, 1095–1111.

Lanari, C., Lamb, C.A., Fabris, V.T. *et al.* (2009) The MPA mouse breast cancer model: evidence for a role of progesterone receptors in breast cancer. *Endocrine Related Cancer*, **16**, 333–350.

Lange, C.A. (2008) Integration of progesterone receptor action with rapid signaling events in breast cancer models. *Journal of Steroid Biochemistry and Molecular Biology*, **108**, 203–212.

Lange, C.A., Shen, T. and Horwitz, K.B. (2000) Phosphorylation of human progesterone receptors at serine-294 by mitogen-activated protein kinase signals their degradation by the 26S proteasome. *Proceedings of the National Academy of Sciences, USA*, **97**, 1032–1037.

Lange, C.A. Sartorius, C.A., Abdel-Hafiz, H. *et al.* (2008) Progesterone receptor action: translating studies in breast cancer models to clinical insights. *Advances in Experimental Medicine and Biology*, **630**, 94–111.

Lewis, M.J., Wiebe, J.P. and Heathcote, J.G. (2004) Expression of progesterone metabolizing enzyme genes (AKR1C1, AKR1C2, AKR1C3, SRD5A1, SRD5A2) is altered in human breast carcinoma. *BMC Cancer*, **4**, 27.

Losel, R. and Wehling, M. (2003) Nongenomic actions of steroid hormones. *Nature Reviews. Molecular Cell Biology*, **4**, 46–56.

Lydon, J.P., DeMayo, F.J., Funk, C.R. *et al.* (1995) Mice lacking progesterone receptor exhibit pleiotropic reproductive abnormalities. *Genes and Development*, **9**, 2266–2278.

Lydon, J.P., Ge, G., Kittrell, F.S. *et al.* (1999) Murine mammary gland carcinogenesis is critically dependent on progesterone receptor function. *Cancer Research*, **59**, 4276–4284.

McKenna, N.J., Lanz, R.B. and O'Malley, B.W. (1999) Nuclear receptor coregulators: cellular and molecular biology. *Endocrne Reviews*, **20**, 321–344.

Migliaccio, A., Piccolo, D., Castoria, G. *et al.* (1998) Activation of the Src/p21ras/Erk pathway by progesterone receptor via cross-talk with estrogen receptor. *Embo Journal*, **17**, 2008–2018.

Moore, M.R., Conover, J.L. and Franks, K.M. (2000) Progestin effects on long-term growth, death, and Bcl-xL in breast cancer cells. *Biochemical and Biophysical Research Communications*, **277**, 650–654.

Moore, N.L., Narayanan, R. and Weigel, N.L. (2007) Cyclin dependent kinase 2 and the regulation of human progesterone receptor activity. *Steroids*, **72**, 202–209.

Mote, P.A., Balleine, R.L., McGowan, E.M. and Clarke, C.L. (1999) Colocalization of progesterone receptors A and B by dual immunofluorescent histochemistry in human endometrium during the menstrual cycle. *Journal of Clinical and Endocrinology and Metabolism*, **84**, 2963–2971.

Mote, P.A., Bartow, S., Tran, N. and Clarke, C.L. (2002) Loss of co-ordinate expression of progesterone receptors A and B is an early event in breast carcinogenesis. *Breast Cancer Research and Treatment*, **72**, 163–172.

Mulac-Jericevic, B., Mullinax, R.A., DeMayo, F.J. *et al.* (2000) Subgroup of reproductive functions of progesterone mediated by progesterone receptor-B isoform. *Science*, **289**, 1751–1754.

Mulac-Jericevic, B., Lydon, J.P., DeMayo, F.J. and Conneely, O.M. (2003) Defective mammary gland morphogenesis in mice lacking the progesterone receptor B isoform. *Proceedings of the National Academy of Sciences, USA*, **100**, 9744–9749.

Musgrove, E.A., Davison, E.A. and Ormandy, C.J. (2004) Role of the CDK inhibitor p27 (Kip1) in mammary development and carcinogenesis: Insights from knockout mice. *Journal of Mammary Gland Biology and Neoplasia*, **9**, 55–66.

Narayanan, R., Adigun, A.A., Edwards, D.P. and Weigel, N.L. (2005a) Cyclin-dependent kinase activity is required for progesterone receptor function: novel role for cyclin A/Cdk2 as a progesterone receptor coactivator. *Molecular and Cellular Biology*, **25**, 264–277.

Narayanan, R., Edwards, D.P. and Weigel, N.L. (2005b) Human progesterone receptor displays cell cycle-dependent changes in transcriptional activity. *Molecular and Cellular Biology*, **25**, 2885–2898.

Osborne, C.K., Schiff, R. and Arpino, G. *et al.* (2005) Endocrine responsiveness: understanding how progesterone receptor can be used to select endocrine therapy. *Breast*, **14**, 458–465.

Owen, G.I. Richer, J.K., Tung, L. *et al.* (1998) Progesterone regulates transcription of the p21(WAF1) cyclin- dependent kinase inhibitor gene through Sp1 and CBP/p300. *Journal of Biological Chemistry*, **273**, 10696–10701.

Pierson-Mullany, L.K. and Lange, C.A. (2004) Phosphorylation of progesterone receptor serine 400 mediates ligand-independent transcriptional activity in response to activation of cyclin-dependent protein kinase 2. *Molecular and Cellular Biology*, **24**, 10542–10557.

Pierson-Mullany, L.K., Skildum, A., Faivre, E. and Lange, C.A. (2003) Cross-talk between growth factor and progesterone receptor signaling pathways: implications for breast cancer cell growth. *Breast Disease*, **18**, 21–31.

Poole, A.J., Li, Y., Kim, Y., Lin, S.C. *et al.* (2006) Prevention of Brca1-mediated mammary tumorigenesis in mice by a progesterone antagonist. *Science*, **314**, 1467–1470.

Proietti, C., Salatino, Ro M., Semblit, C. *et al.* (2005) Progestins induce transcriptional activation of signal transducer and activator of transcription 3 (Stat3) via a Jak- and Src-dependent mechanism in breast cancer cells. *Molecular and Cellular Biology*, **25**, 4826–4840.

Proietti, C.J., Beguelin, W., Flaque, M.C. *et al.* (2011) Novel role of signal transducer and activator of transcription 3 as a progesterone receptor coactivator in breast cancer. *Steroids*, **76** (4), 381–392.

Qiu, M. and Lange, C.A. (2003) MAP kinases couple multiple functions of human progesterone receptors: degradation, transcriptional synergy, and nuclear association. *Journal of Steroid Biochemistry and Molecular Biology*, **85**, 147–157.

Richer, J.K., Lange, C.A., Wierman, A.M. *et al.* (1998) Progesterone receptor variants found in breast cells repress transcription by wild-type receptors. *Breast Cancer Research and Treatment*, **48**, 231–241.

Richer, J.K., Jacobsen, B.M., Manning, N.G. *et al.* (2002) Differential gene regulation by the two progesterone receptor isoforms in human breast cancer cells. *Journal of Biological Chemistry*, **277**, 5209–5218.

Roemer, S.C., Donham, D.C., Sherman, L. *et al.* (2006) Structure of the progesterone receptor-deoxyribonucleic acid complex: novel interactions required for binding to half-site response elements. *Molecular Endocrinology*, **20**, 3042–3052.

Roemer, S.C., Adelman, J., Churchill, M.E. and Edwards, D.P. (2008) Mechanism of high-mobility group protein B enhancement of progesterone receptor sequence-specific DNA binding. *Nucleic Acids Research*, **36**, 3655–3666.

Saitoh, M., Ohmichi, M., Takahashi, K. *et al.* (2005) Medroxyprogesterone acetate induces cell proliferation through up-regulation of cyclin D1 expression via phosphatidylinositol 3-kinase/Akt/nuclear factor-kappaB cascade in human breast cancer cells. *Endocrinology*, **146**, 4917–4925.

Salatino, M., Beguelin, W., Peters, M.G. *et al.* (2006) Progestin-induced caveolin-1 expression mediates breast cancer cell proliferation. *Oncogene*, **25**, 7723–7739.

Santen, R.J., Song, R.X., Zhang, Z. *et al.* (2005) Long-term estradiol deprivation in breast cancer cells up-regulates growth factor signaling and enhances estrogen sensitivity. *Endocrine Related Cancer*, **12** (Suppl 1), S61–S73.

Sartorius, C.A., Melville, M.Y., Hovland, A.R. *et al.* (1994) A third transactivation function (AF3) of human progesterone receptors located in the unique *N*-terminal segment of the B-isoform. *Molecular Endocrinology*, **8** 1347–1360.

Scarpin, K.M., Graham, J.D., Mote, P.A. and Clarke, C.L. (2009) Progesterone action in human tissues: regulation by progesterone receptor (PR) isoform expression, nuclear positioning and coregulator expression. *Nuclear Receptor Signalling*, **7**, e009.

Shen, T., Horwitz, K.B. and Lange, C.A. (2001) Transcriptional hyperactivity of human progesterone receptors is coupled to their ligand-dependent down-regulation by mitogen-activated protein kinase-dependent phosphorylation of serine 294. *Molecular and Cellular Biology*, **21**, 6122–6131.

Skildum, A., Faivre, E. and Lange, C.A. (2005) Progesterone receptors induce cell cycle progression via activation of mitogen activated protein kinases. *Molecular Endocrinology*, **19**, 327–339.

Smith, C.L., Archer, T.K., Hamlin-Green, G. and Hager, G.L. (1993) Newly expressed progesterone receptor cannot activate stable, replicated mouse mammary tumor virus templates but acquires transactivation potential upon continuous expression. *Proceedings of the National Academy of Sciences, USA*, **90**, 11202–11206.

Smith, C.L., Htun, H., Wolford, R.G. and Hager, G.L. (1997) Differential activity of progesterone and glucocorticoid receptors on mouse mammary tumor virus templates differing in chromatin structure. *Journal of Biological Chemistry*, **272**, 14227–14235.

Smith, C.L., Wolford, R.G., O'Neill, T.B. and Hager, G.L. (2000) Characterization of transiently and constitutively expressed progesterone receptors: evidence for two functional states. *Molecular Endocrinology*, **14**, 956–971.

Stoecklin, E., Wissler, M., Schaetzle, D. *et al.* (1999) Interactions in the transcriptional regulation exerted by Stat5 and by members of the steroid hormone receptor family. *Journal of Steroid Biochemistry and Molecular Biology*, **69**, 195–204.

Tang, Q., Chen, Y., Meyer, C. *et al.* (2011) A comprehensive view of nuclear receptor cancer cistromes. *Cancer Research*, **71**, 6940–6947.

Tawfic, S., Yu, S., Wang, H. *et al.* (2001) Protein kinase CK2 signal in neoplasia. *Histology and Histopathology*, **16**, 573–582.

Trembley, J.H., Wang, G., Unger, G. *et al.* (2009) Protein kinase CK2 in health and disease: CK2: a key player in cancer biology. *Cell and Molecular Life Sciences*, **66**, 1858–1867.

Tyagi, R.K., Amazit, L., Lescop, P. *et al.* (1998) Mechanisms of progesterone receptor export from nuclei: role of nuclear localization signal, nuclear export signal, and ran guanosine triphosphate. *Molecular Endocrinology*, **12**, 1684–1695.

Vicent, G.P., Ballare, C., Nacht, A.S. *et al.* (2006a) Induction of progesterone target genes requires activation of Erk and Msk kinases and phosphorylation of histone H3. *Molecular Cell*, **24**, 367–381.

Vicent, G.P., Ballare, C., Zaurin, R. *et al.* (2006b) Chromatin remodeling and control of cell proliferation by progestins via cross talk of progesterone receptor with the estrogen receptors and kinase signaling pathways. *Annals of the New York Academy of Science*, **1089**, 59–72.

Yin, P., Roqueiro, D., Huang, L. *et al.* (2012) Genome-wide progesterone receptor binding: cell type-specific and shared mechanisms in T47D breast cancer cells and primary leiomyoma cells. *PLoS One*, **7**, e29021.

Zhang, Y., Beck, C.A., Poletti, A. *et al.* (1994) Identification of phosphorylation sites unique to the B form of human progesterone receptor. *In vitro* phosphorylation by casein kinase II. *Journal of Biological Chemistry*, **269**, 31034–31040.

Zhang, Y., Beck, C.A., Poletti, A. *et al.* (1997) Phosphorylation of human progesterone receptor by cyclin-dependent kinase 2 on three sites that are authentic basal phosphorylation sites *in vivo*. *Molecular Endocrinology*, **11**, 823–832.

9

Signalling cross-talk

Amanda Harvey
Biosciences, Brunel University, London

9.1 Introduction

So far this book has focused on individual pathways and their roles in cancer formation. Whilst it would be hard to deny the contribution that each pathway plays in the processes underlying tumour development and progression, it is very unlikely that these pathways function in isolation. This is abundantly clear when examining therapeutic responses to targeted therapies and the mechanisms underlying acquired drug resistance. Inhibition of individual pathways, often results in up-regulation of another as a mechanism of compensatory signalling.

The observant reader will also have noticed that a number of classes of adaptor molecules are common to more than one pathway and these have been depicted in pink, green and orange in the relevant chapter figures. This commonality amongst several pathways plays a large role in mediating signalling cross-talk.

Robin Donaldson and Mufty Calder (2010) discuss some of the different types of signalling cross-talk and categorise them into at least five broad classes:

- signal flow cross-talk;
- substrate availability cross-talk;
- receptor function cross-talk;
- gene expression cross-talk;
- intracellular communication cross-talk.

These classes are illustrated in Figure 9.1 and summarised in the figure legend.

These are not the only mechanisms through which cross-talk occurs and both these and more complex examples of other mechanisms involved in intracellular communication cross-talk are discussed in more detail throughout this chapter in

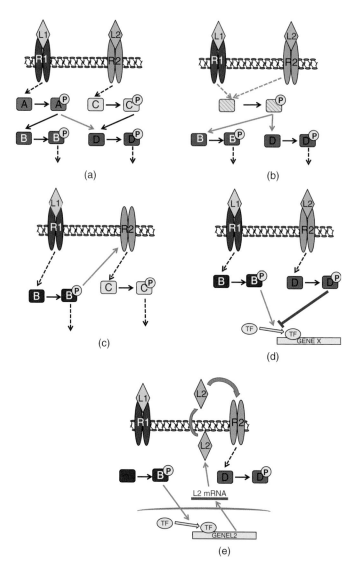

Figure 9.1 Schematic representation on the different types of signalling cross-talk. In signal flow cross-talk (a) a molecule in one pathway affects the rate of activation of signalling molecules in a second pathway. Substrate availability cross-talk (b) occurs when two pathways 'compete' for common components. In receptor function cross-talk (c) an individual receptor's ability to detect a ligand is altered and signalling can occur in ligand absence. When gene expression cross-talk (d) occurs, two pathways have reciprocal effects on transcription factor activation and subsequent gene expression. Lastly, intracellular communication cross-talk (e) occurs when one pathway affects the amount of available ligand for a second pathway. The example given by Donaldson and Calder (2010) focuses on ligand gene expression, although this is not the only mechanism by which ligand levels can be affected.

the context of tumour development and therapeutic responses. It can be seen that one class of cross-talk will then facilitate another, for example increased gene expression cross-talk, results in increased signal flow and intracellular communication. This makes discussing an individual class of cross-talk difficult and the specific examples discussed in the following sections are neither an exhaustive list nor exclusive to an individual cross-talk type.

9.2   Examples of cross-talk

9.2.1   Wnt mediated cross-talk

Wnt and EGFR signalling pathways (Chapters 1 and 4) potentially converge at a number of points. Both pathways have long been known to activate β-catenin in the A431 cell line (Hoschuetzky, 1994). In addition, EGFR antagonises Wnt in development, but they also coordinate in establishing planar cell polarity in *Drosophila*. Together both pathways synergistically induce tumour formation (reviewed in Hu and Li, 2010).

   In tumours induced by TGFα, decreasing the latency period increased the expression of *Wnt-1* and *Wnt-3*, suggesting a link between these two signalling pathways (Schroeder *et al.*, 2000). Over-expression of Wnt1 and Wnt5a in mammary epithelial cells resulted in phosphorylation of EGFR and Erk activation (Civenni *et al.*, 2003). This effect was not observed in the presence of the Wnt antagonist, sFRP-1, or EGFR kinase inhibitors. Inhibition of Wnt signalling in breast cancer cells resulted in a decrease in Erk activity and cell proliferation (Schlange *et al.*, 2007) via a mechanism that was independent of β-catenin activity (reviewed in Collu *et al.*, 2009). Activation of MAPK signalling by Wnt does not come about in response to a direct induction of EGFR ligands, but may be dependent on ligand availability. The metalloproteinase family of enzymes has been linked to this effect (Figure 9.2). TACE cleaves pro-amphiregulin (Gschwind *et al.*, 2003) and G-protein coupled receptors trans-activate EGFR through MMP cleavage of HB-EGF (Prenzel *et al.*, 1999). Cleavage of pro- or bound forms of growth factors increases the availability of ligands for ErbB receptor binding resulting in downstream activation of the pathways.

   This style of intracellular communication cross-talk has implications therapeutically, especially as Wnt expression blocks the anti-proliferative effects of anti-hormone therapy in breast cancer cells through activation of EGFR (Schlange *et al.*, 2007). The use of plant compounds that inhibit both Wnt and EGFR signalling could be useful in combating resistance to selective oestrogen receptor modulators, and compounds such as fisetin have already been shown to inhibit Wnt and EGFR and induce apoptosis and COX2 inhibition in colon cancer cells (Suh *et al.*, 2009). More studies in this research area will surely follow, especially as the consequences of EGFR mutations in the context of Wnt antagonist gene

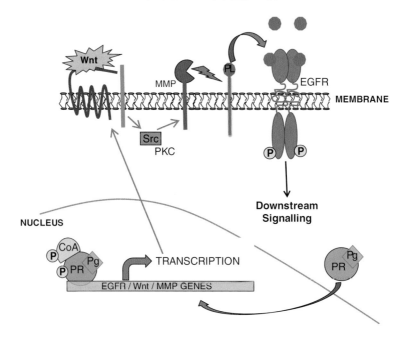

Figure 9.2 Wnt mediated cross-talk. Wnt induces activation of membrane bound MMPs, which then cleave pro-ligands (PL) such as pro-amphiregulin and HB-EGF, releasing them for ErbB receptor activation. An additional layer of cross-talk is added as progestin (Pg) can activate the progestersone receptor (PR) which, with transcriptional co-activators, initiate transcription of genes involved in mediating the cross-talk such as Wnt, EGFR and MMP. Adapted from Faivre and Lange 2007 and Ferguson *et al.*, 2003.

methylation are explored. Currently these are associated with good prognosis and it is hypothesised that they may have some effect on the chemosensitivity of cells to EGFR inhibition (Suzuki *et al.*, 2007).

9.2.2 Growth factors and steroid hormones

Oestrogens and growth factors

Oestrogens are known drivers of breast cancer cells (McGuire, 1975), and one of the underlying mechanisms of increased proliferation may involve sensitisation to IGF, possibly by regulating IGF1R (Stewart *et al.*, 1990). In oestrogen sensitive breast cancer cells there is a link between TGFβ signalling, IGF1 and MMP production that mediates epithelial–mesenchymal transition (EMT) (Walsh and Damjanovski, 2011).

Oestrogens mediate cross-talk through regulating ligand levels. Production of the EGFR ligand, TGFα, is increased and the section of the inhibitory TGFβ is decreased (reviewed in Lippman *et al.*, 1987; Knabbe *et al.*, 1987).

Cross-talk between the oestrogen receptor (ER) and HER2 signalling is partly responsible for the intrinsic resistance to anti-endocrine therapy that exists in many breast cancers. EGFR-mediated signalling down-regulates ER expression (reviewed in Nahta and O'Regan, 2012), although, not surprisingly in the context of cross-talk, the picture is likely to be more complex than this. *ER* expression is actually mediated through both EGFR and IGFR signalling, with each pathway coordinating expression of a specific ER isoform. IGFR increases expression of *ERα*, whereas EGFR regulates expression of *ERβ* (Tsonis *et al.*, 2013). HER2 inhibition increases the transcriptional activity of ER (Sabnis *et al.*, 2009) and HER2 positive tumours are less sensitive to the anti-proliferative effects of tamoxifen (reviewed in Nahta and O'Regan, 2012). Cross-talk exists in a variety of forms and links between receptor availability and substrate availability. The ER has been shown to have a non-genomic aspect to its function. It is proposed, in tamoxifen resistant cells, that in response to oestradiol, the ER can localise to HER2 and increase the coupling of ErbB signalling to PI3K activity. If HER2 activity is inhibited, ErbB signalling will decrease meaning that cells will become more dependent on the genomic actions of the ER allowing tamoxifen to become more effective. Genes such as *TGFα* and *VEGF* are regulated by the ER and are increased in models of trastuzumab resistance (reviewed in Nahta and O'Regan, 2012). Combined inhibition of EGFR, HER2 and ER resulted in complete regression of xenograft models (Wang *et al.*, 2011). Combining inhibition of both ErbBs and ER is more effective than either pathway and individually highlights the effects of cross-talk between the two signalling pathways. Some mechanisms of resistance to ErbB inhibition induce progesterone receptor (PR) activity (Xia *et al.*, 2006) (Chapter 8) and this can result in a feed-forward loop via PR through to Wnt activity (next section).

Progesterone and Wnt

Progesterone receptors (PRs) participate in integrated signalling cross-talk. They up-regulate *Wnt1* expression, which in turn has a knock-on effect on MMP-mediated release of EGFR ligands, resulting in sustained c-src and MAPK activation and increased anchorage independent cell growth (Faivre and Lange, 2007) (Figure 9.2).

9.3   Convergence of signalling at downstream foci

In normal cells under physiological conditions, signalling 'hubs' or foci will control the downstream events and regulate the cellular outcomes in a tightly coordinated manner. However, when components of foci are elevated or hyper-activated, an increased 'flux' in signalling is possible with the ultimate result that the cellular outcomes required for tumour development are also elevated.

9.3.1   mTOR

EGF, IGF and Wnt signalling pathways converge on the highly conserved serine/ threonine kinase mTOR (Chapter 5), which functions as a signalling 'hub'. Cross-talk from mTOR signalling results in activation of STAT3 (Yokogami *et al.*, 2000) and increased Notch signalling via STAT3 (Ma *et al.*, 2010). As this research field grows it is likely that more substrates of mTOR complexes will be identified (Wang and Proud, 2011).

9.3.2   β-Catenin

In addition to EGF and Wnt, β-catenin is also downstream of HGF/c-Met sig-nalling. Phosphorylation of β-catenin in response to receptor activation results in redistribution to the nucleus and enhanced transcription of β-catenin target genes, such as those containing LEF-1 promoters (reviewed in Jamieson *et al.*, 2012) (Chapter 4). Nuclear β-catenin is observed in invasive regions of many cancers including colon carcinomas (Brabletz *et al.*, 2001). Wnt signalling is crucial in normal colon development but is frequently dysregulated in colon carcinomas (Chapter 4) and especially in those cells that are believed to be tumour-initiating cells (sometimes termed cancer stem cells) (Vermeulen *et al.*, 2010). In tumours where Wnt dysregulation is less crucial, β-catenin nuclear localisation could be induced by factors such as EGF and HGF.

9.4   Common signalling components

Common pathway elements could be viewed as alternative signalling foci. This is possible for PI3K activation, although as it is an upstream event in many pathways. It links receptor signalling to downstream events that converge on foci such as mTOR. Along with PI3K, the MAPK cascades tend to be viewed as signalling components that are common to a number of pathways. At least 3 MAPK families have been identified, each with distinct components in their cascades (reviewed in Zhang and Liu, 2002).

9.4.1   MAPK

MAPK signalling cascades are common to a number of different signalling path-ways, notably, EGF, IGF, c-met and VEGF (Chapters 1, 2, 6 and 7). Different cellular stresses or conditions will activate distinct cascades, however there is definite overlap in response to growth factor signalling (Figure 9.3). This gives rise to 'competition' for substrates (substrate availability cross-talk, Figure 9.1b) in response to signalling from different receptor families.

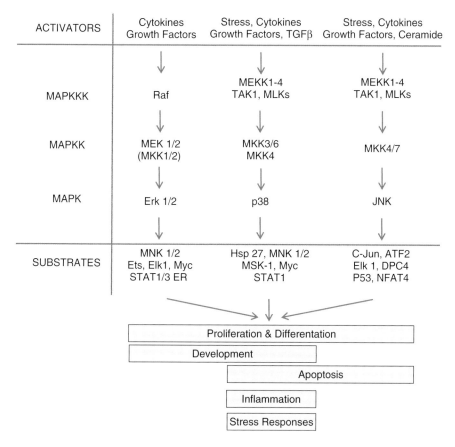

ACTIVATORS	Cytokines Growth Factors	Stress, Cytokines Growth Factors, TGFβ	Stress, Cytokines Growth Factors, Ceramide
	↓	↓	↓
MAPKKK	Raf	MEKK1-4 TAK1, MLKs	MEKK1-4 TAK1, MLKs
	↓	↓	↓
MAPKK	MEK 1/2 (MKK1/2)	MKK3/6 MKK4	MKK4/7
	↓	↓	↓
MAPK	Erk 1/2	p38	JNK
	↓	↓	↓
SUBSTRATES	MNK 1/2 Ets, Elk1, Myc STAT1/3 ER	Hsp 27, MNK 1/2 MSK-1, Myc STAT1	C-Jun, ATF2 Elk 1, DPC4 P53, NFAT4

Proliferation & Differentiation

Development

Apoptosis

Inflammation

Stress Responses

Figure 9.3 **Major components in mammalian MAPK cascades.** The individual cascades are activated by specific stimuli with individual effects on cellular responses. Some of the components of the cascades (for example, MEKK1-4 and MKK4) are common to more than one cascade, potentially allowing for inter-cascades cross-talk. Adapted from Zhang and Liu, 2002.

Outside of conventional growth factor signalling pathways, MAPKs are involved in coordinating both signal flow (Figure 9.1a), gene expression (Figure 9.1d) and intracellular communication (Figure 9.1e) cross-talk.

MAPKs and TGFβ

Both signal flow and gene expression cross-talk exist between the MAPKs and TGFβ signalling (reviewed in Guo and Wang, 2009). Transcription factors that are activated by MAPK initiate gene expression of TGFβ target genes. Cross-talk between signalling pathways increases expression of further signalling molecules that are required for TGFβ-induced migration (Vasilaki *et al.*, 2010). p38MAPK activity is required for the increase in expression of MMPs and their inhibitors in

TGFβ-mediated breast cancer cell migration and invasion (Gomes *et al.*, 2012). In pancreatic cancer cells increased EMT in response to TGFβ is partly dependent on p38MAPK and partly on Smad4 dependent pathways (Han *et al.*, 2012).

This interplay is not limited to tumour cells as fibroblast *TIMP3* expression is regulated by TGFβ in a complex system that is dependant on Erk1/2, Smad3 and p38 pathways (Leivonen *et al.*, 2013).

Cell death regulators are also controlled through cooperation of Smads and MAPK pathways (Ramesh *et al.*, 2008; van der Heide *et al.*, 2011).

Owing to its pleiotropic effects, dysregulation of TGFβ in cancers is complex and much of the signalling that contributes to tumour development is a balance of cross-talk effects. Elevated *TGFβ* expression is detected in invasive tumours (Peters *et al.*, 2009) but it is likely that the anti-proliferative effects associated with TGFβ are lost because MAPK proteins de-activate the R-Smads and degrade Smad 4 (reviewed in Donaldson and Calder, 2010). Another mechanism that supports this theory is via cross-talk from Wnt and MAPK pathways inhibiting SMAD7 inhibition leading to reduced feedback inhibition of the pathway (discussed in Keld and Ang, 2011). An additional layer of complexity is added when the fact that both TGFβ and MAPKs mediate cross-talk with Wnt signalling is considered (reviewed in Donaldson and Calder, 2010, 2012) (Figure 9.4).

MAPKs and oestrogens

17β-oestradiol induces activation of MAPK. This effect is independent of transcriptional and translational regulation, and is preceded by an increase in cytosolic calcium levels (Improta-Brears *et al.*, 1999). Both Erk 1 and Erk2 are activated by oestrogen, even in oestrogen receptor-negative cell lines. As with Wnt cross-talk, this activation is mediated through G-protein coupled receptor homologues that signal the release of HB-EGF, thereby trans-activating EGFR (Filardo *et al.*, 2002).

Conversely, in breast cancer cells MAPK can also mediate the phosphorylation of the oestrogen receptor (ER) resulting in receptor function cross-talk (Figure 9.1c). Thyroid hormone activates MAPK (Lin *et al.*, 1999) promoting cell proliferation through phosphorylation of the ER (Tang *et al.*, 2004).

9.4.2 PI3K and Akt

The PI3K/Akt pathway is synonymous with mTOR activation. A number of different growth factor pathways including EGF, IGF, HGF and VEGF (Chapters 1, 2, 6 and 7) activate PI3K signalling in response to receptor activation. This in turn feeds downstream into mTOR (for EGF, IGF and HGF) or MAPK cascades (for VEGF).

Activation of PI3K is common in many cancers and loss of its negative regulator, PTEN, enhances its activity. Enhanced EGFR signalling can be acquired by

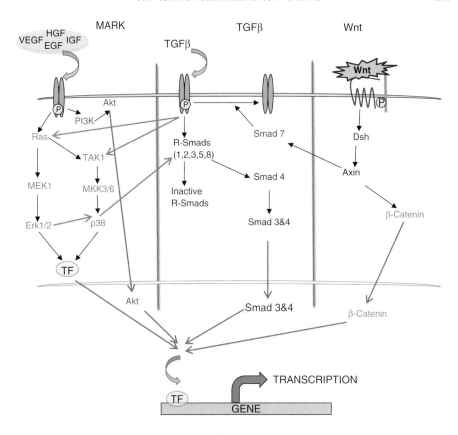

Figure 9.4   **Cross talk between MAPK, TGFβ and Wnt signalling.** A schematic representation of the key components involved in these pathways. As MAPK activation is downstream of several growth factors, cross-talk between MAPK and TGFβ, in reality, results in cross-talk between EGF, IGF, VEGF and HGF signalling. Adapted from Donaldson and Calder, 2010 and Leivonen, 2013.

non-small cell lung carcinomas through mutations of downstream elements such as PI3K (Ghandi *et al.*, 2009) and 70% of breast cancers have mutations in genes that lead to elevated PI3K activity (reviewed in Miller *et al.*, 2011). Increased PI3K/Akt activity is associated with decreased therapeutic responses and increased resistance to anti-endocrine based therapies, as well as HER2 inhibitors (reviewed in Miller *et al.*, 2011). A number of pathway inhibitors are in clinical development and PI3K inhibition has been shown to increase the efficacy of trastuzumab by disrupting the HER2/HER3/PI3K complex (Junttila *et al.*, 2009).

Given the number of receptors that utilise PI3K/Akt to transduce signals, it is hardly surprising that inhibiting one pathway leads to increased substrate availability for another.

9.5   Compensatory signalling

Treatment of a number of different cancers that are driven by aberrant cell signalling pathways has progressed markedly with the introduction of either monoclonal antibodies that prevent ligand binding and receptor dimerisation events, or ATP analogues that act as competitive inhibitors and block ATP from accessing the enzyme's active site. Both approaches result in reduced kinase activity of the targeted signalling pathway. One of the limitations with these approaches is that signalling cross-talk can give rise to a decrease in therapeutic sensitivity to the drug.

As discussed previously, several pathways converge on focal points in the signalling networks. If one path is inhibited, cell signalling to the focal point can simply be re-routed via an alternate pathway to the same hub, a little like a traffic diversion for road works.

The presence of common pathway components means that if one pathway is inhibited, more components are available to transduce signals in another pathway, thereby allowing for increased 'traffic' flow on the different route.

9.5.1   IGFR interplay with EGFR

In HER2 positive breast cancers, IGF-1R was shown to reduce the sensitivity of the breast cancer cells to the anti-HER2 monoclonal antibody therapy trastuzumab (Herceptin), and conversely inhibiting IGF-1R increased the effects of HER2 inhibition. This suggests that IGF-1R signalling can compensate for EGFR family signalling in tumours where the EGFR family could be targeted therapeutically. Therefore targeting both IGFR and HER2/EGFR could have clinical benefit, and IGFR inhibitors are currently in clinical trials as a combination therapy with ErbB kinase inhibitors such as laptinib and gefitinib (reviewed in Nahta, 2012). In addition, given the interplay between IGFR, EGFR and ER, therapy targeted towards IGFR signalling may also be beneficial in patients that have become resistant to endocrine targeted therapies (reviewed in Tinoco *et al.*, 2013).

Throughout this volume the concept of receptor heterodimerisation has been discussed as a mechanism of regulating signalling and inducing activation of different downstream cascades. It has, however, been assumed that heterodimerisation exists within the context of a single growth factor receptor family. To add yet a further layer of complexity to signalling cross-talk, we now know that, at least in the context of therapeutic resistance, this is not the case. Rita Nahta and colleagues have published extensively on mechanisms of resistance to HER2 inhibitor, and they showed that inter-signalling pathway heterodimerisation could contribute to trastuzumab resistance in breast cancer cells. The presence of IGF-1R/HER2 dimers was observed in trastuzumab resistant, but not sensitive, cells (Nahta *et al.*, 2005), lending support to the concept of combined HER2/IGFR inhibition in patients with HER2-targeted therapy-resistant tumours.

9.6 Summary

The examples of signalling cross-talk provided is by no means an exhaustive list, but serves as a starting point for understanding the context through which signalling contributes to tumour development and patient responses to therapy. As has been discussed through the individual chapters of this book, as well as in the sections in this chapter, cross-talk in signalling is crucial in the clinical setting. Future therapeutic strategies for inhibiting signalling in cancer will undoubtedly focus on combining therapies to limit the acquired therapeutic resistance that arises from signalling cross-talk.

Targeting focal points such as mTOR/PI3K will certainly be one way of mitigating some, but certainly not all, cross-talk. In addition, specific inhibition of the broader aspects of signalling, such as the basis behind protein stability, will affect more than one pathway. Inhibition of Hsp90, a chaperone for a number of signalling molecules, has been a central topic in HER2 positive cancers for some time. Recent reports suggest that Hsp90 inhibition could also destabilise MAPK and TGFβ signalling, providing a much broader therapeutic benefit than first envisaged (Haupt *et al.*, 2012).

Future research will also shed further light on the importance of careful planning in the context of the order of drug delivery. Trastuzumab prevents HER2 dimerisation events (Chapter 1) and some patients will become resistant. However, what has emerged in recent years from *in vitro* work (Nahta *et al.*, 2007), and is becoming correlated in the clinic, is that many patients are still sensitive to HER2 kinase inhibitors even though they are resistant to monoclonal antibody therapy targeted at the same molecule.

A topic that has not had much, if any, discussion is the role that the extracellular matrix and tumour microenvironment play in regulating cell signalling and transcriptional responses. This is a growing topic and one to look out for in the future. One thing is certainly clear: cell signalling in cancer is a very complex topic and an area that has attracted much research focus over recent decades. As a scientific community the understanding of potential cross-talk and its consequences in the clinical setting has cultivated an ever-growing knowledge of signalling networks. Whilst this knowledge is far from complete, the impact that it has had so far in improving the prognosis for many cancer patients cannot be underestimated.

References

Alistair, J., Stewart, A.J., Michael, D. *et al.* (1990) Role of insulin-like growth factors and the type I insulin-like growth factor receptor in the estrogen-stimulated proliferation of human breast cancer cells. *Journal of Biological Chemistry*, **265** (34), 21171–21178.

Brabletz, T., Jung, A., Reu, S. *et al.* (2001) Variable β-catenin expression in colorectal cancers indicates tumor progression driven by the tumor environment. *Proceedings of the National Academy of Sciences, USA*, **98**, 10356–10361.

Civenni, G., Holbro, T. and Hynes, N.E. (2003) Wnt1 and Wnt5a induce cyclin D1 expression through erbB1 transactivation in HC11 mammary epithelial cells. *EMBO Reports*, **4**, 166–171.

Collu, G.M., Meurette, O. and Brennan, K. (2009) Is there more to Wnt signalling in breast cancer than stabilisation of β-catenin? *Breast Cancer Research*, **11**, 105.

Donaldson, R. and Calder, M. (2010) Modelling and analysis of biochemical signalling pathway cross-talk. *Electronic Proceedings in Theoretical Computer Science*, **19**, 40–54.

Donaldson, R. and Calder, M. (2012) Modular modelling of signalling pathways and their crosstalk. *Theoretical Computer Science*, **456**, 30–50.

Faivre, E.J. and Lange, C.A. (2007) Progesterone receptors upregulate Wnt-1 to induce epidermal growth factor receptor transactivation and c-Src-dependent sustained activation of Erk1/2 mitogen-activated protein kinase in breast cancer cells. *Molecular and Cellular Biology*, **27** (2), 466–480.

Ferguson, K.M., Mitchell, B., Berger, M.B. *et al.* (2003) EGF Activates Its Receptor by Removing interactions that autoinhibit ectodomain dimerization. *Molecular Cell*, **11**, 507–517.

Filardo, E.J., Quinn, J.A., Bland, K.I. and Frackelton, A.R., Jr., (2001) Estrogen-induced activation of Erk-1 and Erk-2 requires the G protein-coupled receptor homolog, GPR30, and occurs via trans-activation of the epidermal growth factor receptor through release of HB-EGF. *Molecular Endocrinology*, **14**, 1649–1660.

Gandhi, J., Zhang, J., Xie, Y. *et al.* (2009) Alterations in genes of the EGFR signaling pathway and their relationship to EGFR tyrosine kinase inhibitor sensitivity in lung cancer cell lines. *PLoS ONE*, **4** (2), e4576.

Gomes, L.R., Terra, L.F., Rosângela, A.M. and Wailemann, R.A.M. (2012) TGF-β1 modulates the homeostasis between MMPs and MMP inhibitors through p38 MAPK and ERK1/2 in highly invasive breast cancer cells. *BMC Cancer*, **12**, 26.

Gschwind, A., Hart, S., Fischer, O.M. and Ullrich A. (2003) TACE cleavage of proamphiregulin regulates GPCR-induced proliferation and motility of cancer cells. *EMBO Journal*, **22**, 2411–2421.

Guo, X. and Wang, X.F. (2009) Signaling cross-talk between TGF-beta/BMP and other pathways. *Cell Research*, **19** (1), 71–88.

Han, L., Zhang, H.-W., Zhou, W.-P. *et al.* (2012) The effects of genistein on transforming growth factor-β1-induced invasion and metastasis in human pancreatic cancer cell line Panc-1 in vitro. *Chinese Medical Journal*, **125** (11), 2032–2040.

Haupt, A., Joberty, G., Bantscheff, M. *et al.* (2012) Hsp90 inhibition destabilises MAP kinase and TGFβ signalling components. *BMC Cancer*, **12**, 38.

Hoschuetzky, H., Aberle, H. and Kemler, R. (1994) β-Catenin mediates the interaction of the cadherin-catenin complex with epidermal growth factor receptor. *Journal of Cell Biology*, **127**, 1375–1380.

Hu, T. and Li, C. (2010) Convergence between Wnt-β-catenin and EGFR signaling in cancer. *Molecular Cancer*, **9**, 236.

Improta-Brears, T., Whorton, A.R., Codazzi, F. *et al.* (1999) Estrogen-induced activation of mitogen-activated protein kinase requires mobilization of intracellular calcium. *Proceedings of the National Academy of Sciences, USA*, **96** (8), 4686–4691.

Jamieson, C., Sharma, M. and Henderson, B.R. (2012) Wnt signaling from membrane to nucleus: β-catenin caught in a loop. *International Journal of Biochemistry and Cell Biology*, **44** (6), 847–850.

Junttila, T.T., Akita, R.W. and Parsons, K. *et al.* (2009) Ligand-independent HER2/HER3/PI3K complex is disrupted by trastuzumab and is effectively inhibited by the PI3K inhibitor GDC-0941. *Cancer Cell*, **15**, 429–440.

Keld, R.R. and Ang, Y.S. (2011) Targeting key signalling pathways in oesophageal adenocarcinoma: A reality for personalised medicine. *World Journal of Gastroenterology*, **17** (23), 2781–2790.

Knabbe, C., Lippman, M.E., Wakefield, L.M. *et al*. (1987) Evidence that transforming growth factor-beta is a hormonally regulated negative growth factor in human breast cancer cells. *Cell*, **48** (3), 417–428.

Leivonen, S.-K., Lazaridis, K., Decock, J. *et al*. (2013) TGFβ-elicited induction of tissue inhibitor of metalloproteinases (TIMP)-3 expression in fibroblasts involves complex interplay between Smad3, p38a, and ERK1/2. *PLoS ONE*, **8** (2), e57474.

Lin, H.-Y., Davis, F.B., Gordinier, J.K. *et al*. (1999) Thyroid hormone induces activation of mitogen-activated protein kinase in cultured cells. *American Journal of Physiology*, **276**, C1014–C1024.

Lippman, M.E., Dickson, R.B., Gelmann, E.P. *et al*. (1987) Growth regulation of human breast carcinoma occurs through regulated growth factor secretion. *Journal of Cellular Biochemistry*, **35** (1), 1–16.

Ma, J., Meng, Y., Kwiatkowski, D.J. *et al*. (2010) Mammalian target of rapamycin regulates murine and human cell differentiation through STAT3/p63/Jagged/Notch cascade. *Journal of Clinical Investigation*, **120** (1), 103–114.

McGuire, W.L. (1975) Current status of estrogen receptors in human breast cancer. *Cancer*, **36** (2), 638–644.

Miller, T.W., Rexer, B.N. Garrett, J.T. and Arteaga, C.L. (2011) Mutations in the phosphatidylinositol 3-kinase pathway: role in tumor progression and therapeutic implications in breast cancer. *Breast Cancer Research*, **13** (6), 224.

Nahta, R. (2012) Deciphering the role of insulin-like growth factor-I receptor in trastuzumab resistance. *Chemotherapy Research and Practice*. doi:10.1155/2012 /648965.

Nahta, R., Yuan, L.X.H., Zhang, B. *et al*. (2005) Insulin-like growth factor-I receptor/ human epidermal growth factor receptor 2 heterodimerization contributes to trastuzumab resistance of breast cancer cells. *Cancer Research*, **65**, 11118–11128.

Nahta, R., Yuan, L.X.H., Du, Y. *et al*. (2007) Lapatinib induces apoptosis in trastuzumab-resistant breast cancer cells: effects on insulin-like growth factor I signaling. *Molecular Cancer Therapeutics*, **6**, 667–674.

Nahta, R. and O'Regan, R.M. (2012) Therapeutic implications of estrogen receptor signaling in HER2-positive breast cancers. *Breast Cancer Research and Treatment*, **135**, 39–48.

Peters, C.R., Hardwick, J., Hardwick, R. *et al*. (2009) On behalf of the OCCAMS study group, A seven gene signature outperforms clinical features at predicting survival in oesophageal adenocarcinoma. World Congress of Gastroenterology/UEGW, London, 2009.

Prenzel, N., Zwick, E., Daub, H. *et al*. (1999) EGF receptor transactivation by G-protein-coupled receptors requires metalloproteinase cleavage of proHB-EGF. *Nature*, **402**, 884–888.

Ramesh, S., Qi, X.-J., Wildey, G.M. *et al*. (2008) TGFβ-mediated BIM expression and apoptosis are regulated through SMAD3-dependent expression of the MAPK phosphatase MKP2. *EMBO Reports*, **9**, 990–997.

Sabnis, G., Schayowitz, A., Goloubeva, O. *et al*. (2009) Trastuzumab reverses letrozole resistance and amplifies the sensitivity of breast cancer cells to estrogen. *Cancer Research*, **69**, 1416–1428.

Schlange, T., Matsuda, Y., Lienhard, S., *et al*. (2007) Autocrine WNT signaling contributes to breast cancer cell proliferation via the canonical WNT pathway and EGFR transactivation. *Breast Cancer Research*, **9**, R63.

Schroeder, J.A., Troyer, K.L. and Lee, D.C. (2000) Cooperative induction of mammary tumorigenesis by TGFalpha and Wnts. *Oncogene*, **19**, 3193–3199.

Suh, Y., Afaq, F., Johnson, J.J. and Mukhtar, H. (2009) A plant flavonoid fisetin induces apoptosis in colon cancer cells by inhibition of COX2 and Wnt/EGFR/NF-kB-signaling pathways. *Carcinogenesis*, **30** (2), 300–307.

Suzuki, M., Shigematsu, H., Nakajima, T. *et al.* (2007) Synchronous alterations of Wnt and epidermal growth factor receptor signaling pathways through aberrant methylation and mutation in non−small Cell lung cancer. *Clinical Cancer Research*, **13**, 6087–6092.

Tang, H.-Y., Lin, H.-Y., Zhang, S. *et al.* (2004) Thyroid hormone causes mitogen-activated protein kinase-dependent phosphorylation of the nuclear estrogen receptor. *Endocrinology*, **145** (7), 3265–3272.

Tinoco, G., Warsch, S., Glück, S. *et al.* (2013) Treating breast cancer in the 21st century: emerging biological therapies. *Journal of Cancer*, **4** (2), 117–132.

Tsonis, A.I., Afratis, N., Gialeli, C. *et al.* (2013) Evaluation of the coordinated actions of estrogen receptors with epidermal growth factor receptor and insulin-like growth factor receptor in the expression of cell surface heparan sulfate proteoglycans and cell motility in breast cancer cells. *FEBS Journal*, **280** (10), 2248–2259.

van der Heide, L.P., van Dinther, M., Moustakas, A. and ten Dijke, P. (2011) TGFβ activates mitogen- and stress-activated protein kinase-1 (MSK1) to attenuate cell death. *Journal of Biological Chemistry*, **286** (7), 5003–5011.

Vasilaki, E., Papadimitriou, E., Tajadura, V. *et al.* (2010) Transcriptional regulation of the small GTPase RhoB gene by TGFβ-induced signaling pathways. *FASEB Journal*, **24**, 891–905.

Vermeulen, L., Melo, F.S.E., Heijden, M. *et al.* (2010) Wnt activity defines colon cancer stem cells and is regulated by the microenvironment. *Nature Cell Biology*, **12** (5), 468–477.

Walsh, L.A. and Damjanovski, S. (2011) IGF-1 increases invasive potential of MCF 7 breast cancer cells and induces activation of latent TGF-β1 resulting in epithelial to mesenchymal transition. *Cell Communication and Signaling*, **9**, 10.

Wang, X. and Proud, C.G. (2011) mTORC1 signaling: what we still don't know. *Journal of Molecular Cell Biology*, **3** (4), 206–220.

Wang, Y.C., Morrison, G., Gillihan, R. *et al.* (2011) Different mechanisms for resistance to trastuzumab versus lapatinib in HER2-positive breast cancers – role of estrogen receptor and HER2 reactivation. *Breast Cancer Research*, **13**, R121.

Xia, W., Bacus, S., Hegde, P. *et al.* (2006) A model of acquired auto-resistance to a potent ErbB2 tyrosine kinase inhibitor and a therapeutic strategy to prevent its onset in breast cancer. *Proceedings of the National Academy of Sciences*, **103** (20), 7795–7800.

Yokogami, K., Wakisaka, S., Avruch, J. and Reeves, S.A. (2001) Serine phosphorylation and maximal activation of STAT3 during CNTF signaling is mediated by the rapamycin target mTOR. *Current Biology*, **10** (1), 47–50.

Zhang, W. and Liu, H.T. (2002) MAPK signal pathways in the regulation of cell proliferation in mammalian cells. *Cell Research*, **12** (1), 9–18.

Index

Page numbers in *italics* refer to Figures; those in **bold** to Tables

---

Cancer Cell Signalling, First Edition. Edited by Amanda Harvey.
© 2013 John Wiley & Sons, Ltd. Published 2013 by John Wiley & Sons, Ltd.